AF544912

Complications of GLAUCOMA THERAPY

Editors
Mark B. Sherwood, MD
George L. Spaeth, MD

SLACK Incorporated, 6900 Grove Road, Thorofare, New Jersey 08086

SLACK International Book Distributors

In Europe, the Middle East and Africa:
John Wiley & Sons Limited
Baffins Lane
Chichester, West Sussex P019 1UD
England

In Canada:
McGraw-Hill Ryerson Limited
330 Progress Avenue
Scarborough, Ontario
M1P 2Z5

In Australia and New Zealand:
MacLennan & Petty Pty Limited
P.O. Box 425
Artarmon, N.S.W. 2064
Australia

In Japan:
Igaku-Shoin, Ltd.
Tokyo International P.O. Box 5063
1-28-36 Hongo, Bunkyo-Ku
Tokyo 113
Japan

In Asia and India:
PG Publishing Pte Limited.
36 West Coast Road, #02-02
Singapore 0512

Foreign Translation Agent

John Scott & Company
International Publishers' Agency
417-A Pickering Road
Phoenixville, PA 19460
Fax: 215-988-0185

Managing Editor: Lynn C. Borders
Designer: Susan Hermansen
Production Manager: David Murphy
Publisher: Harry C. Benson

Copyright © 1990 by SLACK Incorporated

All rights reserved. No part of this book may be reproduced, stored in a retrieval system or transmitted in any form or by any means, electronic, mechanical, photocopying, recording or otherwise, without written permission from the publisher, except for brief quotations embodied in critical articles and reviews.

Printed in the United States of America

Library of Congress Catalog Card Number: 85-052377

ISBN: 1-55642-174-5

Published by: SLACK Incorporated
6900 Grove Road
Thorofare, NJ 08086

Last digit is print number: 10 9 8 7 6 5 4 3 2 1

Dedication

This book is dedicated to our wives, Ruth and Ann

Contributors

George L. Spaeth, M.D.
Professor of Ophthalmology, Jefferson Medical College
Director, Glaucoma Service, Wills Eye Hospital
Philadelphia, Pennsylvania

Richard Starita, M.D.
Clinical Assistant Professor, Southwestern Medical School
Dallas, Texas

Ronald L. Fellman, M.D.
Clinical Assistant Professor, Southwestern Medical School
Dallas, Texas

Joseph Caprioli, M.D.
Associate Professor, Yale University
Director, Glaucoma Service
New Haven, Connecticut

Louis W. Schwartz, M.D.
Attending Surgeon, Wills Glaucoma Service
Clinical Associate Professor of Ophthalmology, Jefferson Medical College
Philadelphia, Pennsylvania

Marlene R. Moster, M.D.
Associate Surgeon, Glaucoma Service, Wills Eye Hospital
Clinical Assistant Professor, Jefferson Medical College
Philadelphia, Pennsylvania

Ralph S. Sando, M.D., FRCS
Attending Surgeon in Glaucoma, Wills Eye Hospital
Associate Professor, Jefferson Medical College
Director, Philadelphia Ophthalmologic Association
Philadelphia, Pennsylvania

Richard P. Wilson, M.D.
Attending Surgeon in Glaucoma, Wills Eye Hospital
Associate Professor, Jefferson Medical College
Philadelphia, Pennsylvania

Steven T. Simmons, M.D.
Director, Glaucoma Service
Assistant Professor, Albany Medical College
Albany, New York

Louis B. Cantor, M.D.
Assistant Professor of Ophthalmology
Director, Glaucoma Service, Indiana University Hospitals
Indianapolis, Indiana

L. Jay Katz, M.D.
Associate Surgeon, Glaucoma Service, Wills Eye Hospital
Assistant Professor, Jefferson Medical College
Philadelphia, Pennsylvania

Robert D. Fechtner, M.D.
Clinical Instructor of Glaucoma
Department of Ophthalmology, University of California, San Diego

Dan A. Nichols, M.D.
Clinical Assistant Professor
Department of Ophthalmology, University of Minnesota
Minneapolis, Minnesota

Mark B. Sherwood, M.D.
Assistant Professor of Ophthalmology
Director, Glaucoma Service, University of Florida College of Medicine
Gainesville, Florida

Roger A. Hitchings, F.R.C.S., F.C.Ophth
Director of Glaucoma
Consultant Ophthalmologist
Moorfields Eye Hospital
London, England

James McAllister, F.R.C.S., F.C.Ophth
Consultant Ophthalmologist
Prince Charles Eye Unit, King Edward VII Hospital
Windsor, Berkshire, UK

Jody R. Piltz-Seymour, M.D.
Department of Ophthalmology
University of British Columbia
Vancouver, British Columbia
Canada

Nina Tolat, M.D.
Research Fellow
Temple University Hospital
Philadelphia, PA

Contents

CHAPTER 1

Introduction

George L. Spaeth, MD

The burden of suffering caused by glaucoma is great. Treatment can be effective in alleviating and potentially effective in eliminating the condition. But treatments, both medical and surgical, unfortunately cause their own suffering: blurred vision, discomfort, blindness, systemic illness, even death. This is the dilemma that faces the physician as he or she tries to be of greatest benefit to the patient.

The goal of treatment is always to have the greatest benefit at the least risk. But the matter is not so simple as it sounds. In many instances those treatments that benefit most are also associated with the greatest risk, whereas those that have less risk are also less beneficial.

The present text concentrates on the complications of the medical and surgical therapy of glaucoma. The purpose of this is not merely to provide a litany of the misfortunes that beset the patient, though practitioners and patients alike should appreciate fully the problems associated with treatment. The major emphasis rather, is on prevention of the complications. Especially with regard to surgery, it is far better to avoid complications than to try to correct them. Even the physician as wise as Solomon and as competent as Harvey Cushing cannot totally avoid complications. A major difference distinguishing the great from the mediocre physician is that the great actively searches out problems, recognizes them, and knows how best to correct for them. This takes remarkable intellectual and emotional honesty combined with extensive knowledge. While it is unlikely that this small volume will change a physician's character, we hope it provides a more complete knowledge of the art and science of glaucoma therapy, with the intent that patients will be better served.

One of the first chapters written on complications of glaucoma surgery pointed out that the success of glaucoma surgery is strongly affected by the quality of the preoperative preparation and the postoperative management of the patient.[1] This is even more true today than it was 50 years ago.

Increased understanding of the natural history of glaucoma, better methods of surgery, and the availability of a wide variety of techniques to alter the response to surgery have made possible manipulations of the surgical event that were not feasible before. The responsible surgeon needs to be knowledgeable regarding the advantages and disadvantages of these techniques, both old and new, in order to assure that his or her patient will have the best obtainable result.

An additional reason for becoming knowledgeable regarding the management of surgical complications in patients with glaucoma relates to the increasing frequency with which surgery is being performed. There is a growing disenchantment with using medication to treat chronic glaucoma. While it is still not clear whether the continued deterioration of function that occurs in some patients with glaucoma is inevitable, most physicians caring for patients with glaucoma appear to believe that the likely explanation for continuing deterioration is the failure of medical therapy to lower intraocular pressure *enough* to prevent progressive nerve damage from occurring. Recent information shows that surgery is a more effective method of lowering intraocular pressure than medications.

Another factor is the increasing longevity of the general population. In years past it was rarely necessary to continue glaucoma medications for most people simply did not live that long. Further, glaucoma is probably being diagnosed in more patients at a younger age; such patients may need to continue medications for 40 or 50 years! It is unusual for patients to use an epinephrine product for this long without developing hypersensitivity.[2] After 10 or 15 years of pilocarpine the pupil has become permanently miotic; the blood vessels seem to become hypertrophic and leaky, the pupillary sphincter definitely becomes fibrotic, and the lens may become prematurely cataractous.[3,4,5] The effect on the eye of long-term use of topical medications and of suppression of aqueous formation is not well established, but there are suggestions that the glaucoma medications may predispose to surgical failure and to premature deterioration of the trabecular meshwork.[6,7,8,9]

Performing glaucoma surgery on an eye that has received drops for 20 years is far more difficult than operating on any eye that has been virtually untreated. In the former instance the eye bleeds more, the iris is flaccid, and posterior synechiae almost always develop postoperatively. The eye is far more inflamed in the postoperative period, and Tenon's capsule cysts are more likely to form. In general the surgery is an unpleasant event in eyes that have received long-term topical medications, with a surgical outcome less favorable than either the patient or surgeon would hope. In contrast, the glaucomatous eye that has not been extensively treated has a reaction to surgery similar to that of the normal eye.

Nor are the unpleasant effects of topical and systemic medications employed for glaucoma limited to the eye. Every medication causes substantive systemic problems. While these are relatively infrequent with the sympathetic and parasympathetic agonists, they are frequent and may be severe with the beta blockers and the carbonic anhydrase inhibitors. The systemic side effects of topical glaucoma medications are problematical because neither the patient nor the physician is likely to relate the side effects to the use of eye drops. Patients simply do not attribute their impotency to instilling a watery drop in their eye twice a day. As medical therapy for glaucoma has been used longer in more patients it has become even more apparent that the treatment itself is consistently troublesome and occasionally fatal.

There appear to be three possible causes of persistent deterioration of visual function or progressive optic nerve damage in the patient considered to have glaucoma: 1) The patient really does not have glaucoma and the deterioration is caused by some other condition; 2) the optic neurons are mortally wounded and will die in the future no matter what is done (the structural defect is so severe that the cause for nerve death cannot be alleviated) or 3) the intraocular pressure is higher than the eye can tolerate.

With careful diagnosis and thoughtful, periodic reevaluation, the first of these possibilities can be kept to an acceptable minimum. In patients with far advanced glaucomatous nerve damage, it may be that nothing can prevent further deterioration. Nevertheless, cases in which vision remains stable even after the development of advanced visual field loss are not rare. Indeed, some patients with extraordinarily far-advanced disease appear to be well stabilized for years when their IOP has been markedly lowered. *In the overwhelming majority of cases, the reason that patients with glaucoma get worse appears to be that the intraocular pressure is too high.*

Successful, persistent, marked lowering of intraocular pressure through mechanical means is the logical treatment for patients with glaucomatous disease. Were it possible to achieve such mechanical lowering of intraocular pressure safely, there would be little use for the expensive, troublesome, and often ineffective eye drops which now so interfere with daily living for many patients.

Glaucoma management is plagued by the frequency and severity with which substantial complications are associated with both glaucoma medications and glaucoma surgery. A thorough understanding of how to prevent them as effectively as possible is absolutely essential for all those supervising the care of patients with glaucoma.

The purpose of this text is to provide a comprehensive analysis of the complications associated with the medical and surgical therapy of glaucoma. The purpose is not to change the fundamental indication for glaucoma surgery, which is documented or anticipated progression of glaucomatous optic nerve damage or visual field loss due to glaucoma (despite maximal tolerated medical therapy) occurring at a rate that would diminish the patient's quality of life. It is well understood today that intraocular pressure above the statistically defined limits of normal is not necessarily an indication for the medical treatment of glaucoma. Similarly, progressive glaucomatous nerve damage or progressive visual field loss is not necessarily an indication for the surgical treatment of glaucoma. An elderly person with a fairly healthy appearing optic disc and cataract is often best treated conservatively despite mild progressive visual field loss. Such decisions involve the art of medicine. Treating any individual by formula will not result in the best patient care for that individual. Each case is unique and must be treated uniquely.

Today, glaucoma surgery is often delayed because both the surgeon and the patient fear that the surgery will make the patient worse. Phrased differently, the major reason for deferring glaucoma surgery is fear of a surgical complication. In some cases this fear is related to a lack of knowledge about avoiding complications and treating them appropriately if they occur. If this text results in improved understanding of the complications of glaucoma surgery, so that the experienced surgeon is able to treat his or her patient better, and the fearful surgeon, equipped with better understanding, no longer withholds surgery from those patients who in fact are appropriate candidates, we will have more than justified this publication.

References

1. Spaeth EB. Reoperations and complications following glaucoma operations. In Fasanella RM (ed): Management of Complications in Eye Surgery. Philadelphia, W.B. Saunders Co., 1957, pp. 187-208.
2. Becker B. Topical epinephrine in the treatment of glaucoma. In Symposium of Glaucoma, Transactions of New Orleans Academy of Ophthalmology. St. Louis, C.V. Mosby, 1967, pp. 152, 162.
3. Benjamin KW. Toxicity of ocular medications. In Spaeth GL (ed): Early Primary Open-Angle Glaucoma: Diagnosis and Management, International Ophthalmology Clinics, Spring 1979, Vol. 19, No. 1. Boston, Little, Brown Co., p. 204.
4. Havener WH. Ocular Pharmacology. St. Louis, C.V. Mosby, 1966, pp. 228, 233.
5. Levene RZ. Uniocular miotic therapy. Trans Am Acad Ophthalmol Otolaryngol 1978;79:376.
6. Grierson I, Lee WR, Abraham S. The effects of topical pilocarpine on the morphology of the outflow apparatus of the baboon (Papio cynocephalus). Invest Ophthalmol Vis Sci 1979; 18:346-355.
7. Lutjen-Drecoll E, Kaufman PL. Echothiophate-induced structural alterations in the anterior chamber angle of the cynomolgus monkey. Invest Ophthalmol Vis Sci 1979; 18:918-929.
8. Lutjen-Drecoll E. Ultrastructural changes in the monkey eye following long-term treatment with pilocarpine. Invest Ophthalmol Vis Sci (Suppl) 1981; 20:30.
9. Sherwood MB, Grierson I, Miller L. et al. Long-term morphologic effects of antiglaucoma drugs on conjunctiva and Tenon's capsule in glaucomatous patients. Ophthalmology 96(3): 327, 1989.

SECTION I

Medical Treatment — Side Effects of Drugs Used in Glaucoma

CHAPTER 2

Ocular and Systemic Side Effects of Topical Cholinergic and Anticholinesterase Drugs

Ronald L. Fellman, MD
Richard J. Starita, MD

Introduction

It is a challenging task to improve the quality of life for glaucoma patients. The primary goal is to educate them about their disease and the need for intervention. Patients must be informed about the efficacy and side effects of their medications before treatment is initiated. Properly informed patients are more likely to accept minimal drug-induced life changes and are aware that alternatives exist when these changes are unacceptable. Ophthalmologists have a rare opportunity to enhance the quality of life for their patients by informing, educating, and exploring new avenues of treatment when relentless side effects destroy a satisfactory quality of life. Such communication between the patient and doctor creates a long- lasting rapport that is necessary for a lifetime disease.

Ophthalmologists have used the miotic family of topical cholinergic drugs such as pilocarpine, and anticholinesterase drugs such as physostigmine (Eserine), for more than 100 years.[1] However, periodic reminders about the mechanism of action and side effects of these century old medications is essential. A good start begins with the autonomic nervous system.

The sympathetic and parasympathetic subsystems of the autonomic nervous system govern the constancy of the internal environment of man. Acetylcholine is the neurotransmitter of the entire parasympathetic nervous system and even transmits certain sympathetic signals. The term cholinergic is derived from acetylcholine and refers to agents that simulate the effect of acetylcholine.[2] The direct-acting cholinergic and indirect-acting anticholinesterase drugs mimic and amplify the parasympathetic nervous system and are known as parasympathomimetic agents.[3] These drugs prolong cholinergic activity and thus augment the parasympathomimetic response.

Enhancing the parasympathetic side of the autonomic nervous system upsets the delicate balance of bodily functions. Because the autonomic nervous system is concerned primarily with visceral functions such as cardiac output, blood flow to various organs, digestion, elimination, and respiration, a multitude of patient complaints might arise because of alteration in these organ systems.[4]

Pre- and postjunctional cholinergic receptors are of two types: muscarinic and nicotinic.[5] Nicotinic receptors are subdivided into N_1 found in autonomic ganglionic synapses and N_2 found in striated muscle. Muscarinic receptors are found mainly in the smooth muscle of various organ systems (gastrointestinal, genitourinary, cardiac, pulmonary) and secretory glands. There are also cholinoceptive sites in the brain.

Pilocarpine, a direct-acting cholinergic drug, has only muscarinic activity. However, phospholine, which is an indirect acting parasympathomimetic agent, stimulates both nicotinic and muscarinic receptors.

Historical Perspective

The parasympathomimetics have been used since 1875 in the treatment of glaucoma. Investigation into the trials by ordeal using the Calabar bean eventually led to the use of physostigmine in ophthalmology.[1] Argyll Robertson and Laquer were the first ophthalmologists to use physostigmine therapeutically in glaucoma. In the same year the ocular actions of pilocarpine were discovered by Weber. It's appropriate that toxicologists were the first to describe the use and abuse of topical miotic medications.

The toxic nerve gases developed during World War II spawned the long-acting anticholinesterases. Initially, diisopropyl fluorophosphate and demecarium bromide (Humorsol) were evaluated, followed by the more popular compound, echothiophate (phospholine iodide).[6,7] Echothiophate was used therapeutically for glaucoma in 1957.[8] However, its popularity waned in the mid- 1960s when its cataractogenic potential finally was appreciated. This led to the recommendation that long-acting organophosphates be used mainly in aphakic patients.

Carbachol was first introduced in the early 1930s. Velhagen found carbachol to be an effective agent for lowering IOP and suggested its use to augment the range of miotics in the conservative treatment of glaucoma[9,10]

Mechanism of Action

All of the miotic medications work by a similar mechanism. Normally, aqueous humor leaves the eye through two pathways. The most familiar and important is the conventional route through the trabecular meshwork. Cholinergic stimulation increases outflow of fluid through this pathway. The unconventional or uveoscleral route is through the iris root and ciliary body musculature leading to the suprachoroidal space with drainage through the sclera. This pathway can account for 5 to 20% of total aqueous humor drainage.[11,12,13] Cholinergic stimulation decreases the outflow of fluid through this route.[14]

The cholinergic drugs can be classified as direct acting, indirect acting, or dual acting.

1. Pilocarpine is a direct-acting parasympathomimetic drug that duplicates the muscarinic effect of acetylcholine but not its nicotinic effect. Cholinergic stimulation of the ciliary body by pilocarpine results in traction on the scleral spur. The shortened, longitudinal fibers of the ciliary body displace the scleral spur altering the configuration of the trabecular meshwork and Schlemm's canal leading to enhanced outflow and reduced IOP.[15,16] In addition to lowering IOP, pilocarpine dampens the diurnal curve in both normal and glaucomatous eyes.[17] The maximal pressure fall from pilocarpine occurs at two hours. The magnitude and duration of this fall can be dependent on concentration; 1%, 2% and 4% show a dose-related response. Increasing the concentration to 8% does not change the magnitude of IOP reduction but might extend the duration of the fall.[18] Some patients show very little pressure reduction regardless of concentration used. In other cases, the pressure lowering effect is not related to traction on the scleral spur. Pilocarpine can produce a definite lowering in IOP without an increase in facility of outflow.[17] It has been suggested that cholinergic agents have an inhibitory effect on aqueous secretion.[11,19] In primary angle closure without pupillary block, pilocarpine can reduce IOP by direct stimulation of the pupillary sphincter pulling the peripheral iris from the obstructed trabecular meshwork.
2. The indirect-acting parasympathomimetic drugs bind to acetylcholinesterase, preventing the breakdown of acetylcholine at neuroeffector sites. The muscarinic ocular effects, because of a buildup of acetylcholine at receptor sites, follows the same mechanism of action for direct-acting cholinergic drugs; however, their responses are more exaggerated. Systemic absorption of anticholinesterase drugs leads to a buildup of acetylcholine and amplifies both muscarinic and nicotinic side effects.[20] Physostigmine and neostigmine are short-acting cholinesterase inhibitors, while echothiophate iodine, isoflurophate, and demecarium bromide are longer-acting agents.[21] Drance demonstrated .25% phospholine iodide lowered IOP in normal human eyes with a marked fall in IOP starting at 12 hours and persisting for 3 to 5 days; 57 of the 59 glaucomatous eyes were controlled with adequate pressure.[22] He also compared 4% pilocarpine to .06% phospholine iodide. Seventy percent of pilocarpine treated eyes showed peaks of IOP over 24mm Hg, whereas only 20% of the phospholine iodide treated eyes showed similar peaks.[23] Numerous investigators demonstrated the efficacy of phospholine iodide.[24-26]

3. Carbachol is a dual action parasympathomimetic for its has direct-acting cholinergic muscarinic activity and simultaneously inhibits acetylcholinesterase, allowing a buildup of acetylcholine at receptor sites. Thus, carbachol has both muscarinic and nicotinic activity. However, carbachol has poor corneal penetration and requires an additive such as benzalkonium chloride to achieve effective treatment levels.

There are several mechanisms by which miotics can elevate IOP rather than lower it. Six possible methods by which cholinergic stimulation can affect IOP adversely are listed (Table 2-1) :

Table 2-1. Paradoxical Pressure Response to Topically Applied Parasympathomimetic Drugs

Decreased uveoscleral outflow
Uveitis because of breakdown of blood aqueous barrier
Increased pupil block with closure of the angle
Phacomorphic obstruction of the chamber angle because of axial thickening of the crystalline lens
Forward shift of the lens because of ciliary body congestion with subsequent closure of the angle
Ciliolenticular obstruction of aqueous with aqueous misdirection syndrome

1. Failure to enhance trabecular outflow along with miotic induced loss of uveoscleral outflow might lead to a paradoxical rise in IOP.[27] In eyes with severely compromised trabecular outflow the IOP might actually decrease by using anticholinergic agents (cycloplegics) that enhance uveoscleral outflow.
2. Cholinergic drugs cause dilation of anterior segment blood vessels. Muscarinic-induced anterior segment vasodilation leads to increased blood flow to the iris and ciliary body with resultant swelling.[28] Congestion of the ciliary body and its processes can lead to anterior rotation, secondary angle closure, and elevated IOP.
3. Contraction of the ciliary body musculature and/or congestion of ciliary processes can increase ciliolenticular and/or iridovitreal block precipitating misdirection of aqueous fluid resulting in malignant glaucoma.
4. The presence of flare and cells in the anterior chamber might indicate a breakdown of the blood aqueous barrier because of cholinergic vasodilation of uveal arterioles. Clearly, eyes with preexisting inflammation can experience increased uveitis by miotic induced breakdown of the blood aqueous barrier with protein and cells spilling into the anterior chamber causing trabecular dysfunction/obstruction.[29]
5. Just as acute miosis might help pull the peripheral iris out of the chamber angle during an angle closure attack, chronic miosis might lead to increased pupil block with silent closure of the angle. This is most commonly seen in eyes with narrow angles devoid of peripheral iridectomies.

6. When the circular muscle of the ciliary body contracts, the axial thickness of the crystalline lens increases in a dose-related response with concomitant shallowing of the chamber angle. Cholinergic drugs might therefore induce a phacomorphic component of aqueous obstruction.

Preparations and Distributions

There is a wide variety of topical parasympathomimetic drugs available for ophthalmic use. Whether pilocarpine is used as a nitrate or hydrochloride salt, the pressure reduction is the same.[30] Also, there is no substantial evidence that one particular drug vehicle is therapeutically superior to another.[31]

Topically applied pilocarpine is degraded in the cornea with only a small amount entering the anterior chamber. Then, apparently, pilocarpine is absorbed by uveal pigment and gradually released to muscarinic receptor sites. Ocular pigmentation hinders penetration of topically applied cholinergic drugs to receptor sites causing a shift in the dose response curve.[32-34] Maximal miosis and accommodation occur at 30 and 60 minutes respectively;[35,36] however, maximal IOP reduction does not occur until approximately two hours.

Carbachol is a very stable parasympathomimetic, 100 times more effective than acetylcholine and 200 times more effective than pilocarpine as an intraocular cholinomimetic.[37] It usefulness, however, is limited for it is a water soluble choline ester with limited corneal penetration. Wetting agents dramatically increase the drug absorption of carbachol.[38] Once carbachol is absorbed through the cornea, it acts as a direct muscarinic agonist, simultaneously inhibiting acetylcholinesterase, and thereby allowing a buildup of acetylcholine. This results in its longer duration of action when compared to pilocarpine.

The three most commonly used anticholinesterases include isoflurophate,[39] demecarium, and echothiophate. The majority of anticholinesterase research has been with echothiophate. Because of the hygroscopic properties of echothiophate, discard solutions after 2 to 3 months. Within two hours after topical .06% echothiophate, profound inhibition of cholinesterase occurs in the entire anterior segment of the eye.[40] Cholinesterase activity is decreased in the cornea, conjunctiva, iris, subcapsular lens epithelium, and ciliary body.

The necessity for multiple applications of pilocarpine led to pilocarpine-impregnated, soft contact lenses. However, these soft lenses contain only a relatively short-term pilocarpine repository dispensing 90% of the pilocarpine within four hours.[41]

The Ocusert (Alza Corp.) is a membrane-controlled delivery system with zero order pharmacokinetics. This approximately 13 x 6 mm system is placed in the conjunctival cul-de-sac and delivers a constant rate of 20 micrograms per hour (Ocusert P-20) or 40 micrograms per hour (Ocusert P-40) equivalent to 1 to 2% and 4% pilocarpine respectively.[42-46] The system delivers one-fifth the amount of medicine required by drops for a comparable pressure reduction.

Pilocarpine also can be administered in a high-viscosity, acrylic vehicle designed to be used once daily.[47,48] Fifty microliters of pilocarpine hydrochloride gel contains 2 mg. of pilocarpine and is equivalent to a 50 microliter drop of 4% pilocarpine solution (2 mg per 50 microliter).

Adverse Effects of Topical Parasympathomimetic Agents

When parasympathomimetic drops are applied to the eye, ocular and systemic adverse reactions can, depending on the strength of the drug used, and whether it is a direct-acting or indirect-acting parasympathomimetic (Table 2-2). Ocular side effects are far more common than adverse systemic reactions.

Table 2-2. Adverse Effects of Parasympathomimetic Drugs

Common	Uncommon
External Adverse Ocular Effects	
Common:	*Uncommon:*
Hyperemia	Epithelial toxicity
Superficial corneal haze*	Contact dermatitis
	Pseudo-pemphigoid†
	Punctal occlusion†
Intraocular Adverse Effects	
Common:	*Uncommon:*
Miosis	Acute angle closure
Accommodative spasm-myopia	Aqueous misdirection
Breakdown of blood aqueous barrier	Retinal detachment
Iris and ciliary body congestion	
Increased pupil block with peripheral anterior synechiae	
Posterior synechiae	
Cataracts (anterior subcapsular)†	
Iris cysts†	
Systemic Adverse Effects	
Common:	*Uncommon:*
Headache	Nausea
Brown ache	Diarrhea
	Abdominal cramps
	Sweating
	Salivation
	Asthma, dyspnea
	Bradycardia
	Anxiety, restlessness, confusion
	Weakness, muscular twitching, pallor†
	Cholinesterase depletion†

*Pilocarpine gel, incidence 20%
†Only reported with indirect-acting parasympathomimetics

External Ocular Effects

Miotic drugs can cause a transient hyperemia of the conjunctiva because of vasodilation of conjunctival vessels. Local allergic sensitivity to the topical parasympathomimetic drugs is relatively uncommon, and if present, a different preservative can be tried.

In 20% of patients using pilocarpine gel for more than 8 weeks, diffuse asymptomatic superficial cornea haze develops. The long-term consequences of this corneal haze are unknown.[49]

The cholinesterase inhibitors can cause stenosis of the lacrimal punctum resulting in epiphora.

Intraocular Effects

The majority of intraocular adverse effects stem from altered muscarinic ocular activity.

Enhanced cholinergic activity of the pupillary sphincter muscle and circular ciliary body muscle results in miosis and accommodative spasm. These are undesired but expected intraocular effects, and result in dim vision, myopia, and a typical brow ache.

Younger persons are more severely affected by ciliary spasm, and typically complain of headaches, myopia, blurred vision, and nyctalopia. Initial discomfort from miotics in phakic patients is least with pilocarpine, moderate with carbachol, and severe with the anticholinesterases. Analgesics taken 30 minutes before topical cholinergic drugs dissipate some of the undesirable brow ache.

Contraction of the ciliary muscle results in axial thickening of the crystalline lens, with a concomitant shallowing of the chamber angle.[50] Topical parasympathomimetics might thereby induce a phacomorphic closure of the trabecular meshwork. Sometimes, the beneficial effect of miosis (pulling the peripheral iris out from the chamber angle) is overcome by relentless miosis leading to increased pupil block and angle closure disease (either acute, subacute, or chronic). Silent closure of the chamber angle might occur in eyes previously described as open because increase pupil block and phacomorphic closure of the chamber angle. Comparative ultrasonography by Francois and colleagues demonstrated that accommodative myopia and lens thickening are much less pronounced with the Ocusert P-20 system compared to 2% pilocarpine drops.[51]

Prolonged and intense miosis produced by the anticholinesterase drugs might lead to iris cysts.[52] These cysts are most common in children and can occlude the pupil and cause visual distortion. Iris cysts are most frequent with isoflurophate and echothiophate. Fortunately, iris cysts resolve when therapy is discontinued. Simultaneous use of phenylephrine 2.5 to 10% will help prevent the formation of iris cysts and as expected, will not hinder therapeutic response.[53]

Cholinergic induced dilation of anterior segment vessels can lead to breakdown of the blood aqueous barrier and ciliary body congestion. Clearly, the strong miotics cause more vascular breakdown and ciliary body congestion. Any topical miotic can cause breakdown of the blood aqueous barrier with resultant iritis, synechiae formation, and elevated IOP. Congestion of the ciliary body and its processes can lead to shallowing of the chamber angle or misdirection of aqueous with elevated IOP. Aqueous misdirection syndrome can be precipitated by miotic medications without ocular surgery.[54]

Unfortunately, anterior subcapsular cataracts are characteristic of indirect-acting parasympathomimetic drugs. In 1960, Harrison was the first to describe lens opacity because of the anticholinesterases.[55] It was found that over a two-year period 50% of echothiophate-treated eyes and 10% of pilocarpine-treated eyes developed lens opacities.[56,57] By late 1969 it was emphasized that anticholinesterases should be used mainly in aphakic glaucoma and other desperate type cases.[58] The cataractogenic potential of the anticholinesterase drugs might be related to inhibition of acetylcholinesterase found in the lens capsule.

It is unknown whether miotic medications truly cause retinal detachment. Pape and Forbes suggested detachment prone eyes might be at increased risk with miotic use; however, Havener presents a convincing argument that there is no causal relationship between miotic use and retinal detachment.[59-61] Whichever is true, it is wise to dilate eyes and examine the peripheral retina before miotic medications are instituted. High risk patients placed on miotic therapy should be educated about the symptoms of vitreoretinal pathology.

Systemic Effects

Topically applied parasympathomimetic drugs are absorbed into the systemic circulation through the nasopharyngeal and gastrointestinal surfaces and produce muscarinic and nicotinic poisoning; the mode of poisoning depends on the type and strength of the parasympathomimetic.

As little as 5 mg. of pilocarpine given subcutaneously causes diaphoresis, and less than 1 mg. of carbachol causes flushing of the face, perspiration, salivation, increased pulse rate, decreased blood pressure, and increased basal metabolic rate. One 50 microliter drop of 10% pilocarpine solution contains 5 mg. of pilocarpine, and a similar size drop of 3% carbachol contains 1.5 mg. of carbachol. The anticholinesterase drugs, which are derivatives of insecticides and war gases, are absorbed rapidly and are extremely potent. Havener points out that these drugs are very dangerous when ingested orally; the contents of a single bottle could kill a child easily.[62]

Excessive doses of pilocarpine might cause muscarinic poisoning. Stimulation of the smooth muscle of various organ systems might cause asthma, diarrhea, salivation, bradycardia, diaphoresis, nausea, and vomiting. This is most likely to occur during treatment for an attack of angle closure when multiple doses of pilocarpine are applied.[63] All of these signs and symptoms occur with increased frequency and intensity with the anticholinesterase drugs, with the added problem of nicotinic poisoning of striated muscle, sympathetic ganglion, and neurologic sequelae. Nicotinic reactions include weakness, muscular twitching, cramps, elevated blood pressure, pallor, and central nervous system reactions of anxiety, tension, restlessness, headaches, tremor, and confusion.[64-69] Severe overdose leads to coma with loss of reflexes.

Anticholinesterases inhibit both tissue acetylcholinesterase and plasma cholinesterase.[70,71] Plasma cholinesterase is required to breakdown succinylcholine. Glaucoma patients treated with anticholinesterases might experience prolonged apnea necessitating ventilatory assistance if succinylcholine is used for induction during general anesthesia. Communication between the patient, anesthesiologist, and ophthalmologist is imperative in the preoperative assessment of glaucoma patients receiving the anticholinesterase drugs. Topically applied anticholinesterase eyedrops or exposure to organophosphate insecticides can reduce the amount of plasma pseudocholinesterase, creating a potentially fatal hazard for surgical patients receiving succinylcholine. Anticholinesterase agents should be discontinued six weeks prior to surgery.[72]

Topical parasympathomimetic drugs have been reported to aggravate an undetected dementia and worsen a preexisting degenerative dementia. Pilocarpine drops can alter cholinoceptive sites in the brain and worsen dementia.[73]

Recommendations

Pilocarpine and carbachol might be helpful to ophthalmologists in a variety of clinical settings. Theoretically, improving outflow that is decreased in the glaucomatous eye seems more appealing than decreasing inflow; this has never been proven. The direct acting parasympathomimetics enhance trabecular outflow and are the time honored drugs for the treatment of primary open angle glaucoma. The long-term use of miotics is also beneficial in patients with primary angle closure glaucoma post iridectomy, especially if at least 180° of the chamber angle is still open. Patients with developmental glaucoma with abnormal trabecular outflow might not respond to parasympathomimetic drugs. Many patients do not tolerate multiple daily dosing of powerful miotics. A more gradual approach is required, especially in younger patients. Starting a weak miotic such as pilocarpine 0.5% once or twice daily can improve compliance and tolerance. Concentration and frequency can be increased in incremental steps until the desired therapeutic response is achieved. If this approach fails, alternative delivery systems such as pilocarpine 4% gel can be offered. Ocuserts give a much lower and constant dose of pilocarpine and are ideal for the younger patient. The insertion and maintenance of a weekly, membrane-controlled delivery system limits its usefulness in the elderly population.

During chronic miotic treatment, periodic gonioscopy is essential to make certain parasympathomimetic induced angle closure does not occur. Shallowing of the chamber angle during miotic treatment might be because of increased pupil block, axial thickening of the lens, ciliary body congestion, or misdirection of aqueous.

All of the miotics can cause breakdown of the blood aqueous barrier with resultant iritis. These drugs might induce iridocyclitis in a previously uninflammed or predisposed eye (e.g., early post-op). If careful slit lamp biomicroscopy reveals increasing flare or cell, the strength or the concentration of the miotic should be reduced. Patients with active uveitis and elevated IOP do not benefit from further breakdown of the blood aqueous barrier because of parasympathomimetic drugs.

Miotics should be used cautiously in patients with vitreoretinal pathology. Some studies suggest patients with vitreoretinal disease are at a higher risk for retinal detachment following miotic treatment, while other authorities believe that there is no definite causal relationship. Depending on the physician's viewpoint, high risk patients should be informed about the presence of vitreoretinal pathology, and how it can alter the therapeutic approach. It is suggested that a peripheral retinal examination be performed when possible. If vitreoretinal pathology is found, such as lattice degeneration and/or retinal holes, treatment of the underlying condition must be considered before miotic therapy is initiated.

If possible, miotics should be discontinued several days before scheduled surgery in order to decrease postoperative inflammation. Severe inflammation, iris cysts, anterior subcapsular cataracts, and angle closure disease can all occur with the powerful indirect-acting parasympathomimetics, such as echothiophate, demecarium bromide, or DFP. The indirect-acting parasympathomimetics are most commonly used in aphakic glaucoma, but iris cysts, inflammation and vitreoretinal pathology might still be a problem.

The physician always must be on the lookout for the systemic muscarinic and nicotinic side effects from these potent indirect- acting parasympathomimetic drugs. Muscarinic side effects include nausea, vomiting, abdominal cramps, diarrhea, bronchial constriction, rhinorrhea, bradycardia, sweating, salivation, and lacrimation. Nicotinic side effects include weakness, muscular twitching, cramps, pallor, and central nervous system problems such as anxiety, tension, headache, tremor, confusion, and coma. Succinylcholine should be avoided during general anesthesia in glaucoma patients receiving anticholinesterases because of prolonged apnea following extubation.

Ophthalmologists have the unique challenge of preserving not only vision, but also a satisfactory quality of life. Understanding parasympathomimetics is one of the keys to quality physician-patient interaction.

References

1. Rodin FH. Eserine: Its history in the practice of ophthalmology. Am J Ophthalmol 30:19-28, 1947.
2. Taylor P. Cholinergic agonists. In Gilman AG, Goodman LS, Rall TW, Murad F. (eds): The Pharmacological Basis of Therapeutics, 7th ed. New York: McMillan 100-109, 1985.
3. Leopold IH. The use and side effects of cholinergic agents in the management of intraocular pressure. In: Drance SM, Newfeld AH, (eds): Glaucoma: Applied Pharmacology and Medical Treatment. Orlando: Grune and Stratton 357-393, 1984.
4. Weiner N, Taylor P. Drugs acting at synaptic and neuroeffector junctional sites: Neurohumoral transmission: the autonomic and somatic motor nervous systems. In Gilman AG, Goodman LS, Rall TW, Murad F,

(eds): The Pharmacological Basis of Therapeutics, 7th ed. New York: McMillan 66-99, 1985.

5. Mindel JS. Cholinergic pharmacology. In Duane TD, Jaeger EA, (eds): Biomedical Foundation of Ophthalmology, vol. 3. Philadelphia: Harper and Row 26:1-26, 1985.
6. Marr WG. The clinical use of di-isopropyl fluorophosphate (D.F.P.) in chronic glaucoma. Am J Ophthalmol 30:1423-1426, 1947.
7. Becker B, Gage T. Demecarium bromide and echothiophate iodide in chronic glaucoma. Arch Ophthalmol 63:126-131, 1960.
8. Leopold IH, Gold P, Gold D. Use of 217MI in the treatment of glaucoma. Arch Ophthalmol 58:363, 1957.
9. Velhagen K Jr. Die grundlagen der okularen pharmakologie und toxikologie des carbaminoylcholins (Lentin Doryll). Klin Monatsbl Augenheilkd 107:319, 1933.
10. Swan KC. Carbaminoylcholine chloride in petrolatum. Arch Ophthalmol 30:591-592, 1943.
11. Bill A, Walinder PE. The effects of pilocarpine on the dynamics of aqueous humor in a primate (macaca irus). Invest Ophthalmol 5:170-175, 1966.
12. Bill A, Philips CI. Uveoscleral drainage of aqueous humor in human eyes. Exp Eye Res 12:275, 1971.
13. Kaufman PL. Mechanisms of actions of the cholinergic drugs in the eye. In Drance SM, Newfeld AH, (eds): Glaucoma: Applied Pharmacology and Medical Treatment. Orlando: Grune and Stratton 395-427, 1984.
14. Barany EH, Rohen JW. Localized contraction and relaxations in the ciliary muscle of vervet monkey (cercopithecus ethiops). In Rohen JW (ed): The Structure of the Eye, Second Symposium. Stuttgart: Schattauer 287-311, 1965.
15. Barany EH. The mode of action of pilocarpine on outflow resistance in the eye of a primate (cercopitheous ethiops). Invest Ophthalmol 1:712, 1962.
16. Barany EH. The immediate effect on outflow resistance of intravenous pilocarpine in the vervet monkey (cercopitheous ethiops). Invest Ophthalmol 6:373, 1967.
17. Krill AE, Newell FW. Effects of pilocarpine on ocular tension dynamics. Am J Ophthalmol 57:34-40, 1964.
18. Drance SM, Nash PA. The dose response of human intraocular pressure to pilocarpine. Can J Ophthalmol 6:9-13, 1971.
19. Berggren L. The effect of parasympathomimetic and sympathomimetic drugs on secretion in vitro by the ciliary processes of the rabbit eye. Invest Ophthalmol 4:91-97, 1965.
20. Taylor P. Anticholinesterase agents. In Gilman AG, Goodman LS, Rall TW, Murad F (eds): The Pharmacological Basis of Therapeutics, 7th ed. New York: McMillan 110-129, 1985.
21. Shields MB. Textbook of Glaucoma. Baltimore: Williams and Wilkins 374-386, 1987.

22. Drance SM, Carr F. Effects of phospholine iodide (217MI) on intraocular pressure in man. Am J Ophthalmol 49:470-474, 1960.
23. Pratt-Johnson JA, Drance SM. Comparison between pilocarpine and echothiophate for chronic simple glaucoma. Arch Ophthalmol 72:485-488, 1964.
24. Kellerman L, King AD. Preliminary observations on the use of new concentrations of echothiophate iodide in the treatment of glaucoma. Am J Ophthalmol 62:278-280, 1966.
25. Krishna N, Leopold H. Echothiophate (phospholine) iodide (217MI) in treatment of glaucoma. Arch Ophthalmol 62:300-313, 1959.
26. Atchoo PD, Vogel HP. Phospholine iodide (.03%) in the therapy of glaucoma. Am J Ophthalmol 62:1044-1048, 1966.
27. Bleiman BS, Schwartz AL. Paradoxical intraocular pressure response to pilocarpine: A proposed mechanism and treatment. Arch Ophthalmol 97:1305-1306, 1979.
28. Alm A, Bill A, Young FA. The effects of pilocarpine and neostigmine on the blood flow through the anterior uveae in monkeys: A study with radioactively labelled microspheres. Exp Eye Res 15:31-36, 1973.
29. Stocker FW. Experimental studies on the blood aqueous barrier. Arch Ophthalmol 37:583-590, 1947.
30. Richardson KT. Parasympathetic Physiology and Pharmacology. Selected Readings in Ophthalmology: Comparison Source Manual. Rochester: American Academy of Ophthalmology and Otolaryngology 209-224, 1975.
31. Harbin, TS, Kaback MB, Podos SM. Comparative intraocular pressure effects of absorbocarpine and isoptocarpine. Ann Ophthalmol 10:59-61, 1978.
32. Harris LS, Galin MA. Effect of ocular pigmentation on hypotensive response to pilocarpine. Am J Ophthalmol 72:923-925, 1971.
33. Lyons JS, Krohn DL. Pilocarpine uptake by pigmented uveal tissue. Am J Ophthalmol 75:885-888, 1973.
34. Melikian HE, Lieberman TW, Leopold IH. Ocular pigmentation and outflow response to pilocarpine and epinephrine. Am J Ophthalmol 72:70-73, 1971.
35. Lowenstein O. The Argyll Robertson pupillary syndrome. Am J Ophthalmol 42:105, 1956.
36. Abramson DH, Chang S, Coleman J. Pilocarpine therapy in glaucoma: Effects on anterior chamber depth, lens thickness, in patients receiving long-term therapy. Arch Ophthalmol 94:914-918, 1976.
37. Havener WH. Ocular Pharmacology. St. Louis: C.V. Mosby, 319, 1983.
38. O'Brien CS, Swann CK. Carbaminoylcholine chloride in the treatment of glaucoma simplex. Arch Ophthalmol 27:253, 1942.
39. Havener WH. Ocular Pharmacology. St. Louis: C.V. Mosby 349-358, 1983.
40. Laties AM. Localization in cornea and lens of topically applied irreversible cholinesterase inhibitors. Am J Ophthalmol 68:848, 1969.

41. Podos SM, Becker B, Asseff G, Hartstein J. Pilocarpine therapy with soft contact lenses. Am J Ophthalmol 73:336, 1972.
42. Macoul KL, Pavan-Langston D. Pilocarpine ocuserts system for sustaining control of ocular hypertension. Arch Ophthalmol 93:587-590, 1975.
43. Friedrich RL. The pilocarpine ocuserts, a new drug delivery system. Ann Ophthalmol 6:1279-1284, 1974.
44. Armally MF, Rao KR. The effects of pilocarpine ocusert with different release rates on ocular pressure. Invest Ophthalmol 12:491-496, 1973.
45. Worthen DM, Zimmerman TJ, Wind CA. An evaluation of the pilocarpine ocuserts. Invest Ophthalmol 13:296-299, 1974.
46. Drance SM, Mitchell DWA, Schulzer M. The duration of action of pilocarpine ocusert on the intraocular pressure in man. Can J Ophthalmol 10:450-452, 1975.
47. Goldberg I, Ashburn FS, Cass MA, Becker B. Efficacy in patient acceptance of pilocarpine gel. Am J Ophthalmol 88:843-846, 1979.
48. March WF, Stewart RM, Mandell AL, Bruce LA. Duration of effects of pilocarpine gel. Arch Ophthalmol 100:1270-1271, 1982.
49. Johnson DH, Epstein DL, Allen RC, et al. A one year multicenter clinical trial of pilocarpine gel. Am J Ophthalmol 97:723-729, 1984.
50. Abramson DH, Chang S, Coleman J, Smith ME. Pilocarpine induced lens changes: an ultrasonic biometric evaluation of dose response. Arch Ophthalmol 92:464-469, 1974.
51. Francois J, Goes F, Zagoriski Z. Comparative ultrasonographic study of the effect of pilocarpine 2% and ocusert P-20 on the eye components. Am J Ophthalmol 86:233-238, 1978.
52. Abraham SV. Intraepithelial cyst of the iris. Am J Ophthalmol 37:327, 1954.
53. Newell, FW. The 1963 AOS Meeting. Am J Ophthalmol 56:311-312, 1963.
54. Rieser JC, Schwartz B. Miotic-induced malignant glaucoma. Arch Ophthalmol 87:706-712, 1972.
55. Harrison R. Bilateral lens opacities: associated with use of di-isopropyl fluorophosphate eyedrops. Am J Ophthalmol 50:153-156, 1960.
56. Shaffer RN, Hetherington J. Anticholinesterase drugs and cataracts. Am J Ophthalmol 62:613-618, 1966.
57. DeRoetth A. Lens opacities in glaucoma patients on phospholine iodide therapy. Am J Ophthalmol 62:619-628, 1966.
58. Morton WR, Drance SM, Fairolough M. The effect of echothiophate iodide on the lens. Am J Ophthalmol 63:1003-1010, 1969.
59. Pape LG, Forbes M. Retinal detachment and miotic therapy. Am J Ophthalmol 85:558-566, 1978.
60. Alpar JJ. Miotics and retinal detachment: A survey and case report. Ann Ophthalmol 11:395-401, 1979.
61. Havener WH. Ocular Pharmacology. St. Louis: C.V. Mosby 370-373, 1983.
62. Havener WH. Ocular Pharmacology. St. Louis: C.V. Mosby 357, 1983.

63. Epstein E, Kaufman I. Systemic pilocarpine toxicity from overdose. Am J Ophthalmol 59:109, 1965.
64. Ellis PP. Systemic effects of locally applied anticholinesterase agents. Invest Ophthalmol 5:146-151, 1966.
65. Hiscox PEA, McCullough C. Cardiac arrest occurring in a patient on echothiophate iodide therapy. Am J Ophthalmol 60:425, 1965.
66. Wahl JW, Tyner GS. Echothiophate iodide: The effect of 0.625% solution on blood cholinesterases. Am J Ophthalmol 60:419, 1965.
67. Klendshoj NC, Olmsted EP. Observation of dangerous side effects of phospholine iodide in glaucoma therapy. Am J Ophthalmol 56:247-250, 1963.
68. Humpreys JA, Holmes JH. Systemic effects produced by echothiophate iodide in the treatment of glaucoma. Arch Ophthalmol 69:737-743, 1963.
69. Drance SM. Comparison of action of cholinergic and anticholinesterase agents in glaucoma. Ophthalmol 5:130-135, 1966.
70. DeRoetth HA, Wong A, Dettbarn WD, et al. Blood cholinesterase activity of glaucoma patients treated with phospholine iodide. Am J Ophthalmol 62:834, 1966.
71. Friberg TR, Thomas JV, Dressel TD. Serum cholinesterase, serum lipase, and serum amylase levels during long-term echothiophate iodide therapy. Am J Ophthalmol 91:530-533, 1981.
72. Leopold IH, Krishna N, Lehman RA. The effects of anticholinesterase agents on the blood cholinesterase levels of normal and glaucoma subjects. Trans Am Ophthalmol Soc 57:63, 1959.
73. Reyes P, et al. Mental status changes induced by eye drops in dementia of the Alzheimer type (letter). J of Neurology, Neurosurgery and Psychiatry 50:113-115, 1987.

CHAPTER 3

Ocular and Systemic Side Effects of Topical Epinephrine and Dipivefrin

Richard J. Starita, MD
Robert D. Fechtner, MD
Ronald L. Fellman, MD

Introduction

Epinephrine (adrenaline) is the major hormone of the adrenal medulla, accounting for 80% of stored catecholamines. It is produced by N-methylation of norepinephrine and released intravascularly by exocytosis. It binds directly to adrenergic receptors resulting in stimulatory activity. Circulating hormone is inactivated by hepatic catechol-O-methyltransferase. Subsequent action of monamine oxidase allows excretion in the urine. Drugs that mimic the action of this hormone at sympathetic receptors are called adrenergic agonists.

Adrenergic receptors are divided into two types, alpha and beta. Alpha receptors are subdivided into α_1 and α_2. Classically the α_1 subtype is postsynaptic mediating vasoconstriction, and the α_2 type is presynaptic inhibiting the release of norepinephrine from sympathetic nerve terminals. Beta receptors are generally thought of as postsynaptic and are subdivided into β_1 and β_2. The β_1 subtype predominates in cardiac tissue mediating inotropic and chronotropic activity, and β_2 is in lung and glandular tissues causing relaxation of smooth muscle. In addition, presynaptic β_2 receptors mediating the release of norepinephrine have been identified. Epinephrine is potentially active at all of these sites.[1]

Historical Perspective

Epinephrine was first used in ophthamology by Darier in 1900. Early clinical trials and research were conducted by a number of physicians; however, Hamburger is given credit for calling attention to this drug as an antiglaucomatous medication in the 1920s. Enthusiasm waned when it was found to precipitate an acute glaucoma attack in a small percentage of patients. Two factors limited its usefulness; the failure to differentiate angle closure from open angle glaucoma, and the unavailability of a stable form of drug in high concentrations for topical use. By 1950, these problems had been overcome and topical epinephrine became an accepted treatment for open angle glaucoma.[2-5]

Epinephrine can decrease IOP as much as 10 to 30% depending on the initial pressure reading and the dose of the drug.[6-10] Fifty to eighty-five percent of ocular hypertensive and primary open angle glaucoma patients using topical epinephrine have their IOP lowered.[11-13] Rarely, a paradoxical elevation of pressure can occur despite a gonioscopically open angle.[14]

Studies of the dose-response relationship of epinephrine treatment have shown that 0.06% solution produces an ocular hypotensive effect with a 1% solution representing the top of the curve. Higher concentrations are needed occasionally. IOP reduction is maximal at 2 to 6 hours with a duration of 12 to 24 hours following topical administration.[3,9,15-17]

Mechanism of Action

Epinephrine is a nonspecific (alpha and beta), direct-acting sympathomimetic drug. Ocular adrenergic pharmacology is complex, and the mechanism of epinephrine-induced pressure reduction is not fully understood. Recent evidence points to an improvement in outflow as the predominant feature of this effect, rather than decreased aqueous production as once thought. A unified concept regarding the action of epinephrine on aqueous dynamics has been postulated.[18,19] The increase in outflow facility with chronic use seems to be mediated mainly by beta adrenergic receptors.

Immediately following instillation, epinephrine stimulates inflow.[20-23] Increased aqueous humor formation is minimal, short-lived, and variable. This can be mediated by beta-adrenergic receptors in the ciliary processes and can result in a transient increase in IOP. Simultaneously, it is believed that alpha-adrenergic stimulation causes vasoconstriction, mydriasis, and an increase in outflow facility.[1,6] Decrease in blood flow and ultrafiltration lead to reduced aqueous production and IOP.[24] These effects are transient and do not significantly affect IOP long term.

Hours after administration, the alpha adrenergic effects are gone and a clinically more significant, intermediate phase of increased facility of outflow can be demonstrated by fluorophotometry. Concomitant tonographic studies suggest an increase in uveal scleral outflow as well.[21,22] The increased facility of outflow can be blocked by timolol (β_1- , β_2-antagonist),[23] but not by betaxolol (β_1- antagonist)[25] nor thymoxamine (α-antagonist),[26] suggesting that this effect is mediated by β_2 adrenergic receptors. Pretreatment with indomethacin (a cyclo-oxygenase inhibitor),[27] leads to inhibition of the epinephrine-induced decrease in IOP, which suggests that prostaglandins play some role in mediating the effect. The exact mechanism remains speculative.

Following chronic administration, continued increase in the facility of outflow occurs.[11,28] This is possibly because of changes in glycosaminoglycan chemistry at the level of the trabecular meshwork,[18,29] or supersensitivity to epinephrine following prolonged use.[30]

Preparations and Distributions

Topical epinephrine is available commercially as hydrochloride, borate salt, or bitartrate (Table 3-1). Borate salt has a higher pH and has been reported to cause less irritation.[31] The bitartrate is available alone or as a 1% solution in combination with variable amounts of pilocarpine. The amount of active bitartrate is proportional to the amount of free base available, and is about half of the stated percentage of commercial concentration. Epinephrine hydrochloride 1%, epinephryl borate 1%, and epinephrine bitartrate 2% are essentially equal in their pressure lowering effects.[32]

Table 3-1. Commercially Available Preparations

Compound	pH	Concentration (%)
Epinephrine hydrochloride	3.5	0.25, 0.5, 1.0, 2.0
Epinephryl borate	7.4	0.5, 1.0, 2.0
Epinephrine bitartrate	4.0	1.0, 2.0
Dipivefrin	4.0	0.1

Epinephrine is also available as the prodrug, dipivefrin (dipivalyl epinephrine). The addition of two pivalic acid groups to epinephrine creates a compound that is far more lipophilic and therefore increases corneal penetration by 17- to 53-fold. This results in about ten times the ocular absorption compared to an equivalent dose of epinephrine.[33-35] Dipivefrin is hydrolized to epinephrine after absorption into the eye, primarily in the cornea (Figure 3-1). While this drug has been shown to be equal to 1% epinephrine in effectiveness, it offers theoretical advantages, such as reduced local and systemic toxicity.[36-39]

When topical epinephrine is applied to an eye, significant uptake occurs in the iris and ciliary body, and to a lesser degree in the choroid and optic nerve. Measurable amounts of the drug can be identified in similar tissues of the untreated eye. In phakic eyes, there is no significant uptake by the retina. However, in aphakia, retinal uptake does occur and choroidal concentration is 2.5 times greater than that found in the phakic eye.[40]

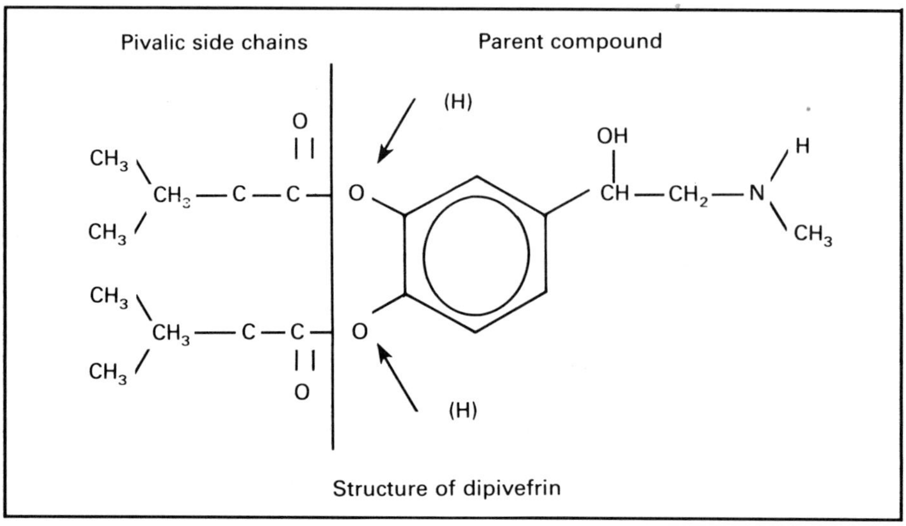

Pivalic side chains

Parent compound

Structure of dipivefrin

Figure 3-1. Structure of dipivefrin: hydrolysis of the ester bonds of dipivefrin results in formation of the parent compound (epinephrine) and two molecules of pivalic acid.

Adverse Effects of Topical Adrenergic Agonists

Adverse effects can be classified as external ocular, intraocular, and systemic effects (Table 3-2).

Table 3-2. Adverse reactions to adrenergic agonists

Common Side Effects		Uncommon Side Effects
	External ocular	
Hyperemia		Bulbar follicular reaction
Blepharoconjunctivitis		Nasolacrimal duct obstruction
Adrenochrome deposition		Pseudo-pemphigoid
		Reactivation of herpes simplex
		Madarosis (loss of lashes)
	Intraocular	
Transient visual blur		Cystoid macular edema
Mydriasis		Visual field loss
	Systemic	
Headache		Vascular hypertension
Anxiety		Cardiac arrhythimas
Palpitations		Tremor

External Ocular Effects

Instillation of topical epinephrine results in transient vasoconstriction with blanching of the conjunctiva followed a few hours later by a reactive hyperemia that can persist for several hours. Patients frequently complain of red eyes while on topical ephinephrine therapy, but might not associate the two because of the delay between application of the drug and onset of hyperemia.

Ocular hypersensitivity to epinephrine is a well-known phenomenon.[41] A blepharoconjunctivitis with or without periocular skin involvement can mimic an atopic reaction or dermatitis.[42] Isolated madarosis (loss of lashes) can also occur.[43] Typically, the conjunctivitis is a toxic follicular type, not allergic as it is commonly labelled. The mechanism is an irritative rather than a hypersensitive one. This reaction is specific to epinephrine compounds, not preservatives, and usually presents from months to years after starting therapy. After discontinuing the drug, symptoms can take weeks to months to fully resolve. In patients taking the medication for the first time, approximately 20% will have persistent ocular irritation from topical epinephrine compounds.[38] In one series, adverse effects involving the external eye (foreign body sensation, tearing, chemosis, and follicles), occurred in two-thirds of the patients within five years. The drug was discontinued in 80% of these patients because of adverse local and systemic effects.[44]

Dipivefrin can cause an external ocular irritation similar to that of epinephrine, but might be tolerated better in many individuals. In a double blind cross-over study, 23.5% of the patients complained of ocular irritation with epinephrine compared to 2.9% with dipivefrin.[38] While the blepharoconjunctivitis from dipivefrin can be as severe as that with epinephrine, there are patients intolerant of epinephrine who can be successfully managed on dipivefrin therapy.[45-47] Dipivefrin also has been associated with bulbar conjunctival follicles similar to those seen with topical antiviral agents.[48]

Many adverse effects of epinephrine have been related to its metabolism into adrenochrome and melanin or melanin-like compounds. Deposition of these pigments has been reported in a variety of ocular tissues. Deposits in the conjunctiva have been reported in up to 30% of patients being treated for more than nine months, and can appear as early as five months.[49-51] Tarsal conjunctival deposits have been implicated in recurrent erosion of the underlying cornea.[52] There have been several reports of black cornea from deposition of pigment. Several of these eyes were thought to have melanomas and were enucleated before the phenomenon was recognized.[51,54-59] Adrenochrome staining has been reported with soft contact lenses. As yet, this has not been noted when using dipivefrin.[60-62] Nasolacrimal duct obstructions have been caused by collections of pigmented debris in several patients.[63,64]

Squamous metaplasia and epidermalization have been noted rarely in the conjunctiva following instillation of epinephrine compounds[65] and have resulted in punctal occlusion.[66] Epinephrine has been implicated as a cause of a drug-induced "pseudo-pemphigoid," with a slowly progressive cicatricial process of the conjunctiva and symblepharon formation.[67-69]

As has been demonstrated in animal models, iontophoresis of epinephrine can cause virus shedding and reactivation of herpes simplex infection of the eye.[70-72] The recommendation is to avoid the use of this drug in patients with a history of herpes simplex.

Intraocular effects

A rather bothersome result of topically administered epinephrine is a sudden decrease in visual acuity that occurs five to fifteen minutes after instillation, and lasts two to four hours. Investigation of this effect usually fails to determine the exact etiology and the mechanism remains unknown.

Mydriasis is an expected, undesired consequence of epinephrine administration. It can precipitate an episode of angle closure and the drug is to be avoided in the predisposed eye. Concomitant timolol therapy potentiates this mydriatic effect.[39,73-75] Careful gonioscopic examination should be performed prior to initiating epinephrine therapy.

Commercially prepared epinephrine has been shown to produce corneal endothelial damage in animal models and cell cultures.[76,77] This is thought to be related to the buffer capacity of the solution.[78] Decreased endothelial cell counts have been reported in human following long-term therapy with topical epinephrine.[79]

Macular edema is a well-recognized complication of epinephrine therapy in the aphakic eye.[80] Fluorescein angiography shows an occurrence rate of 28% with therapy versus 13% for controls. Cystoid macular edema appears within weeks to months of initiating therapy and resolves in 90% of the cases on discontinuation of treatment. Resolution can take six to twelve months and is not related to the length of drug use.[81-84] In animal studies, an intact lens provided an effective barrier to epinephrine penetration of the retina and choroid.[40] Dipivefrin was implicated in one case of cystoid macular edema in a phakic eye, pretreated with timolol, and concurrently treated with pilocarpine. Cessation of dipivefrin resulted in a rapid resolution, and a monocular rechallenge did not induce recurrence.[85]

In a small group of ocular hypertensive patients treated with topical epinephrine hydrochloride in one eye, the untreated contralateral eye developed visual field defects in 32% and glaucomatous cupping in 53%, a much higher incidence than is usually expected in these patients. As first suggested by Jonathan Herschler, it is possible that the epinephrine was deleteriously affecting the circulation of both optic nerves but the treated eye might have been protected from damage by the IOP lowering effect of ephinephrine.[86,87]

Systemic effects

In glaucoma, it is common to use one drop in each eye twice daily. Assuming a drop size of 50 microliters, two drops of epinephrine 1% is a dose of 1 mg., approximately twice the dose administered subcutaneously for the treatment of asthma. The massive doses required for the topical use of epinephrine are a result of relatively poor corneal penetration of this drug. Only about 1% of catecholamines applied topically to the eye is found in ocular contents.[1,34] In animals, 55-65% of topically applied drug was absorbed systemically, reaching peak blood levels in about one and a half hours.[88]

Surprisingly, systemic side effects of topical epinephrine therapy are relatively uncommon.[12,89-92] Frequent complaints seem to be of pain in the area about the eyes or head. In some cases the pain can be severe, causing great anxiety and stress. The pain can come on quickly, usually within minutes, and can last for hours. This is not to be confused with that of stinging on administration. The mechanism of the headache pain described might be related to sudden vasoconstriction and decreased blood flow to the eye.

Patients might also note an increase in anxiety or occasional palpitations. Systemic effects such as elevated blood pressure and cardiac arrhythmias are the most worrisome and can be severe in susceptible patients.[91] When topical epinephrine drugs are being used in hypertensive patients or patients with preexisting cardiac arrhythmias, vital signs should be closely monitored during initiation of therapy. Dipivefrin, which is administered in low concentration and is inactive until hydrolysis, markedly decreases the incidence of systemic side effects.

Drug Interactions

Several of the antidepressant drugs affect adrenergic physiology. Epinephrine is inactivated mainly through uptake by adrenergic neurons or through the action of catechol-O-methyltransferase. The tricyclic antidepressants interfere with the neuronal uptake of epinephrine. These drugs potentiate the presser response to epinephrine and can predispose patients to hypertensive crisis and cardiac arrhythmias. While the interaction between monoamine oxidase inhibitors and indirectly acting sympathomimetic drugs is well known, the MAO inhibitors would not be expected to potentiate the effect of the directly acting adrenergic drugs to a clinically significant extent.[93]

The action of epinephrine can be enhanced by catecholamine-depleting drugs (e.g., reserpine, guanethidine) or blocked by cyclo-oxygenase inhibitors (e.g., indomethacin).[27]

Many inhaled anesthetic agents interact with systemically administered epinephrine to produce cardiac arrhythmias.[94] It is possible that topically administered epinephrine can have a similar effect.

In a single-dose, double blind study, the cardiovascular effects of epinephrine and dipivefrin in patients using timolol was reported. Of the epinephrine-treated patients with cardiovascular disease, 90% demonstrated premature atrial or ventricular contractions (PACs, PVCs) in the two hours of monitoring after application of the test drops and had a significant but modest increase in the mean diastolic blood pressure 10 minutes after instillation. Of the patients without cardiovascular disease, 83% had PACs or PVCs after the administration of epinephrine. The use of dipivefrin did not significantly modify the blood pressure or cause arrhythmias.[95]

A potentially serious adverse interaction between beta-blockers and epinephrine exists. When a patient whose beta-receptors are blocked is exposed to epinephrine, the normal cardiac response of increased rate and force of contradiction is blocked while the α-adrenergic mediated vasconstriction can cause a profound increase in peripheral resistance and elevated blood pressure. This can be followed by carotid baroreceptor mediated vagal showing of the heart leading to bradycardia and hypotension. This sequence of events has been reported in patients taking systemic beta-blockers who received local anesthetic solutions containing epinephrine.[96,97] Bradycardia and hypotension following retrobulbar and eyelid blocks in a patient receiving timolol eye drops has been reported and might have been because of the sympathetic discharge associated with the stress of surgery and beta-blockade from the timolol.[98]

Disease Interactions

In the absence of a patent iridectomy, epinephrine compounds should be used with caution in patients with narrow angles or chronic angle closure glaucoma. By topical administration of these drugs, dilation of the pupil can precipitate an acute angle closure attack or exacerbate relative pupillary block. In high risk patients, an iridectomy is recommended prior to use of these drugs. Pilocarpine does not protect the patient from angle closure problems and might make them worse (see Chapter 2). Cataract development can cause progressive angle compromise over time.[73] In these cases, gonioscopy is recommended at regular intervals.

Epinephrine compounds should be used with caution in patients with hypertensive cardiovascular disease or coronary artery disease.[91, 95] Mean diastolic blood pressure can be increased transiently. Cardiac arrhythmias such as PACs and PVCs can be precipitated or exacerbated by topical administration. Dipivefrin is the epinephrine compound of choice in these cases. Consultation with the patient's medical physician might be required in high risk cases when therapy is initiated (e.g., Holter monitor).

Thyrotoxicosis imposes a variety of burdens upon the heart. Cardiac work and cardiac output are increased. Atrial irritability is enhanced, leading to atrial fibrillation. In patients with a normal heart, exogenous epinephrine might be tolerated. In the patient with underlying heart disease, the use of exogenous epinephrine might precipitate or aggravate cardiac insufficiency.

Recommendations

Topical epinephrine compounds have been in use for the medical treatment of glaucoma for many years. There is evidence that they prevent visual field loss and glaucomatous cupping in glaucoma suspects with a low incidence of side effects.[44,86] The risk of serious systemic adverse reactions is lower with epinephrine than with beta-blockers. The use of dipivefrin increases the margin of safety by reducing the amount of drug absorbed systemically.

Although the one year failure rate of epinephrine is greater than that of timolol, and the IOP lowering effect averages less than that of timolol,[99] epinephrine is a considerably safer drug that can effectively lower intraocular pressure in some patients and should be considered as a first-line drug in the treatment of glaucoma.[100] Many patients on single drug therapy with either epinephrine or timolol will eventually require additional medications or other therapy. After the first year of successful IOP reduction, the failure rate is the same for both medications.[99]

Prior to initiation of epinephrine therapy a careful medical and drug history should be obtained. Several possible drug interactions have been discussed. Certain systemic diseases might be exacerbated by exogenous catecholamine; their use in the presence of unstable hypertensive disease, advanced coronary artery disease, cardiac arrhythmias, and hyperthyroidism should be monitored closely. In high risk patients, consultation with their general medical physician is advisable and dipivefrin should be selected if an epinephrine compound is to be used. A thorough pretreatment ophthalmic examination should be performed including gonioscopy as topical instillation of epinephrine can be potentially harmful to a patient with narrow angles or chronic angle closure disease. If an epinephrine compound is used in an aphakic or pseudophakic eye, macular function must be monitored carefully.

Epinephrine can have a delayed pressure lowering effect.[11,28] A reasonable trial of therapy is probably between one and three months. Any patient who has not responded to epinephrine within three months is unlikely to do so.[99] Epinephrine is a safe and effective medication for the treatment of glaucoma. Use of dipivefrin increases the margin of safety. These drugs should be considered as first line therapy in the treatment of primary open angle glaucoma.[100] The presence of ocular and systemic side effects should be reevaluated at each patient visit. Late failures of therapy are common due to intolerance or loss of effectiveness.

References

1. Sears ML. Autonomic nervous system: adrenergic agonist. In Sears ML (ed): Pharmacology of the Eye. New York: Springer-Verlag pp 193-248, 1984.
2. Duke-Elder S. Pharmacological agents - II: systemic effectors. In: Duke-Elder S. System of Ophthalmology. St. Louis, MI: C.V. Mosby 7:570-579, 1962.
3. Drance SM, Ross RA. The ocular effects of epinephrine. Surv Ophthalmol 14:330-335, 1970.
4. Goldmann H. Abflussdruck, minutenvolumen und widerstand der kammerwassershomung des menshen. Doc Ophthalmol 5-6:278-356, 1951.
5. Weekers R, Delmarcelle Y, Gustin J. Treatment of ocular hypertension by adrenaline and diverse sympathomimetic amines. Am J Ophthalmol 40:666-672, 1955.
6. Kronfeld PC. Dose-effect relationships as an aid in the evalutation of ocular hypotensive drugs. Invest Ophthalmol Vis Sci 3:258-265, 1964.
7. Krill AE, Newell FW, Novack M. Early and long-term effects of levo-epinephrine on ocular tension and outflow. Am J Ophthalmol 59:833-839, 1965.
8. Galin MA, Baras I, Glenn J. L-epinephrine and intraocular pressure. Invest Ophthalmol Vis Sci 5:120-124, 1966.
9. Kitazawa Y. Dose responsive analysis of ocular hypotensive effects of epinephrine and norepinephrine. Jpn J Ophthalmol 16:30-38, 1972.

10. Kass MA, Mandell AI, Goldberg I, Paine JM, Becker B. Dipivefrin and epinephrine treatment of elevated intraocular pressure. A comparative study. Arch Ophthalmol 97:1865-1866, 1979.
11. Becker B, Pettit TH, Gay AJ. Topical epinephrine therapy of open-angle glaucoma. Arch Ophthalmol 66:219-225, 1961.
12. Becker B, Montgomery SW, Kass MA, Shin DH. Increased ocular and systemic responsiveness to epinephrine in primary open-angle glaucoma. Arch Ophthalmol 95:789-790, 1977.
13. Drance SM, Saheb NE, Schulzer M. Response to topical epinephrine in chronic open-angle glaucoma. Arch Ophthalmol 96:1001-1002, 1978.
14. Lee PF. The influence of epinephrine and phenylephrine on intraocular pressure. Arch Ophthalmol 60:863-867, 1958.
15. Garner LL, Johnstone WW, Ballintine EJ, Carroll NE. Effect of 2% levo-rotary epinephrine on the intraocular pressure of the glaucomatous eye. Arch Ophthalmol 62:230-238, 1959.
16. Obstbaum SA, Kolker AE, Phelps CD. Low-dose epinephrine. Effect on intraocular pressure. Arch Ophthalmol 92:118-120, 1974.
17. Harris LS, Galin MA, Lerner R. The influence of low-dose l-epinephrine on the intraocular pressure. Ann Ophthalmol 2:253- 257, 1970.
18. Sears ML, Neufeld AH. Adrenergic modulation of the outflow of aqueous humor. Invest Ophthalmol Vis Sci 14:83-86, 1975.
19. Neufeld AH. The mechanisms of action of adrenergic drugs in the eye. In Drance SM, Neufeld AH (eds): Glaucoma: Applied Pharmacology in Medical Treatment. Orlando: Grune and Stratton pp 277-301, 1984.
20. Nagataki S, Brubaker RF. Early effect of epinephrine on aqueous formation in the normal human eye. Ophthalmology 88:278- 282, 1981.
21. Townsend DJ, Brubaker RF. Immediate effect of epinephrine on aqueous formation in the normal human eye as measured by fluorophotometry. Invest Ophthalmol Vis Sci 19:256-266, 1980.
22. Schenker HI, Yablonski ME, Podos SM, Linder L. Photometric study of epinephrine and timolol in human subjects. Arch Ophthalmol 99:1212-1216, 1981.
23. Higgins RG, Brubacker RF. Acute effect of epinephrine on aqueous humor formation in the timol-treated normal eye as measured by fluorophotometry. Invest Ophthamol Vis Sci 19:420- 423, 1980
24. Alm A. The effect of topical l-epinephrine on regional ocular blood flow in monkeys. Invest Ophthalmol Vis Sci 19:487-491, 1980.
25. Allen RC, Epstein DL. Additive effect of betaxolol and epinephrine in primary open-angle glaucoma. Arch Ophthalmol 104:1178-1184, 1986.
26. Lee DA, Brubaker RF, Nagataki S. Acute effect of thymoxamine on aqueous humor formation in the epinephrine-treated normal eye as measured by fluorophotometry. Invest Ophthalmol Vis Sci 24:165-168, 1983.
27. Camras CB, Feldman SG, Podos SM, et al. Inhibition of the epinephrine-induced reduction of intraocular pressure by systemic indomethacin in humans. Am J Ophthalmol 100:169-175, 1985.

28. Ballintine EJ, Garner LL. Improvement of the coefficient outflow in glaucomatous eyes. Prolonged treatment with epinephrine. Arch Ophthalmol 66:48-51, 1961.
29. Armaly MF, Wang Y. Demonstration of acid mucopolysaccharides in the trabecular meshwork of the Rhesus monkey. Invest Ophthalmol Vis Sci 14:507-516, 1975.
30. Flach AJ, Kramer SG. Supersensitivity to the topical epinephrine after long-term epinephrine therapy. Arch Ophthalmol 98:482-483, 1980.
31. Vaughan D. Shaffer R, Riegelman S. A new stabilized form of epinephrine for the treatment of open-angle glaucoma. Arch Ophthalmol 66:108-111, 1961.
32. Criswick VG, Drance SM. Comparative study of four different epinephrine salts on intraocular pressure. Arch Ophthalmol 75:768-770, 1966.
33. Mandell AI, Stentz F, Kitabchi AE. Dipivalyl epinephrine: a new prodrug in the treatment for glaucoma. Ophthalmology 85:268- 275, 1978.
34. Wei C, Anderson JA, Leopold I. Ocular absorption and metabolism of topically applied epinephrine and a dipivalyl ester of epinephrine. Invest Ophthalmol Vis Sci 17:315-321, 1978.
35. Mishima S. Clinical pharmacokinetics of the eye. Invest Ophthalmol Vis Sci 21:504-541, 1981.
36. Kaback MB, Podos SM, Harbin TS, Mandell A, Becker B. The effects of dipivalyl epinephrine on the eye. Am J Ophthalmol 81:768-772, 1976.
37. Kass MA, Mandell AI, Goldberg I, Paine M, Becker B. Dipivefrin and epinephrine treatment of elevated intraocular pressure. A comparative study. Arch Ophthalmol 97:1865-1866, 1979.
38. Kohen AN, Moss AP, Hargett NA, et al. Clinical comparison of dipivalyl and epinephrine in the treatment of glaucoma. Am J Ophthalmol 87:196-201, 1979.
39. Goldberg I, Ashburn FS, Palmberg PF, Kass MA, Becker B. Timolol and epinephrine. A clinical study of ocular interactions. Arch Ophthalmol 98:484-486, 1980.
40. Kramer SG. Epinephrine distribution after topical administration to phakic and aphakic eyes. Trans Am Ophthalmol Soc 78:947-982, 1980.
41. Aronson SB, Wyamamoto EA. Ocular hypersensitivity to epinephrine. Invest Ophthalmol Vis Sci 5:75-80, 1966.
42. Byron HM. Conjunctival reaction due to l-epinephrine bitartrate (Epitrate). Arch Ophthalmol 63:567-570, 1960.
43. Kass MA, Stamper RL, Becker B. Madarosis and chronic epinephrine therapy. Arch Ophthalmol 88:429-432, 1972.
44. Becker B, Morton WR. Topical epinephrine in glaucoma suspects. Am J Ophthalmol 62:272-277, 1966.
45. Yablonski ME, Shin DH, Kolker AE, et al. Dipivefrin use in patients with intolerance to topically applied epinephrine. Arch Ophthalmol 95:2157-2158, 1977.

46. Theodore J, Leibowitz HM. External ocular toxicity of dipivalyl epinephrine. Am J Ophthalmol 88:1013-1016, 1979.
47. Wandel T, Spinak M. Toxicity of dipivalyl epinephrine. Ophthalmology 88:259-260, 1981.
48. Liesegang TJ. Bulbar conjunctival follicles associated with dipivefrin therapy. Ophthalmology 92:228-233, 1985.
49. Corwin ME, Spencer WH. Conjunctival melanin depositions. A side-effect of topical epinephrine therapy. Arch Ophthalmol 69:317-321, 1963.
50. Mooney D. Pigmentation after long-term topical use of adrenaline compounds. Br J Ophthalmol 54:823-826, 1970.
51. Cashwell LF, Shields MB, Reed JW. Adrenochrome pigmentation. Arch Ophthalmol 95:514-515, 1977.
52. Pardos GJ, Krachmer JH, Mannis MJ. Persistent corneal erosion secondary to tarsal adrenochrome deposits. Am J Ophthalmol 90:870-871, 1980.
53. Reinecke RD, Kuwabara T. Corneal deposits secondary to topical epinephrine. Arch Ophthalmol 70:170-172, 1963.
54. Ferry AP, Zimmerman LE. Black cornea, a complication of topical use of epinephrine. Am J Ophthalmol 58:205-210, 1964.
55. Cleasby G, Donaldson DD. Epinephrine pigmentation of the cornea. Arch Ophthalmol 78:74-75, 1967.
56. Green WR, Kaufer GJ, Dubroff S. Black cornea: a complication of topical use of epinephrine. Ophthalmologica 154:88-95, 1967.
57. Krejci L, Harrison R. Corneal pigment deposits from topically administered epinephrine. Experimental production. Arch Ophthalmol 82:836-839, 1969.
58. Madge GE, Geeraets WJ, Guerry D. Black cornea secondary to topical epinephrine. Am J Ophthalmol 71:402-405, 1971.
59. McCarthy RW, LeBlanc R. "Black Cornea" secondary to topical epinephrine. Can J Ophthalmol 11:336-340, 1976.
60. Sugar J. Adrenochrome pigmentation of hydrophilic lenses. Arch Ophthalmol 91:11-12, 1974.
61. Miller D, Brooks SM, Mobilia E. Adrenochrome staining of soft contact lenses, Ann Ophthalmol 8:65-67, 1976.
62. Newton MJ, Nesburn AB. Lack of hydrophilic lens discoloration in patients using dipivalyl epinephrine for glaucoma. Am J Ophthalmol 87:193-195, 1979.
63. Spaeth GL. Nasolacrimal duct obstruction caused by topical epinephrine. Arch Ophthalmol 77:355-357, 1967.
64. Barishak R, Romano A, Stein R. Obstruction of lacrimal sac caused by topical epinephrine. Ophthalmologica 159:373-379, 1969.
65. Wright. Squamous metaplasia or epidermalization of the conjunctiva as an adverse reaction to topical medication. Trans Ophthalmol Soc UK 99:244-246, 1979.
66. Romano A, Barishak R, Stein R. Obstruction of lacrimal puncta caused by topical epinephrine. Ophthalmologia 166:301-305, 1973.

67. Norn MS. Pemphigoid related to epinephrine treatment. Am J Ophthalmol 83:138, 1977.
68. Fraunfelder FT. Interim report: national registry of possible drug-induced ocular side-effects. Ophthalmology 87:87-90, 1980.
69. Blanchard DL. Adrenergic-associated symblepharon. Glaucoma 9:18-20, 1987.
70. Kwon BS, Gangarosa LP, Burck KD, DeBack J, Hill JM. Induction of ocular herpes simplex virus shedding by iontophoresis of epinephrine to rabbit cornea. Invest Ophthalmol Vis Sci 21:442- 449, 1981.
71. Shimomura Y, Gangarosa LP, Kataoka M, Hill JM. HSV-1 shedding of iontophoresis of 6-hydroxydopamine followed by topical epinephrine. Invest Ophthalmol Vis Sci 24:1588-1594, 1983.
72. Hill JM, Shimomura Y, Kwon BS, Gangarosa LP. Iontophoresis of epinephrine isomers to rabbit eyes induced HSV-1 ocular shedding. Invest Ophthalmol Vis Sci 26:1299-1303, 1985.
73. Van Buskirk EM. Hazards of medical glaucoma therapy in the cataract patient. Ophthalmology 89:238-241, 1982.
74. Öhrstrom A, Pandolfi M. Regulation of intraocular pressure and pupil size by beta-blockers and epinephrine. Arch Ophthalmol 98:2182-2184, 1980.
75. Keates EU, Stone RA. Safety and effectiveness of concomitant administration of dipivefrin and timolol maleate. Am J Ophthalmol 91:243-248, 1981.
76. Hull BS, Chemotti MT, Edelhauser HF, Van Horn DL, Hyndiuk RA. Effect of epinephrine on the corneal endothelium. Am J Ophthalmol 79:245-250, 1975.
77. Krejci L, Harrison R. Epinephrine effects on corneal cells and tissue culture. Arch Ophthalmol 83:451-454, 1970.
78. Edelhauser HF, Hyndiuk RA, Zeeb A, Schultz RO. Corneal edema and the intraocular use of epinephrine. Am J Ophthalmol 93:327- 333, 1982.
79. Waltman SR, Yarian D, Hart W, Becker B. Corneal endothelial changes with long-term topical epinephrine therapy. Arch Ophthalmol 95:1357-1358, 1977.
80. Kolker AE, Becker B. Epinephrine maculopathy. Arch Ophthalmol 79:552-562, 1968.
81. Michels RG, Maumenee E. Cystoid macular edema associated with topically applied epinephrine in aphakic eyes. Am J Ophthalmol 80:379-388, 1975.
82. Thomas JV, Gragoudas ES, Blair NP, Lapus JV. Correlation of epinephrine use and macular edema in aphakic glaucomatous eyes. Arch Ophthalmol 96:625-628, 1978.
83. Obstbaum SA, Galin MA, Poole TA. Topical epinephrine and cystoid macular edema. Ann Ophthalmol 8:455-458, 1976.
84. Mackool RJ, Muldoon T, Fortier A, Nelson D. Epinephrine- induced cystoid macular edema in aphakic eyes. Arch Ophthalmol 95:791-793, 1977.

85. Mehelas TJ, Kollarits CR, Martin WG. Cystoid macular edema presumably induced by dipivefrin hydrocholoride (Propine). Am J Ophthalmol 94:682, 1982.
86. Shin DH, Kolker AE, Kass MA, Kaback MB, Becker B. Long-term epinephrine therapy of ocular hypertension. Arch Ophthalmol 94:2059-2060, 1976.
87. Kramer SG. Considerations on epinephrine therapy in glaucoma. Ann Ophthalmol 10:1077, 1978.
88. Anderson JA. Systemic absorption of topical ocularly applied epinephrine and dipivefrin. Arch Ophthalmol 98:350-353, 1980.
89. Ballin N, Becker B, Goldman ML. Systemic effects of epinephrine applied topically to the eye. Invest Ophthalmol Vis Sci 5:125-129, 1966.
90. Kerr CR, Hass I, Drance SM, Walters MB, Schultzer M. Cardiovascular effects of epinephrine and dipivalyl epinephrine applied topically to the eye in patients with glaucoma. Br J Ophthalmol 66:109-114, 1982.
91. Lansche RK. Systemic reactions: to topical epinephrine and phenylephrine. Am J Ophthalmol 61:95-98, 1966.
92. Shaffer RN. Autonomic ocular drugs: desirable and undesirable effects. Invest Ophthalmol Vis Sci 3:498-503, 1964.
93. Boakes AJ, Laurence DR, Teoh PC, et al. Interaction between sympathomimetic amines and antidepressant agents in man. Br Med J 1:311-315, 1973.
94. Katz RL, Epstein RA. The interaction of anesthetic agents in adrenergic drugs to produce cardiac arrhythmias. Anesthesiology 29:763-784, 1968.
95. Blondeau P, Cote M. Cardiovascular effects of epinephrine and dipivefrin in patients using timolol. Can J Ophthalmol 19:2932, 1984.
96. Foster CA, Aston SJ. Propranolol-epinephrine interaction: a potential disaster. Plast Reconstr Surg 72:74-78, 1983.
97. Brummett RE. Warning to otolaryngologists using local anesthetics containing epinephrine: potential serious reaction occurring in patients treated with beta-adrenergic receptor blockers. Arch Otolaryngol 110:561, 1984.
98. Caprioli J, Sears ML. Caution of the preoperative use of topical timolol. Am J Ophthal 95:561-562, 1983.
99. Alexander DW, Berson FG, Epstein DL. A clinical trial of timolol and epinephrine in the treatment of primary open-angle glaucoma. Ophthalmology 95:247-251, 1988.
100. Podos SM, Ritch R. Epinephrine as the initial therapy in selective cases of ocular hypertension. Surv Ophthalmol 25:188-194, 1980.

CHAPTER 4

Ocular and Systemic Side Effects of Topical Beta Adrenergic Antagonists

Ronald L. Fellman, MD
Richard J. Starita, MD

Introduction

There are three topical beta blockers available for ophthalmic use in the United States. The ophthalmic and medical literature concerning these beta blockers is voluminous, confusing, conflicting, and controversial. Trying to interpret this pharmacologic and neurobiologic drug data and to incorporate it into the routine practice of medicine is becoming an increasingly difficult task. Many of the side effects of beta blockers can be deduced from a working knowledge of normal sympathetic nervous system functions. The receptors that regulate sympathetic activity at various organ systems are known as alpha and beta adrenoceptors. Beta receptors are classified as β_1 or β_2 based on their affinity for defined pharmacologic agents. Drugs that mimic the actions of norepinephrine and epinephrine are known as sympathomimetics or alpha/beta agonists. Drugs that bind to beta receptors but do not activate them are known as beta antagonists, or simply beta blockers.[1,2] Beta blockers occupy the beta receptor and prevent normal sympathetic beta transmission. However, if the concentration of beta agonists is high enough, the competitive beta blocker is displaced from the receptor and normal sympathetic transmission is resumed. To make this even more complex, certain beta blockers cause partial activation of a receptor. This is known as intrinsic sympathomimetic activity.

At times, we might feel hopelessly lost in the therapeutic jungle of beta blockers. Commercially available beta blockers are described in terms of their specificity for β_1- or β_2- receptors. Timolol and levobunolol are nonselective, binding with equal affinity to both receptors. Betaxolol is considered a relatively selective β_1-blocker. From these agents, the ophthalmologist must select the appropriate beta blocker to fit the individual patient's clinical profile. The following information should help the ophthalmologist to decide which topical beta blocker is best for his/her patients.

Historical Perspectives

Twenty years ago, investigators believed that both alpha and beta adrenergic receptors mediated ocular outflow. Supposedly, the facility of outflow was increased by alpha stimulation and decreased by beta stimulation. By inhibiting beta tone in the outflow channels, investigators hoped to find an increase in outflow with a resultant decrease in IOP. Therefore, the advent of beta blockers afforded the unique opportunity to simulate that part played by beta activity.

In 1964 propranolol was introduced as the first clinically significant, nonselective, beta adrenergic antagonist. During a preliminary investigation giving intravenous followed by oral propranolol, Phillips and colleagues found a lowering of IOP in patients with glaucoma.[3] This observation was confirmed with either oral or intravenous administration.[4,5]

Early reports with topical propranolol revealed a reduction of IOP in normal and glaucomatous eyes.[6,7] However, ocular stinging, irritation, and local anesthetic effect on the cornea limited its usefulness.[8] It was known that cardiac beta blockade did not depend on local anesthetic activity. The ocular hypotensive response of topical practolol, a β_1 selective antagonist with no local anesthetic activity, was similar to propranolol (4-mm Hg drop).[9] This suggested that the lowering of ocular tension was mediated by a blocking effect on β-adrenergic receptors, rather than membrane stabilization, which accounts for the anesthetic effect.

The problems of minimal IOP reduction and local ocular irritation led to the conclusion that topical beta blockers were of little importance therapeutically in the treatment of glaucoma.[10] Further studies with oral beta blockers demonstrated more significant IOP reductions, but with increased systemic side effects.[11,12,13] Investigators continued to try to find an optimal topical beta blocker that would lower IOP significantly with minimal side effects. The breakthrough came in the 1970s when timolol maleate became available. This potent, nonselective beta blocker, which lacked both intrinsic sympathomimetic and local anesthetic activity,[14] was tested topically in normal volunteers.[15] In primary open angle glaucoma, it caused a far greater reduction in IOP (13 mm Hg drop) at one hour than other investigational agents.[16] The multiple studies that followed established its overall safety and efficacy in IOP reduction.[17-23] In 1978, FDA approval was granted and timolol became the predominant topical agent for the chronic treatment of glaucoma. More recently, betaxolol received FDA approval for topical use, followed shortly by levobunolol. Discussion of these three agents will be the main focus in this chapter.

Mechanism of Action

Timolol, levobunolol, and betaxolol lower IOP by decreasing aqueous humor production. Flurophotometric studies demonstrate convincingly that topical beta blockers suppress the flow of aqueous humor by approximately 30 to 50%. This response is not altered by sex or eye color.[24,25,26] How these agents reduce aqueous inflow is unknown. Theories include blockade of β_2 receptors in ciliary processes, inhibition of cAMP synthesis, and dissipation of mitochondrial oxidative phosphorylation in the nonpigmented ciliary epithelium.[27,28,29] It is possible that β_2 receptors can be blocked with a β_1 selective antagonist such as betaxolol. After topical instillation, the concentration achieved in the anterior segment is so high that cross-receptor blocking can occur.[30] These three topical beta blockers lack both intrinsic sympatomimetic and local anesthetic activity.

Topical beta blockers have enough lipophilicity to cross the cornea and gain entrance into the anterior chamber. Following instillation in human eyes, a peak concentration is obtained within 60 to 70 minutes.[31] In animal studies, topical beta blockers bind to eye pigment and are not metabolized by ocular tissues.[32] Topically administered ophthalmic medications are absorbed systemically through the nasal mucosa.[33] Since intestinal absorption is not active, first-pass hepatic clearance does not occur. Nasal absorption of an eye drop thus mimics intravenous therapy and results in varying degrees of systemic beta blockade. For example, systemic absorption might cause a noticeable pressure decrease in the untreated, fellow eye with long-term, monocular timolol therapy.[34]

Neurobiologically speaking, beta blockers can interfere with noradrenergic transmission in the brain, a pathway implicated already in some depressions. Central nervous system adrenoreceptors are thought to be mainly β_1. Utilizing topical timolol in normal volunteers, a strong trend toward decreasing vigor and increasing fatigue was found subjectively when compared to placebo. This observation could not be confirmed by psychological profiles; no statistically significant difference was documented between the timolol treated and placebo groups.[35]

When called upon, the sympathetic nervous system is responsible for increasing heart rate and myocardial contractility. The β_1 adrenoceptors located in the heart are responsible for the appropriate chronotropic and inotropic cardiovascular functions. Vascular smooth muscle tone is regulated also by adrenoceptors. Stimulation of alpha receptors increases arterial resistance, whereas β_2 receptor stimulation promotes smooth muscle relaxation. Clinical response to beta blockade includes slowing of sinus rate, depression of atrioventricular conduction, decreased cardiac output at rest and on exercise, reduction of systolic blood pressure on exercise, general reduction of blood pressure in both supine and standing positions, inhibition of isoproterenol induced tachycardia, and reduction of reflexive orthostatic tachycardia.[1,2] Clearly, the sympathetic compensatory system is inhibited by beta blockade.

The autonomic nervous system is responsible for maintaining open bronchial airways. Parasympathetic stimulation causes bronchospasm while sympathetic stimulation produces bronchodilation. Sympathetic bronchodilation is mediated mainly by β_2 adrenoceptors. It is possible for beta blockers to aggravate or induce bronchospasm at any age.[36] Nonselective beta blockers are more likely to cause bronchospasm than betaxolol because of their inability to selectively bind to β_1 receptors.[37]

Preparations and Distributions

Timolol maleate is a nonselective beta blocker, 6 to 10 times more potent than propranolol.[14] Dose response analysis with varying topical concentrations (0.1 to 1%) reveals 0.25 and 0.5% timolol give the maximal ocular hypertensive effect that lasts up to 24 hours.[17,18] Both concentrations are available commercially. Timolol administered once daily lowers IOP by about 20% and achieves adequate control in approximately 50% of cases. Increasing the dosage to twice daily results in a slightly greater reduction of IOP and adequate control in 70 to 80% of cases.[38,39] The majority of patients respond to 0.25% twice daily;[22,23] increasing to 0.5% might not result in further pressure reduction.[40] If no response is obtained, however, or if IOP control is lost with time, increasing the concentration to 0.5% can be beneficial.[21,41-43] The initial one hour pressure response to timolol is not predictive of future pressure measurements.[41] Timolol is maximally effective in the first few days after initiating therapy; however, the IOP tends to stabilize over the ensuing weeks. An upward drift by 2 to 4 mm Hg per year might occur.

The systemic absorption of topically applied timolol is clinically significant and is estimated to be 80% in the absence of lid closure and/or nasolacrimal occlusion.[33] Only 10% of timolol binds to plasma protein, which leaves the majority of the drug available for receptor activity. The usual intravenous dose of timolol (.025 mg/kg) for a 70 kg individual is 1.75 mg. This amount results in a plasma concentration of 10 ng/ml at 2 hours.[44] Significant beta adrenoceptor blockade has been observed at timolol plasma concentration above 3 to 4 ng/ml.[45] Following 2 drops of 0.5% timolol in adults, plasma levels range from 5 to 9.6 ng/ml;[46,47] and one hour after bilateral instillation from .87 to 2.45 ng/ml. Children might have a more marked elevation.[48] The absolute values are probably higher since timolol plasma levels are already decreasing at one hour.[49] Systemic beta blockade and resultant side effects (such as reduction in resting heart rate) are dose dependent.[19,38]

Like timolol, levobunolol is a nonselective beta blocker with six times the potency of propranolol.[50] Levobunolol is subject to hepatic metabolism and is converted mainly to dihydrobunolol, which has beta blocker activity similar to levobunolol. The plasma half-life of levobunolol is six hours and that of dihydrobunolol seven hours.[51] Levobunolol and its derivatives are excreted primarily in the urine. It is commercially available only in a concentration of 0.5%. The maximal ocular hypotensive response to levobunolol occurs between two and six hours after instillation. Physicians using topical 0.5%

levobunolol can expect adequate IOP control in approximately 65 to 75% of patients. Ten to 15% of patients will not have a meaningful IOP reduction, and another 10% will terminate the drug because of adverse effects.[52-55]

Overall results with this drug are comparable to twice daily timolol.[43,56] However, the mean reduction in IOP using once daily levobunolol 0.5% might not increase further with twice daily therapy (7.0 versus 7.03 mm Hg).[57] It has been suggested that overall reduction in IOP using 0.5% once daily might be greater with levobunolol than with timolol at 24 hours.[57] The effect of once versus twice daily levobunolol on the diurnal pressure curve in glaucoma patients remains unknown. Recent studies have shown the ocular hypotensive efficacy of 0.25% twice daily levobunolol to be comparable to timolol, but greater than betaxolol if measurements are taken 12 hours following instillation.[43,58] Mean plasma levels of levobunolol at one hour are similar to those reported for timolol.[59]

Betaxolol is the first, selective, topical beta blocker approved for use in this country. It blocks mainly β_1 receptors, and is thus called a cardioselective beta blocker. Betaxolol has more than a 100-fold greater affinity for β_1 receptors than for β_2 receptors. This means that 100 times more betaxolol is needed to block β_2 receptors than to block β_1 receptors.[60] Equally effective cardiac blockade occurs with 0.25 mg/kg of intravenous timolol, .150 mg/kg of intravenous betaxolol, and .200 mg/kg of intravenous propranolol.[61] Thus the beta blocking potency of betaxolol is equivalent to propranolol, and is roughly 1/6 that of timolol and levobunolol. Although betaxolol binds 100 times preferentially to the β_1 receptor, this is one tenth that of timolol.[62] This exemplifies the importance of grasping the concepts of receptor selectivity and affinity before understanding the side effects of beta blockers. β_1 selectivity is relative and not absolute. Larger doses of betaxolol might inhibit all beta adrenergic receptors. Betaxolol is broken down into inactive metabolites that are excreted in the urine, with 15% excreted unchanged. Intravascularly, approximately 55% is bound to plasma proteins. The elimination half-life of betaxolol is 14 to 22 hours (compared to 4 to 6 hours for timolol and levobunolol) and might be increased in elderly subjects and in day-old infants.[63,64,65]

Given topically, betaxolol lowers IOP significantly in normal and glaucomatous eyes.[66-69] It is commercially available only in 0.5% concentration. A twice daily administration is recommended, with the IOP lowering effect of a single drop dissipated largely by 24 hours. Statistically, IOP reduction with betaxolol has been shown to be similar to that of timolol.[70,71,72] Other studies have reported that the magnitude of IOP decrease is greater with timolol[72] and levobunolol[58] and that adjunctive therapy is more common with betaxolol.[72] Systemically, betaxolol has less of an effect on resting pulse rate[19,68,73] and pulmonary function in predisposed patients.[37]

Adverse Effects of Topical Beta Adrenergic Antagonists

In the past, ophthalmologists concentrated on ocular side effects because of the constant reminder of visual complaints related to miotic medications and epinephrine compounds. Currently, ocular side effects are minimal with beta blockers; however, a distant body organ might be compromised by systemic absorption of these potent sympathetic antagonists (Table 4-1). Instead of simple ocular problems, patients and ophthalmologists are faced with solving more complex issues concerning general health care and quality of life. Systemic absorption of topical beta blockers results in systemic side effects. Adverse effects are the major reason patients are unable to tolerate topical beta blocker therapy; however, the important point is that the effects of systemic beta blockade are dose-dependent. Following topical instillation of a beta blocker, the major organs affected include the brain, heart, and lungs.[74]

External Ocular Effects

The lipophilic and membrane stabilizing activities of topical beta blockers tend to stabilize the unmyelinated pain fibers of the cornea and produce corneal anesthesia. The majority of investigators have found no significant corneal anesthesia from timolol, levobunolol, or betaxolol.[75,76] However, corneal anesthesia because of topical beta blockers has been reported in isolated cases.[77,78] It might reach clinical significance when combined with a preexisting, superficial punctate keratitis.[77] A reversible, "dry eye" syndrome consisting of punctate staining, reduced tear flow, and shortened tear breakup time has been attributed to topical timolol.[79] This syndrome might be more common in patients with decreased tear production measured by a Schirmer test prior to topical therapy.[78]

Ocular discomfort upon beta blocker instillation is a function of several variables: preservatives, buffers, vehicles, and specific beta blocker molecules. Timolol and levobunolol have a low incidence of burning and stinging on instillation (6 to 9%), while betaxolol is significantly higher (30%).[70] Approximately 3% of patients develop an allergic blepharoconjunctivitis while using topical beta blockers.[30] Changing to a different topical beta blocker might alleviate this problem. Timolol is available as a preservative-free unit dose vial that is useful in patients allergic to the preservative rather than the beta antagonist molecule.

Timolol has been reported to cause reversible blepharoptosis. It was theorized that pharmacologic blockade of Müller's muscle was the mechanism.[80]

Intraocular Effects

Following topical beta blocker usage, patients might describe an ill-defined blurring of vision. Typically, this is not accompanied by a change in refraction. Topical beta blockers can cause a myopic shift (+0.85 diopters) in tonic accommodation by negating the inhibitory sympathetic tone to the ciliary muscle. The far and near points of accommodation are not affected.[81] Although blurred vision is a common complaint, an etiology is identified rarely.

Topical beta blocker therapy has been reported to cause hypotony. Typically, it occurs in previously treated patients who undergo a filtering procedure for glaucoma. When beta blocker therapy is reinstituted months later, a delayed ciliochoroidal detachment can develop.[82]

Systemic Side Effects

Brain As clinical experience with topical beta blockers increases, their ability to adversely alter CNS function is being recognized more frequently. The list of CNS side effects from topical beta blocker therapy is long and impressive: depression, fatigue, lethargy, dizziness, hallucinations, bizarre dreams, memory loss, insomnia, psychosis, confusion, and suicide.[74,78,83-86] Possible CNS side effects occur in 3 to 10% of patients using topical beta blockers[78,83] and account for 21% of the adverse reactions reported to the National Registry of Drug-Induced Ocular Side Effects (Registry).[86] Almost half of the reported side effects are psychiatric in nature, most commonly consisting of depression, psychosis, confusion, and hallucinations. The Registry data includes 20 cases of acute suicidal depression following the use of topical timolol. An acute reversible syndrome characterized by disorientation, memory loss, and inability to concentrate was seen in 13% of patients reporting CNS effects. In several of these patients, this acute confusional state required hospitalization. The syndrome was reversed when the drug was discontinued.[86,87] Episodes of auditory and visual hallucinations, nightmares, and bizarre dreams were reported in 11% of the CNS cases and an additional 3% experienced a psychotic reaction, including depersonalization and dementia.[86] These findings should come as no surprise since they have been associated with oral use as well.[88,89] In addition, the use of tricyclic antidepressants was found to be significantly higher in hypertensive patients taking oral beta blockers (23%) than for patients taking hydralazine or hypoglycemics (both 15%). It was concluded that beta blockers could be an important cause of iatrogenic depression among hypertensive patients.[90]

Sexual dysfunction secondary to topical beta blockers is being appreciated more frequently.[91,92] Decreased libido is the most common complaint although impotence has been reported. In most cases, symptoms reversed after drug therapy was discontinued and reappeared upon drug rechallenge.[91]

A preliminary report suggests that patients who developed CNS side effects (depression, emotional liability, and decreased sexual libido) on topical timolol did significantly better when switched to betaxolol. This finding was supported by a double- masked cross-over study.[92] However, selective β_1-blockers have been implicated as well in CNS side effects, emphasizing the important of individual patient susceptibility.[85,87] Because of their subtle and subjective nature, it is easy to see why CNS side effects are overlooked. Through patient and physician awareness, these side effects may be identified and dealt with properly.

Heart All of the undesirable cardiovascular effects of systemic beta blockade from topical administration can be anticipated. Topical nonselective beta blockers are associated commonly with an asymptomatic decrease in pulse rate.[36,93] Sinus bradycardia and/or cardiac arrythmias significant enough to cause symptoms leads to discontinuation of the drug in 3 to 5% of patients.[83,94] Of the 32 deaths attributed to topical timolol reported to the Registry, 41% were classified as cardiovascular in origin. Approximately 50% of the deaths occurred within 2 to 48 hours after initiation of therapy.[94]

Ophthalmic dosing of 0.5% timolol twice a day causes a statistically significant change in cardiac hemodynamics. Following single drop, bilateral instillation, resting heart rate, and systemic blood pressure are reduced. Chronic therapy reduces cardiac sympathetic tone and ventricular inotropy. Acute and chronic therapy decreases exercise heart rate, oxygen consumption, and blunts the normal sympathetic augmentation of exercise capacity. In these healthy volunteers, this degree of cardiac blockade is uneventful,[36,93] but it might be harmful to patients susceptible to the effects of beta adrenergic blockade.[85,95]

The cardiovascular effects of topical 1% betaxolol and 0.5% timolol were compared to placebo in a double-masked, cross-over, single instillation study. During exercise, no significant differences in heart rate were seen between 1% betaxolol and placebo. When the same subjects were treated with 0.5% timolol, however, there was a significant reduction in exercise tachycardia compared with betaxolol and placebo. No significant differences in mean arterial pressure were detected in any group.[96] Similar findings were reported when levobunolol was included.[97] Betaxolol is marketed as a β_1 cardioselective antagonist, yet the study reveals no significant cardiac beta blockade in normal subjects. It is important to remember that betaxolol has one tenth of the beta blocking potency of timolol and levobunolol.[62] This does not mean that betaxolol cannot cause significant complications in susceptible individuals. Topical betaxolol has been reported to cause sinus arrest[98] and bradycardia with either snycope[85] or amaurosis fugax.[95]

Levobunolol tends to lower resting heart rate slightly more than timolol; whether this is clinically significant depends on patient-drug interaction and detective work by ophthalmologists. The average decrease in heart rate for levobunolol is 5 bpm compared to 4 bpm for timolol and no change for betaxolol.[30] What is average for the population, however, might be meaningless for a patient.

As with oral agents, a rebound phenomenon of reflexive tachycardia (10 bpm) after acute withdrawal has been reported with topical timolol therapy.[99] Theoretically, because beta blockers increase the number of receptor sites, abrupt cessation can make more receptor sites available to circulating sympathetic agonists. As yet, no cases of myocardial infarction or lethal arrythmias have appeared following discontinuation of a topical beta blocker.

Lung Initial clinical trials with timolol excluded all patients with reactive airway disease. One year after the widespread use of timolol, reports appeared in the literature concerning pulmonary compromise with topical beta blockers. It was clear that the risk of respiratory side effects had not been emphasized. Reports from the *New England Journal of Medicine* and *Lancet* stressed that physicians caring for patients with glaucoma appreciate the potential systemic side effects of topical beta blockers and prescribe them with caution for patients with known contraindications to the systemic use of beta blockers.[100,101] By 1986, the Registry was aware of 12 deaths attributed to respiratory compromise precipitated by the use of timolol. More than half of these cases had known histories of pulmonary difficulties.[94]

Despite attempts at education, problems continued to occur.[106] Thirty minutes after the first dose of 0.5% timolol ophthalmic solution, a 67-year-old man with stable chronic obstructive pulmonary disease experienced severe dyspnea leading to respiratory arrest. Unresponsive to metaproterenol inhaler, temporary intubation and mechanical ventilation were required.[103] Patients with asymptomatic bronchial asthma developed severe asthmatic attacks precipitated by topical timolol therapy.[104] Cyanosis, bradycardia, and respiratory distress with diffuse wheezing was precipitated in an 18-month- old girl with congenital glaucoma following twice a day treatment of 0.25% timolol in one eye.[105]

Timolol and betaxolol were compared in a randomized, double-masked, cross-over study in several patients with reactive airway disease. Timolol produced a significant decrease in airflow, measured by FEV_1 (forced expiratory volume at one second). Betaxolol 1% eyedrops caused no decrease in airflow in the same patients with proven airway disease. One patient treated with betaxolol did experience a transient decrease in airflow. It seems that betaxolol could be used safely in a select group of patients who have reactive airway disease and glaucoma.[37] Further studies revealed glaucoma patients with FEV_1/FVC (forced vital capacity) values of at least 40% of normal, tolerated the addition of betaxolol to their glaucoma therapy and benefitted with an 18% further reduction in IOP.[106]

With time, reports in the literature have surfaced concerning respiratory difficulties with betaxolol. Several patients ranging in age from 62 to 82 developed wheezing and dyspnea days to weeks after initiation of betaxolol therapy.[107,108] The Registry has data on 8 cases that required hospitalization for adverse pulmonary effects attributed to betaxolol. Half of the patients had underlying respiratory disease, but all patients improved after the drug was withdrawn.[85] It must be emphasized that betaxolol might not be cardioselective enough to avoid respiratory difficulties entirely.

Miscellaneous

Nursing mothers should be informed that their breast milk can contain significant beta blocker levels. Both timolol and betaxolol have been found in breast milk.[65,109] Alternative therapy seems advisable in nursing mothers since the long-term results of neonatal beta blockade are poorly understood. Beta blockers can also cross the placenta; the effect of fetal beta blockade is unknown. Topical beta blocker therapy might lead to prolonged apnea in neonates possibly because of an immature blood brain barrier and liver enzyme systems.[48,110] In general, because of reduced blood volume, pediatric patients are placed at an increased risk for side effects.

Stress brought on by local or general anesthesia might necessitate considerable changes in the sympathetic nervous system during the intraoperative or postoperative periods. Increased levels of epinephrine usually increase systolic blood pressure and heart rate. In the presence of beta blockade, however, the alpha effects of epinephrine predominate. This can result in peripheral vasoconstriction leading to hypertension with a reflexive increase in vagal tone potentiating bradycardia. The chance of this adverse reaction occurring is enhanced when a local anesthetic containing epinephrine is used.[111] Elderly patients with significant cardiovascular disease might fare better if topical beta blockers are discontinued a day or two before surgery.[112]

Drug Interactions and Additivity

Beta antagonists and epinephrine compounds

In general, topical nonselective beta blockers cause a greater reduction in IOP than epinephrine compounds.[113,114,115] The fact that both sympathetic agonists and antagonists lower IOP seems contradictory. By studying their combined effect, it was hoped that the mechanism of action for each could be better understood.

Short-term studies showed that the additive effect of timolol with epinephrine was transient.[114] The order that the drugs were given[116] and the length of time between administration of the drugs[117] did not change significantly the magnitude of IOP reduction after the first two months. It seemed that timolol blocked the epinephrine-induced increase in facility of outflow. This led to the conclusion that the ocular hypotensive effect of epinephrine is mediated by a beta receptor mechanism located in the trabecular meshwork.[116] Clinically, the majority of patients being treated with either drug are unlikely to have a substantial reduction of IOP with the addition of the second drug.[118] However, the effectiveness of added epinephrine increases with longer follow up time (3 months).[118,119] For the long-term treatment of glaucoma, epinephrine might be partially additive to timolol therapy[119] with one-fifth to one-third of patients having at least a 3-mm reduction in IOP.[117,118] It is postulated that the additive effect is not by a beta-mediated increase in outflow, but through the alpha agonist action of epinephrine that decreases aqueous humor formation.[116,119,120] Concomitant treatment of levobunolol with dipivefrin is equal in both efficacy and safety to combined treatment of timolol with dipivefrin.[120]

The additive effect of betaxolol with epinephrine is similar to that of timolol in total reduction of IOP.[120,121] The mechanism, however, might be different. Epinephrine increases facility of outflow when added to betaxolol but does not when added to timolol.[121] This suggests that the effect of epinephrine on outflow is mediated through β_2-adrenergic receptors.

Theoretically, eyes with significant angle closure would fare better with timolol and epinephrine, while eyes with the majority of the angle open might do better with betaxolol and epinephrine. This has not been evaluated on a clinical basis. Remember that in eyes predisposed to pupillary block, an iridectomy might be indicated prior to epinephrine use. A uniocular trial of combined beta blocker and epinephrine therapy in individual patients might be the only reasonable approach in determining long-term efficacy on IOP control.

Beta antagonists and pilocarpine

Timolol produces a greater reduction in pressure with smaller swings in diurnal IOP than pilocarpine 2%[122] Since beta blockers reduce inflow and miotic agents increase outflow, it is not surprising that concomitant therapy further reduces IOP. Pilocarpine 4% given four times a day reduces IOP by about 20%. The combination of timolol 0.5%-pilocarpine 2% and timolol 0.5%- pilocarpine 4% both given twice a day has been reported to reduce IOP by 25% and 37%, respectively. In these two groups it is of clinical interest that the level of IOP was not meaningfully higher 12 hours after the last instillation when compared to 2 hours after the morning dose.[123] These drug combinations are not only effective, but might improve patient compliance and tolerance in selected cases where a miotic is required. Further study is needed to confirm this observation.

Oral and topical beta antagonists

In glaucoma patients and healthy volunteers, oral beta blockers lower IOP significantly when used alone. In sufficient doses, the magnitude of IOP reduction is equivalent to topical agents.[124,125,126] This raises the question of whether topical beta blockers are beneficial to the patient taking similar drugs orally. The additive effects on the eye and on systemic blockade must be considered.

In normal subjects, the short-term, ocular hypotensive response of concomitant oral propranolol and topical timolol was studied. Timolol reduced the IOP substantially and to the same extent in the subjects who had taken a placebo and in those who had taken 80 mg of propranolol per day. It had no significant additive effect at an oral dose of 160 mg per day.[125] In glaucoma patients, the interaction of oral and topical timolol was studied: similar reductions in IOP were obtained when each drug preparation was given alone. Twenty milligrams of oral timolol administered twice daily reduced IOP an average of 8 mm Hg. The addition of topical timolol did not alter IOP any further.[124]

Systemic beta blockade with topical agents has been discussed. It is easy to understand how it would be enhanced by oral agents. In cases where a medical history was provided, 92% of patients with a reported adverse reaction from topical timolol had preexisting respiratory or cardiovascular disease.[94] In patients on oral beta blockers, caution must be exercised when concomitant, topical therapy is planned. Consider informing the physician who prescribed the oral drug. Ophthalmologists can educate patients to notify them when oral beta blocker therapy is discontinued or initiated because the long-term additivity with their topical counterparts is poorly understood.

Beta antagonists and carbonic anhydrase inhibitors

Used alone, both topical beta blockers and oral CAI lower IOP by significantly reducing aqueous humor information. Knowing this similarity, it is reasonable to consider whether concomitant therapy is of any added benefit. Investigations support the clinical usefulness of combined treatment with timolol/betaxolol and acetazolamide in lowering IOP.[127,128]

Beta antagonists and nonsteroidal anti-inflammatory agents

The vascular antihypertensive effect of systemic beta blockers might be blunted by the concomitant administration of prostaglandin inhibitors. This raises the possibility that the efficacy of topical beta blockers might be attenuated by drugs such as indomethacin. Oral and topical indomethacin have no effect on the ocular hypotensive action of timolol in normal subjects.[129,130]

Beta antagonists and quinidine

Therapeutically, the most valuable action of quinidine is prolonging the refractory period of cardiac muscle by depressing the excitability and conduction velocity in the myocardium. Beta antagonists also prolong the effective refractory period, depress automaticity, and slow atrioventricular node conduction.[131] Theoretically, the reduction in sinus rate by a beta blocker could be exacerbated by the use of quinidine. Clinically, this has been confirmed in an isolated case. A symptomatic, sinus bradycardia developed in a stable patient on quinidine when topical timolol was added. Both drugs were stopped, followed by return of normal sinus rhythm. Rechallenge with timolol did not cause any systemic side effect. Quinidine was restarted and the symptomatic sinus bradycardia returned.[132]

Beta antagonists and verapamil

Verapamil inhibits the calcium ion influx through slow channels into conductible and contractile myocardial cells and vascular smooth muscle cells. Electrophysiologically, this slows A-V conduction and prolongs the effective refractory period within the A-V node in a rate related manner, thus reducing elevated ventricular rate in supraventricular tachycardia. As with quinidine, the addition of a beta blocker can cause a significant reduction in sinus rate. A severe bradycardia because of interaction of topical timolol and oral verapamil has been reported.[133] Hemodynamically, verapamil reduces afterload and myocardial contractility. In most cases, the negative inotropic action is countered by reduction of afterload. Thus the cardiac index is not reduced. In patients taking beta blockers, however, acute worsening of heart failure can occur.[131]

Beta antagonists and cardiac glycosides

The direct effects of digitalis derivatives include increasing the force of myocardial contraction (positive inotropic action), increasing the refractory period of the A-V node, and increasing total peripheral resistance. These drugs also depress the sinoatrial node and prolong conduction to the A-V node via vagal stimulation. The addition of a beta blocker can enhance S-A node dysfunction leading to significant bradycardia, or delay A-V node conduction leading to greater degrees of heart block. On the other hand, the positive inotropic action of digitalis might be reduced by the negative inotropic effect of beta blockade precipitating cardiac failure.[131]

Beta antagonists and catecholamine-depleting drugs

Catecholamine-depleting drugs such as reserpine and guanethidine exert their antihypertensive effects by depletion of norepinephrine through inhibition of catecholamine storage in postganglionic adrenergic nerve endings. This effect is accompanied often by bradycardia. These drugs can have an additive effect with beta blockers. When the second drug is initiated, the patient should be observed closely for evidence of excessive reduction of sympathetic tone. Hypotension and/or excessive bradycardia can result and produce symptoms of vertigo, syncope, and postural hypotension.[131]

Disease Interactions

CNS and psychiatric disorders

The majority of patients under treatment for glaucoma are elderly. The common use of topical beta blockers in this group has particular significance because the chance of a preexisting alteration in mental status is increased. The classic signs of dementia are short-term memory loss, inability to concentrate, disorientation, confusion, and mood change. In more advanced cases, there might be paranoid ideas, delusions, and hallucinations. All of these signs have been reported using topical beta blockers with reversibility on discontinuation.[86] If the patient has an underlying organic brain syndrome, a functional base line should be established. The assistance of informed family members and/or other physicians can be extremely helpful. If symptoms are exacerbated, a trial off beta blockers is recommended to ensure that they contributed to worsening of the preexisting disease. The same approach should be taken in patients with psychiatric histories or disorders. Depression is a common psychiatric condition and also is the most common CNS side effect reported with topical beta blockers.[86,92] It seems reasonable to consider that the addition of such agents might exacerbate preexisting symptomatology. In these cases, betaxolol might be less likely to aggravate symptoms.[92]

Cardiovascular, cerebrovascular, peripheral vascular disease

Topical beta blockers should not be used in the presence of cardiogenic shock, uncontrolled congestive heart failure, known sick sinus syndrome, or symptomatic bradycardia. They should be used with extreme caution in patients with a history of CHF, overt cardiac conduction defects, any degree of heart block, or significant bradycardia ($\leq$55 bpm).

Topical beta blockers can decrease both standing and supine blood pressure. They can exacerbate symptomatology in patients with preexisting orthostatic hypotension, cerebrovascular insufficiency, and peripheral vascular disease.

Studies in healthy volunteers show that topical betaxolol, unlike timolol and levobunolol, does not cause any significant cardiac blockade.[96,97] Betaxolol has only one tenth the β_1 receptor binding affinity of timolol.[62] This suggests that betaxolol might be a better choice in patients at high risk because of cardiovascular compromise. Despite these theoretical advantages, significant adverse cardiovascular reactions have been reported with betaxolol in susceptible individuals.[85,98]

Respiratory disease

Nonselective beta blockers should never be used in the presence of active bronchospastic disease and with extreme caution if suggested vaguely by history. Pulmonary beta blockade can exacerbate symptomatology in patients with chronic obstructive pulmonary disease such as chronic bronchitis, emphysema, bronchiectasis, and cystic fibrosis. In general, nonselective beta blockers should be avoided when restrictive or obstructive pulmonary disease is suspected. If an adverse reaction is precipitated, bronchodilation by exogenous, catecholamine stimulation of β_2 receptors can be blocked. Aminophylline might be less effective because part of its action depends on inhibition of phosphodiesterase that produces β-adrenergic stimulation.[131]

In patients with pulmonary problems, betaxolol is the topical beta blocker of choice.[37,106] It must be emphasized that its β_1 cardioselectivity is relative and respiratory difficulties occur in certain susceptible and/or high risk patients.[85,107,108]

Thyroid disease

Deleterious effects from the long-term use of topical beta blockers in patients with thyroid disease has not been documented. Experience with oral beta blockers and thyrotoxicosis, however, can be extrapolated to topical agents. They can mask the tachycardia associated with hyperthyroidism giving a false impression of control or improvement. If CHF is present, beta blockers have the potential to aggravate it. Abrupt withdrawal of beta blockers can exacerbate symptoms of hyperthyroidism and precipitate a thyroid storm.[131]

Diabetes mellitus

Oral beta blockers might prevent the appearance of premonitory signs and symptoms of acute hypoglycemia because they are mediated by catecholamines. This has been reported with topical use of timolol.[134] Nonselective, oral beta blockers might potentiate insulin-induced hypoglycemia and reduce the release of insulin in response to hyperglycemia.[131] Based on these facts, topical beta blockers should be used with caution in labile diabetic patients.

Myasthenia gravis

Twenty-four hours after initiating timolol therapy, a patient with myasthenia gravis reported a notable deterioration with severe dysarthria, difficulty swallowing, double vision, and marked ptosis. One day after stopping timolol therapy, the patient was back to his original base line state. Even though myasthenia gravis is a problem of the cholinergic neuromuscular junction, beta blockade further aggravates this disease process.[135]

Recommendations

Typically, it takes several years of drug usage before information on side effects can be analyzed and disseminated. Although the medical literature is informative, patients remain one of our best sources of education. They taught us that topical beta blocker therapy could cause bronchospasm and arrhythmias resulting in death within hours following a single instillation.[94] Physicians underestimated the effect of an eye drop on distant organ systems. In retrospect, the key was simple: medication loss from nasolacrimal drainage is significant.[33] Topically applied beta blockers enter the bloodstream through the nasopharyngeal mucosa avoiding first-pass liver metabolism. Thus, this route mimics intravenous administration. Once this is appreciated, it is easy to understand that all of the adverse reactions to oral beta blockers are due to systemic absorption and should be anticipated following topical use. The initial problem was that ophthalmologists did not realize the ramifications of systemic beta blockade. Now, ophthalmologists are expected not only to know the risks and benefits of topical beta blocker therapy, but to inform the patient that an undesirable reaction could occur.[136]

Even though all topical beta blockers lower IOP, they are not the same. Considering there has never been a double-masked, cross-over study with timolol, levobunolol, and betaxolol, it is impossible to comment accurately on which beta blocker causes the greatest reduction in IOP. More importantly, the goal of glaucoma therapy is not to lower IOP but to stabilize or improve visual function. Unfortunately, reports on topical beta blockers and their effects on long-term visual field preservation are scarce.[30] At this time, it seems that timolol and levobunolol are equally effective in stabilizing visual field at two years.[52] In the same regard, timolol is as effective as epinephrine.[115] No long-term data on betaxolol and visual field performance has appeared. Therefore, the clinician must continue individual clinical trials to find the beta blocker that best lowers IOP, maintains quality of life, and prevents progressive glaucomatous disease for the patients.

The selection of the appropriate beta blocker depends on the severity of glaucomatous disease and general health of the patient. Proper patient selection will increase compliance and decrease systemic side effects significantly. A careful review of possible drug interactions along with a review of the patient's medical profile enhances the physicians ability to select the appropriate beta blocker. Ophthalmologists should communicate with the patient's medical physician concerning possible adverse reactions in high risk cases (Table 4-1).

Fortunately, there is some meaningful information regarding systemic side effects of beta blockers. Nonselective beta blockers, such as timolol and levobunolol, cause more undesired effects on the cardiovascular and pulmonary systems and possibly the CNS than a selective beta blocker such as betaxolol. Patients with healthy cardiopulmonary systems usually have no significant systemic side effects from nonselective beta blockade. However, when adaptive, sympathetic tone is necessary to compensate for diseased hearts and lungs, reducing this compensatory sympathetic tone with beta blockers might alter severely the internal harmony of man.

Table 4-1. Adverse Reactions to Beta Blockers

Ocular side effects

External: Corneal anesthesia, punctate keratitis, discomfort on instillation, blepharoconjunctivitis, blepharoptosis

Intraocular: Blurred vision, delayed ciliochoroidal detachment

Systemic side effects

CNS: Depression, fatigue, lethargy, dizziness, weakness, hallucinations, memory loss, confusion, apnea in neonates, sexual dysfunction

Cardiovascular: Bradycardia, hypotension, decreased exercise tolerance, withdrawal reflex tachycardia, cardiac arrhythmia/syncope

Pulmonary: Bronchospasm, dyspnea, respiratory arrest

Miscellaneous: Presence in breast milk, masked hypoglycemic symptoms

Disease Interactions

Cardiac conduction or dysfunction, congestive heart failure, asthma, pulmonary insufficiency, chronic bronchitis, emphysema, bronchiectasis, cystic fibrosis, myasthenia gravis

Drug Interactions

Verapamil (calcium channel blockers), digitalis (cardiac glycosides), oral beta blockers, quinidine

Once it is decided that a topical beta blocker is the best treatment alternative, the minimal dose of drug should be used for the desired clinical effect. A therapeutic trial in one eye is useful to determine if the drug can be tolerated. It is of limited value in estimating the magnitude of IOP reduction because of significant cross-over effect in the untreated fellow eye.[34] Betaxolol 0.5% is best given twice a day. Timolol 0.25% can be started once a day and increased to twice daily; if this is inadequate 0.5% can be tried. Levobunolol 0.5% is best started at once a day; if inadequate little is gained by increasing the dose to twice a day.[57,137] About 20% of patients will not respond to a topical beta blocker.[41,70,137] If the first one chosen is ineffective, a second one can be substituted before they are abandoned or adjunctive therapy added.

Patients should be taught the proper use of eye drops. Five minutes of either nasolacrimal occlusion or eyelid closure decreases systemic drug absorption significantly (65 to 67%).[138] The IOP should be evaluated for efficacy and tachyphylaxis, and the patient should be periodically reevaluated for medical changes. Blood pressure and pulse should be evaluated before and after beta blocker therapy. Patients should be educated concerning the ocular and systemic side effects of beta blockade and instructed to notify their ophthalmologists if changes take place.

Clearly, ophthalmologists can make a difference in the quality of glaucoma care by selecting the appropriate beta blockers for their patients. Awell informed patient will be more compliant and realize the limitations of medical therapy. On this foundation the patient-physician relationship is built.

References

1. Weiner N. Drugs that inhibit adrenergic nerves and block adrenergic receptors. In Goodman LS, Gilman AG, (eds): "The pharmacological basis of therapeutics. 7th edition. New York: Macmillan Publishing Company pp. 192-203, 1985.
2. Hoffman BB: Adrenoceptor-blocking drugs. In Katzung BG (ed): Basic and clinical pharmacology. 3rd edition. Norwalk, Connecticut: Appleton and Lange pp. 95-105, 1987.
3. Phillips CI, Howitt G, Rowlands PJ: Propranolol as ocular hypotensive agent. Br J Ophthalmol 51:222-226, 1967.
4. Cote G, Drance SM. The effect of propranolol on human intraocular pressure. Can J Ophthalmol 3:207-212, 1968.
5. Vale J, Phillips CI. Effect of d- and l-propranolol on ocular tension in rabbits and patients. Exp Eye Res 9:82-90, 1970.
6. Musini A, Fabbri B, Bergamaschi M, Mandelli V, Shanks RG. Comparison of the effect of propranolol, lignocaine, and other drugs on normal and raised intraocular pressure in man. Am J Ophthalmol 72:773-781, 1971.
7. Bietti G. Recent experimental, clinical, and therapeutic research on the problems of intraocular pressure and glaucoma. Am J Ophthalmol 73:475-500, 1972.
8. Vale J, Gibbs ACC, Phillips CI. Topical propranolol and ocular tension in the human. Br J Ophthalmol 56:770-775, 1972.
9. Vale J, Phillips CI. Practolol (Eraldin) eye drops as an ocular hypotensive agent. Br J Ophthalmol 57:210-214, 1973.
10. Holland MG. Section IV: Sympatholytic and sympathetic blocking agents—alpha adrenergic antagonists and beta adrenergic antagonists. Ann Ophthalmol (Nov):1139-1142, 1974.
11. Wettrel K, Pandolfi M. Early dose response analysis of ocular hypotensive effect of propranolol in patients with ocular hypertension. Br J Ophthalmol 60:680-683, 1976.
12. Ohrström A, Pandolfi M: Long-term treatment of glaucoma with systemic propranolol. Am J Ophthalmol 86:340-344, 1978.
13. Wettrel K, Pandolfi M. Propranolol versus acetazolamide: A long term double masked study of the effect on intraocular pressure and blood pressure. Arch Ophthalmol 97:280-283, 1979.
14. Ulrych M, Franciosa J, Conway J. Comparison of a new beta- adrenergic blocker (MK-950) and propranolol in man. Clin Pharmacol Ther 3:332, 1972.
15. Katz IM, Hubbard WA, Gitson AJ, Gould AL. Intraocular pressure decrease in normal volunteers following timolol ophthalmic solution. Invest Ophthalmol 15:489-492, 1976.
16. Zimmerman TJ, Kaufman HE. Timolol: A β-adrenergic blocking agent for the treatment of glaucoma. Arch Ophthalmol 95:601-604, 1977.
17. Zimmerman TJ, Kaufman HE. Timolol: dose response and duration of action. Arch Ophthalmol 95:605-607, 1977.

18. Zimmerman TJ. Timolol maleate—a new glaucoma medication? Invest Ophthal and Vis Sci 16:687-688, 1977.
19. Zimmerman TJ, Kass MA, Yablonski ME, Becker B. Timolol maleate: efficacy and safety. Arch Ophthalmol 97:656-658, 1979.
20. Boger WP, Puliafito CA, Steinert RF, Langston DP. Long term experience with timolol ophthalmic solution in patients with open angle glaucoma. Trans Am Acad Ophthalmol Otolaryngol 85:259-267, 1978.
21. Lin LL, Galin MA, Ostbaum SA, Katz I. Long-term timolol therapy. Surv Ophthalmol 23:377-380, 1979.
22. Ostbaum SA, Galin MA, Katz JM. Timolol: effect on intraocular pressure in chronic open-angle glaucoma. Ann Ophthalmol 10:1347- 1351, 1978.
23. Radius RL, Diamond GR, Pollack IP, Longham ME. Timolol: a new drug for management of chronic simple glaucoma. Arch Ophthalmol 96:1003-1008, 1978.
24. Cookes RL, Brubaker RF. The mechanism of timolol in lowering intraocular pressure; in the normal eye. Arch Ophthalmol 96:2045-2048, 1978.
25. Reiss GR, Brubaker RF. The mechanism of betaxolol, a new ocular hypotensive agent. Ophthalmology 90:1369-1372, 1983.
26. Yablonski ME, Novak GD, Burke PJ, et al. The effect of levobunolol on aqueous humor dynamics. Exp Eye Res 44:49-54, 1987.
27. Neufeld AH, Bartels SP, Liu JHK. Laboratory and clinical studies on the mechanism of action of timolol. Surv Ophthalmol 28:286-290, 1983.
28. Bartels SP, Roth O, Jumblatt MM, Neufeld AH. Pharmacological effects of topical timolol in the rabbit eye. Invest Ophthal Vis Sci 19:1189-1197, 1980.
29. Araki M, Takahashi H: Mechanism of beta-adrenergic blocking agent in suppression of aqueous formation: the effect of timolol on the mitochondral function. In ACTA: XXIV International Congress of Ophthalmology. Philadelphia: J.B. Lippincott pp 691- 694, 1982.
30. Novak GD. Ophthalmic beta-blockers since timolol. Surv Ophthalmol 31:307-327, 1987.
31. Phillips CI, Bartholomew RS, Levy AM, Grove J, Vogel R. Penetration of timolol eye drop into human aqueous humour: the first hour. Br J Ophthalmol 69:217-218, 1985.
32. Putterman GJ, Davidson J, Albert J. Lack of metabolism of timolol by ocular tissues. J Ocular Pharm 1:287-295, 1985.
33. Shell JW. Pharmacokinetics of topically applied ophthalmic drugs. Surv Ophthalmol 26:207-218, 1982.
34. Kwitko GM, Shin DH, Ahn BH, Hong YJ. Bilateral effects of long-term monocular timolol therapy. Am J Ophthalmol 104:591-594, 1987.
35. Forte EJ, Weber PA. Psychologic effects of topical timolol maleate. Contemp Ophthalmic Forum 5:11-18, 1987.
36. Burggraf GW, Munt PW. Topical timolol therapy and cardiopulmonary function. Can J Ophthalmol 15:159-160, 1980.

37. Schoene RB, Abuan T, Ward RL, Beasley CH. Effects of topical betaxolol, timolol, and placebo on pulmonary function in asthmatic bronchitis. Am J Ophthalmol 97:86-92, 1984.
38. Soll DB. Evaluation of timolol in chronic open-angle glaucoma, once a day versus twice a day. Arch Ophthalmol 98:2178- 2181, 1980.
39. Yalon M, Urinowsky E, Rothkoff L, Treister G, Blumenthal M. Frequency of timolol administration. Am J Ophthalmol 92:526-529, 1981.
40. Mills KB. Blind randomized non-crossover long-term trial comparing topical timolol .25% with timolol .5% in the treatment of simple chronic glaucoma. Br J Ophthalmol 67:216-219, 1983.
41. Krupin T, Singer PR, Perlmutter J, Kolker AE, Becker B. One- hour intraocular pressure response to timolol. Lack of correlation with long-term response. Arch Ophthalmol 99:840-841, 1981.
42. Krieglstein GK. Longzeituntersuchungen sur avgendrucksenkerden wirkuz von Timolol-avgentropfin. Klin Noratsbl Augenheilkd 175:627, 1979.
43. Boozman FW, Carriker R, Foerster R, et al. Long-term evaluation of 0.25% levobunolol and timolol for therapy for elevated intraocular pressure. Arch Ophthalmol 106:614-618, 1988.
44. Wilson TW, Firor WB, Johnson GE, et al. Timolol and propranolol: bioavailability, plasma concentration, and beta blockade. Clin Pharmacol Ther 32:676-685, 1982.
45. Bobik A, Jennings GL, Ashley P, Korner PI. Timolol pharmacokinetics and effects on heart rate and blood pressure after acute and chronic administration. Eur J Clin Pharmacol 16:243-249, 1979.
46. Affrime MB, Leiventhal DT, Tabert JA, et al. Dynamics and kinetics of ophthalmic timolol. Clin Pharmacol Ther 27:471-477, 1980.
47. Alvon G, Calissendorff B, Seidman P, Widmark K, Widmark G. Absorption of ocular timolol. Clin Pharmacokinetics 5:95-100, 1980.
48. Passo MS, Palmer EA, Van Buskirk EM. Plasma timolol in glaucoma patients. Ophthalmology 91:1361-1363, 1984.
49. Kaila T, Salminen L, Huupponen R. Systemic absorption of topically applied ocular timolol. J Ocular Pharmacol 1:79-83, 1985.
50. Robson RD, Kaplan HR. The cardiovascular pharmacology of bunolol, a new beta adrenergic blocking agent. J Pharmacol Exper Ther 175:157-167, 1970.
51. DiCarlo FJ, Leinweber FJ, Szpiech JM, Davidson IWF. Metabolism of l-bunolol. Clinical Pharm and Therap 22:858-863, 1977.
52. The Levobunolol Study Group: Levobunolol: a beta-adrenoceptor antagonist effective in the long-term treatment of glaucoma. Ophthalmology 92:1271-1276, 1985.
53. Benson FG, Cohen HB, Foerster RB, et al. Levobunolol compared with timolol for the long-term control of elevated intraocular pressure. Arch Ophthalmol 103:379-382, 1985.
54. Cinotti A, Cinotti D, Grant W, et al. Levobunolol versus timolol for open angle glaucoma and ocular hypertension. Am J Ophthalmol 99:11-17, 1985.

55. Ober M, Scharrer A, David R, et al. Long term ocular hypotensive effect of levobunolol: results of a one-year study. Br J Ophthalmol 69:593-599, 1985.
56. Duzman E, Ober M, Scharrer A, Leopold IH: A clinical evaluation of the effects of topically applied levobunolol and timolol on increased intraocular pressure. Am J Ophthalmol 94:318-327, 1982.
57. Wandel T, Charap AD, Leims RD, et al. Glaucoma treatment with once-daily levobunolol. Am J Ophthalmol 101:298-304, 1986.
58. Long DA, Johns GE, Mullen RS, et al. Levobunolol and betaxolol: A double-masked controlled comparison of efficacy and safety in patients with elevated intraocular pressure. Ophthalmology 95:735-741, 1988.
59. Novak G, Tang-Liu D, Glavinos EP, Duzman E. Plasma levels of levobunolol following topical administration (abstract). Invest Ophthalmol Vis Sci 26(3):125, 1985.
60. Guidicelli JF, Chauvin M, Thuillex C, et al. β-adrenoreceptor blocking effects and pharmacokinetics of betaxolol (SL 75212) in man. Br J Clin Pharmacol 102:41-49, 1980.
61. Warrington SJ, Turner P, Kilborn JR, Bianchetti G, Morselli PL. Blood concentrations and pharmacodynamic effects of betaxolol (SL 75212) a new β-adrenoreceptor antagonist after oral and intravenous administration. Br J Clin Pharmac 10:449-452, 1980.
62. DeSantis L, Chandler M. Cardiac beta blockade after ocular instillation of beta adrenergic blockers in alert cynomolgus monkeys: safety profile for betaxolol (abstract). Invest Ophthalmol Vis Sci 26(suppl):227, 1985.
63. Giudicelli JF, Chauvin M, Thuillez C, et al. B-adrenoreceptor blocking effects and pharmacokinetics of betaxolol (SL 75212) in man. Br J Clin Pharmacol 1041-1049, 1980.
64. Cadigan PJ, London DR, Pentecost BL, et al. Cardiovascular effects of single oral doses of the new β-adrenoreceptor blocking agent betaxolol (SL 75212) in healthy volunteers. Br J Clin Pharmacol 9:569-575, 1980.
65. Beresford R, Heel RC. Betaxolol: A review of its pharmodynamics and pharmacokinetic properties, and therapeutic efficacy in hypertension. Drugs 31:6-28, 1986.
66. Berrospi AR, Leibowitz HM. Betaxolol: a new β-adrenergic blocking agent for treatment of glaucoma. Arch Ophthalmol 100:943-946, 1982.
67. Radius RL. Use of betaxolol in the reduction of elevated intraocular pressure. Arch Ophthalmol, 101:898-900, 1983.
68. Caldwell DR, Salisbury CR, Guzek JP. Effects of topical betaxolol in ocular hypertensive patients. Arch Ophthalmol 102:539-540, 1984.
69. Feghali JG, Kaufman PL. Decreased intraocular pressure in the hypertensive human eye with betaxolol, a β_1-adrenergic antagonist. Am J Ophthalmol 100:777-782, 1985.
70. Berry DP, Van Buskirk M, Shields MB. Betaxolol and timolol. A comparison of efficacy and side effects. Arch Ophthalmol 102:42-45, 1984.
71. Levy NS, Boone L, Ellis E. A controlled comparison of betaxolol and timolol with long-term evaluation of safety and efficacy. Glaucoma 7:54-62, 1985.

72. Stewart RH, Kimbrough RL, Ward RL. Betaxolol versus timolol. A six month double blind comparison. Arch Ophthalmol 104:46-48, 1986.
73. Allen RC, Hertzmark E, Walker AM, Epstein DL. A double masked comparison of betaxolol versus timolol in the treatment of open- angle glaucoma. Am J Ophthalmol 101:535-541, 1986.
74. Van Buskirk EM. Adverse reactions from timolol administration. Ophthalmology 87:447-450, 1980.
75. Maclure GM. A controlled study of corneal sensitivity and timolol. In ACTA:XXIV International Congress of Ophthalmology. Philadelphia: J.P. Lippincott, 687-690, 1982.
76. Kitazawa Y, Tsuchisaka H: Effects of timolol on corneal sensitivity and tear production. Int Ophthalmol 3:25-29, 1980.
77. Van Buskirk EM. Corneal anesthesia after timolol maleate therapy. Am J Ophthalmol 88:739-743, 1979.
78. Wilson RP, Spaeth GL, Poryzees E. The place of timolol in the practice of ophthalmology. Ophthalmology 87:451-454, 1980.
79. Nielsen NV, Prause JU, Eriksen JS. Lysozyme, alpha-1- antitrypsin, and serum albumin in tear fluid of timolol-treated glaucoma patients with and without symptoms of dry eye. Acta Ophthalmol 59:503-509, 1981.
80. Berstein HP, Henkind P. Additional information on adverse reactions to timolol. Am J Ophthalmol 92:295-296, 1981.
81. Gilmartin B, Hogan RE, Thompson SM. The effect of timolol maleate on tonic accommodation, tonic vergence, and pupil diameter. Invest Ophthalmol Vis Sci 25:763-770, 1984.
82. Vela MA, Campbell DG. Hypotony and ciliochoroidal detachment following pharmacologic aqueous suppressant therapy in previously filtered patients. Ophthalmology 92:50-57, 1985.
83. McMahon CD, Shaffer RN, Hoskins HD, Hetherington J. Adverse effects experienced by patients taking timolol. Am J Ophthalmol 88:736-738, 1979.
84. Spaeth GL. Place of timolol in the treatment of glaucoma. In Symposium on Glaucoma. Transactions of the New Orleans Academy of Ophthalmology. St. Louis:CV Mosby, 368-378, 1981.
85. Nelson WL, Kuritsky JN. Early post-marketing surveillance of betaxolol hydrochloride, September 1985-September 1986. Am J Ophthalmol 103:592, 1987.
86. Shore JH, Fraunfelder FT, Meyer SM. Psychiatric side effects from topical ocular timolol, a beta-adrenergic blocker. J Clin Psychopharmacol 7:264-267, 1987.
87. Orlando RG. Clinical depression associated with betaxolol. Am J Ophthalmol 102:275, 1986.
88. Zimmerman TJ, Leader BJ, Golob DS. Potential side effects of timolol therapy in the treatment of glaucoma. Ann Ophthalmol 133:683-689, 1981.
89. Stephen SA. Unwanted effects of propranolol. Am J Cardiol 18:463-472, 1966.

90. Avorn J, Everitt DE, Weiss S. Increased antidepressant use in patients prescribed β-blockers. JAMA 255:357-360, 1986.
91. Fraunfelder FT, Meyer SM. Sexual dysfunction secondary to topical ophthalmic timolol. JAMA 253:3092-3093, 1985.
92. Lynch MG, Whitson JT, Brown RH, Nguyen H, Drake MM. Topical β-blocker therapy and central nervous system side effects. Arch Ophthalmol 106:908-911, 1988.
93. Leier CV, Baker ND, Weber PA. Cardiovascular effects of ophthalmic timolol. Ann of Internal Med 104:197-199, 1986.
94. Nelson WL, Fraunfelder FT, Sills JM, Arrowsmith JB, Kuritsky JN. Adverse respiratory and cardiovascular events attributed to timolol ophthalmic solution 1978-1985. Am J Ophthalmol 102:606-611, 1986.
95. Coppeto JR. Transient ischemic attacks and amaurosis fugax from timolol. Ann Ophthalmol 17(1):64-65, 1985.
96. Atkins JM, Pugh BR, Timewell RM. Cardiovascular effects of topical beta-blockers during exercise. Am J Ophthalmol 99:173-175, 1985.
97. Hernandez HHY, Cervantes R, Frati A, et al. Cardiovascular effects of topical glaucoma therapies in normal subjects. J Toxicol Cut Ocular Toxicol 2(2&3):99-106, 1983.
98. Zabel RW, MacDonald IM. Sinus arrest associated with betaxolol ophthalmic drops (letter). Am J Ophthalmol 104:431, 1987.
99. Ros EF, Dake CL. Timolol eye drops: bradycardia or tachycardia. Documenta Ophthalmologica 48:283-289, 1979.
100. Ahmad S. Cardiopulmonary effects of timolol eye drops. Lancet 2:1028, 1979.
101. Jones FL. Exacerbation of asthma by timolol. NEJM 301:270, 1979.
102. Schoene RB, Martin TR, Charan NB, French CL. Timolol-induced bronchospasm in asthmatic bronchitis. JAMA 245:1460-1461, 1981.
103. Prince DS, Carbiner NH. Respiratory arrest following first dose of timolol ophthalmic solutions. Chest 84(5):640-641, 1983.
104. Charan NB, Latshminarayan S. Pulmonary effects of topical timolol. Arch Intern Med 140:843-844, 1980.
105. Williams T, Ginther WH. Hazard of ophthalmic timolol. NEJM 306:1485-1486, 1982.
106. Van Buskirk EM, Weinreb RN, Berry DP, et al. Betaxolol in patients with glaucoma and asthma. Am J Ophthalmol 101:531-534, 1986.
107. Harris LS, Greinstein SH, Bloom AF. Respiratory difficulties with betaxolol. Am J Ophthalmol 102:274, 1986.
108. Berger WE. Betaxolol in patients with glaucoma and asthma (corres). Am J Ophthalmol 103:600-601, 1987.
109. Lustgarten JS, Podos SM. Topical timolol and the nursing mother. Arch Ophthalmol 101:1381-1382, 1983.
110. Olson RJ, Bromberg BB, Zimmerman TJ. Apneic spells associated with timolol therapy in a neonate. Am J Ophthalmol 88:120-122, 1979.
111. Brummett R. Warning to otolaryngologists using local anesthetics containing epinephrine: Potential serious reaction occurring in patients treated with beta-adrenergic receptor blockers. Arch Otolaryngol 110:561, 1984.

112. Caprioli J, Sears ML. Caution on the preoperative use of topical timolol. Am J Ophthalmol 95:561-562, 1983.
113. Sonntag JR, Brindley GO, Shields MB, Arafat NT, Phelps CD. Timolol and epinephrine. Ann Ophthalmol 97:273-277, 1979.
114. Goldberg I, Ashburn FS, Palmberg PF, Kass MA, Becker B. Timolol and epinephrine, a clinical study of ocular interactions. Arch Ophthalmol 98:484-486, 1980.
115. Alexander DW, Berson FG, Epstein DL. A clinical trial of timolol and epinephrine in the treatment of primary open-angle glaucoma. Ophthalmology 95:247-251, 1988.
116. Thomas JV, Epstein DL. Timolol and epinephrine in primary open angle glaucoma: transient additive effect. Arch Ophthalmol 99:91-95, 1981.
117. Tsoy EA, Meekins BB, Shields MB. Comparison of two treatment schedules for combined timolol and dipivefrin therapy. Am J Ophthalmol 102:320-324, 1986.
118. Korey MS, Hodapp E, Kass M, et al. Timolol and epinephrine: Long-term evaluation of concurrent administration. Arch Ophthalmol 100:742-745, 1982.
119. Cyrlin MN, Thomas JV, Epstein DL. Additive effect of epinephrine to timolol therapy in primary open angle glaucoma. Arch Ophthalmol 100:414-418, 1982.
120. Allen RC, Robin AL, Long D, et al. A combination of levobunolol and dipivefrin for the treatment of glaucoma. Arch Ophthalmol 106:904-907, 1988.
120. Weinreb RN, Ritch R, Kushner FH. Effects of adding betaxolol to dipivefrin therapy. Am J Ophthalmol 101:196-198, 1986.
121. Allen RC, Epstein DL. Additive effect of betaxolol and epinephrine in primary open angle glaucoma. Arch Ophthalmol 104:1178-1184, 1986.
122. Hass I, Drance SM. Comparison between pilocarpine and timolol on diurnal pressures in open-angle glaucoma. Arch Ophthalmol 98:480-481, 1980.
123. Airaksinen PJ, Valkonen R, Stenborg T, et al. A double- masked study of timolol and pilocarpine combined. Am J Ophthalmol 104:587-590, 1987.
124. Batchelor ED, O'Day DM, Shand DG, Wood, AJ. Interaction of topical and oral timolol in glaucoma. Ophthalmology 86:60-65, 1979.
125. Blondeau P, Côté M, Tetrault L. Effect of timolol eye drops in subjects receiving systemic propranolol therapy. Can J Ophthalmol 18:18-21, 1983.
126. Williamson H, Young JDH, Atta H, Muir G, Kadom H. Comparative efficacy of orally and topically administered beta- blockers for chronic simple glaucoma. Br J Ophthalmol 69:41-45, 1985.
127. Kass MA, Korey M, Gordon M, Becker B. Timolol and acetazolamide: a study of concurrent administration. Arch Ophthalmol 100:941-942, 1982.

128. Smith JP, Weeks RH, Newland EF, Ward RL. Betaxolol and acetazolamide. Combined ocular hypotensive effect. Arch Ophthalmol 102:1794-1795, 1984.
129. Lichter M, Feldman F, Clark L, Cohen L, Cohen MM. Effect of indomethacin on the ocular hypotensive action of timolol maleate. Am J Ophthalmol 98:79-81, 1984.
130. Goldberg HS, Feldman F, Cohen MM, Clark L. Effect of topical indomethacin and timolol maleate on intraocular pressure in normal subjects. Am J Ophthalmol 99:576-578, 1985.
131. Boyd JR, ed. Drug facts and comparisons, 1983 ed. St. Louis: J.B. Lippincott Co., 443, 467, 418, 509, 1983.
132. Dinai Y, Sharir M, Naneh N, Holkin H. Bradycardia induced by interaction between quinidine and ophthalmic timolol. Ann Internal Medicine 103:890-891, 1985.
133. Pringle SD, MacEwen CJ. Severe bradycardia due to interaction of timolol eye drops and verapamil. Br J Ophthalmol 294:155, 1987.
134. Velde TM, Kaiser FE. Ophthalmic timolol treatment causing altered hypoglycemic response in a diabetic patient. Arch Intern Med 143:1627, 1983.
135. Shaivitz SA. Timolol and myasthenia gravis. JAMA 242:1611- 1612, 1979.
136. Bettman JW. A review of 412 claims in ophthalmology. In Bettman JW, Tennenhouse DJ (eds): Medicolegal aspects of ophthalmology. Int Ophthalmol Clin 20:131-142, 1980.
137. Long DL, Zimmerman T, Spaeth G, et al. Minimum concentration of levobunolol required to control intraocular pressure in patients with primary open-angle glaucoma or ocular hypertension. Am J Ophthalmol 99:18-22, 1985.
138. Zimmerman TJ, Kooner KS, Kandarakis AS, Ziegler LP. Improving the therapeutic index of topically applied ocular drugs. Arch Ophthalmol 102:551-553, 1984.

CHAPTER 5

Ocular and Systemic Side Effects of Carbonic Anhydrase Inhibitors

Richard J. Starita, MD
Jody R. Piltz-Seymour, MD
Ronald L. Fellman, MD

Introduction

Of all the medications available for the long-term treatment of glaucoma, the use of a carbonic anhydrase inhibitor presents the greatest challenge. Systemic administration of these agents can reduce IOP dramatically in all forms of glaucoma even when topical medications have failed. It is these agents that ophthalmologists turn to when the necessity of surgery seems imminent and progressive glaucomatous damage is leading to blindness. The successful chronic administration of a CAI requires a careful search for undesired actions. As physicians who are concerned with our patients' quality of life, unpleasant and debilitating side effects must be anticipated and dealt with appropriately. To evaluate adequately the risk-to-benefit ratio of these agents the interaction of the enzyme, carbonic anhydrase, with different organ systems must be recognized.[1] The better our understanding of this enzyme and its inhibition, the easier certain side effects can be identified and managed rationally.

Carbonic anhydrase catalyzes the reversible transformation of carbon dioxide and water into carbonic acid. This enzyme controls both the hydration and dehydration reactions. The dissociation of carbonic acid into a hydrogen ion and a bicarbonate anion is instantaneous and not under enzymatic control. Carbonic anhydrase is distributed widely in the body and different isoenzymes have been described. It is present in erythrocytes and a number of secretory tissues such as ciliary body, gastric mucosa, pancreas, renal tubule, and choroid plexus. In the eye, it has been found in the cornea, lens, retina, and ciliary body, and is involved in aqueous humor production. Within erythrocytes, carbonic anhydrase promotes the elimination of carbon dioxide through the lungs by catalyzing the dehydration of carbonic acid. Within secretory cells, it promotes the formation of fluid rich in bicarbonate anion by catalyzing the hydration of carbon dioxide. Bicarbonate excretion is linked to sodium transport on the basal surface of the cell creating an osmotic gradient. The remaining hydrogen ion is extruded through the apical surface into the blood (choroid plexus) or urine (renal tubule).[1,2,3]

More than 99% of this enzyme has to be inhibited before a physiological effect is achieved.[1] It is not surprising that chronic, systemic administration of such powerful drugs would have far-reaching effects on multiple organ systems. The complexity of the problem increases when other disease processes are present and concomitant medications are prescribed. These medications, however, can be used appropriately by proper patient selection, education, and follow up care. The key factor in preventing toxicity is recognizing the problem.

Historical Perspective

Clinically, the first widely used CAI was accidental. Sulfonilamide, a drug used for its antibacterial properties in the 1930s, was observed to cause a secondary metabolic acidosis that could be attributed to inhibitation of the enzyme, carbonic anhydrase. More potent compounds were developed and noted to have a diuretic effect on the kidney. By the 1950s a powerful CAI—acetazolamide—became available for clinical trials. Its role as a diuretic was disappointing. The urinary changes did not persist. Alternate mechanisms for bicarbonate reabsorption unrelated to carbonic anhydrase were present in the kidney and the physiological reaction catalyzed by carbonic anhydrase were proceeds at a very significant rate without the enzyme.[1] These facts were a blessing in disguise because they allowed for nontoxic, chronic administration and set the stage for its application to ophthalmology.

It was Friedenwald who theorized that aqueous humor formation was an active process linked to bicarbonate production.[4] It seemed that inhibition of this active process might lower IOP.[5] Such speculations were strengthened over time. The identification of carbonic anhydrase in the uveal tract by Wistrand[6] and the demonstration of a large excess of bicarbonate in the posterior chamber by Kinsey[7] added strong experimental support to Friedenwald's original ideas. These facts and others lead Becker to administer acetazolamide to glaucoma patients in 1954.[8] He showed that systemic administration of this drug lowered IOP without any change in the facility of outflow. The ocular response was not dependent on renal action but because of direct action on the ciliary body.[9] These discoveries and others have simulated intensive research into the mechanism of actions of carbonic anhydrase inhibition, and has broadened out understanding of aqueous humor dynamics.[2,3]

Mechanism of Action

A CAI blocks the enzymatic hydration of carbon dioxide into carbonic acid and dehydration of carbonic acid into carbon dioxide. The ionic dissociation of carbonic acid into a hydrogen cation and a bicarbonate anion is not under enzymatic control and thus not affected by carbonic anhydrase inhibition. Before physiological effects are observed, enzyme inhibition must approach 99%. At this level of inhibition the actions on the eye and the kidney are the most important.[1,2,3]

In the eye, carbonic anhydrase II (formerly isoenzyme type c) is located in the cell membrane and cytoplasm of both the inner nonpigmented and outer pigmented epithelia of the ciliary processes.[10,11] Anatomically, both layers of cells lie apex to apex with the basal surface of the nonpigmented epithelia facing the posterior chamber. Normally, HCO_3^- formed by the catalyzed hydration CO_2 is transported actively into the posterior chamber. The residual H^+ is extruded eventually into the blood and buffered mainly by hemoglobin. Sodium cations are pumped into the posterior chamber and linked to HCO_3^- secretion. It is the accession rate of HCO_3^- and Na^+ in the posterior chamber that is the critical factor in fluid production.[12] Rapidly extruded solute creates a net flow of fluid toward the posterior chamber (Figure 5-1). The absolute concentration of these ions is not important and can be confusing since equilibrium between the anterior and posterior chambers is reached very quickly. Inhibition of carbonic anhydrase decreases the rate of appearance of newly formed bicarbonate in aqueous humor. Simultaneously sodium entry into the posterior chamber is blocked by an indirect, poorly understood mechanism. Aqueous fluid production is decreased, outflow facility is unchanged, and IOP is lowered.[2,3]

In the kidney, carbonic anhydrase promotes bicarbonate absorption through the renal tubules (Figure 5-1). Anatomically, the apical surface of the epithelia face the lumen and the basal surface is in contact with the extravascular space. Following the administration of a CAI, sodium and bicarbonate excretion are increased while secretion of titratable acid and ammonia is decreased. Alkalinazation of the urine takes place. Acutely, urine volume and potassium excretion are increased. Because of the effects on the kidney, plasma composition is altered and a metabolic acidosis results. With chronic administration, the diuretic effect is lost and potassium balance is restored. In the presence of metabolic acidosis, the renal response to CAI is reduced. In the eye, systemic acidosis lowers IOP and can enhance further the pressure-lowering effects of CAI.[1,2,3]

Local changes in CO_2 tension can occur with systemic inhibition. In the lung, retention of CO_2 occurs giving rise to increased levels in the tissue. Without compensatory mechanisms, a respiratory acidosis can occur. In the brain, an increase in local CO_2 tension can increase cerebral blood flow, inhibit epileptic activity, or stimulate alevolar ventilation. The exact role of carbonic anhydrase in brain function remains controversial and is poorly understood. However, the mechanism of cerebral spinal fluid formation is similar to that of aqueous production in the eye.[1,2,3]

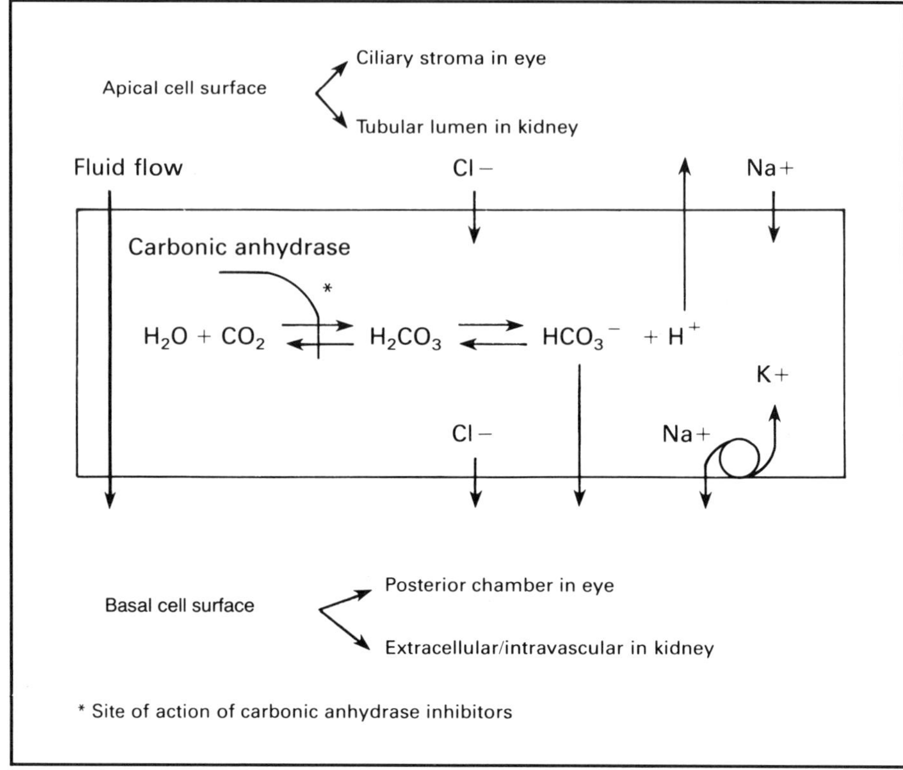

Figure 5-1. Simplified mechanism of action of carbonic anhydrase at the cellular level.

Preparations and Distribution

The two most commonly used drugs are acetazolamide and methazolamide; both have similar ocular effects. Generally speaking, methazolamide is considered less effective in controlling IOP, but induces fewer systemic side effects when compared to acetazolamide.[13] They differ mainly in their cost[14,15] and their effect on the kidney.[2,3] The less commonly used drugs, ethoxzolamide and dichlorophenamide, will not be discussed.

Acetazolamide is relatively inexpensive.[14] It can be administered intravenously, intramuscularly, or orally. An initial dose is typically 5 to 10 mg per kg of body weight. Following intravenous injection, peak effect is reached 15 minutes with continued action for 4 hours. Intramuscular injection can be painful and is usually avoided. The recommended oral dosage for chronic therapy in adults is a 125 or 250 mg table every 6 hours or a 500 mg sustained-release capsule every 12 hours. When tablets are used, the peak effect occurs at 2 hours and lasts up to 6 hours. The maximal effect on IOP can occur with as little as 63 mg per dose. Increasing the dose above 250 mg rarely produces any further reduction in IOP. When capsules are used, the peak effect occurs at 8 hours and lasts for at least 12 hours. A significant reduction in IOP can still be present 23 hours after a single capsule. Regardless of the route of administration, once absorbed acetazolamide has a plasma half-life of 4 hours. It is 95% bound to plasma proteins, excreted 100% unchanged in urine, and is hemodialyzable.[3,16]

Methazolamide is relatively expensive.[15] It is available for oral administration in tablet form only. The recommended oral dosage for chronic therapy in adults is 50 to 100 mg taken 2 to 3 times daily. A dose as small as 25 mg twice daily can produce a significant, sustained reduction in IOP without inducing a metabolic acidosis. Once absorbed, methazolamide has a plasma half-life of 14 hours. It is 55% bound to plasma proteins and only 25% appears unchanged in the urine. It is not actively taken up or secreted by the kidney. The exact metabolism of the drug is unknown.[3,16]

The pharmacologic properties of methazolamide give it increased diffusibility across ocular tissues when compared to acetazolamide. The dose-response curve for ocular and renal effects, while similar for acetazolamide, differ significantly for methazolamide. These facts make methazolamide a good first choice for an ocular CAI.[17]

Adverse Effects of CAI

The chronic administration of a CAI has been associated with a large number of adverse reactions. Most reactions are dose-related and reversible on discontinuation of the drug. Life-threatening situations, however, can develop and persist even when the drug is stopped. Careful consideration must be given to the risks and benefits of these compounds before they are prescribed. The adverse effects of a CAI can be ocular or systemic (Table 5-1) and might induce undesired interactions with other medications (Table 5-2) or disease states (Table 5- 3).

Ocular Effects

Adverse ocular reactions are rare (Table 5-1). The most commonly recognized sensitivity reaction in the eye is bilateral, transient myopia. Typically, it occurs in patients who have already received a CAI or other sulfonilamide derivative without consequence. On restarting the medication, the patient complains of blurred vision, especially at distance, starting within hours and lasting days. Refraction during acute episode reveals several diopters of myopia, unaffected by cycloplegia.[18] Occasionally, vision cannot be corrected and retinal or macular edema might be found.[19] The mechanism leading to an induced myopia is believed to be ciliary body edema resulting in relaxation of zonules, lens thickening, and in marked reaction anterior displacement of the entire lens.[20] In rare cases, anterior chamber shallowing might precipitate an acute or subacute attack of angle closure glaucoma.[21] The treatment is palliative consisting of discontinuation of the drug with the use of miotic and hyperosmotic agents as needed. The anterior chamber returns to its former depth within days. Subsequent administration might or might not cause reoccurrence.

Table 5-1. Adverse Reactions to Carbonic Anhydrase Inhibitors

Common Side Effects

Neurological/Peripheral

Paresthesia: Anticipated reaction; usually transient, involving hands/feet

Neurological/Central

Malaise complex: Insidious reaction, overlooked easily
- fatigue, lethargy, inability to concentrate
- anorexia, weight loss
- depression, indifference to life
- disorientation, increased dementia

Decreased sexual libido: Reaction volunteered rarely
- usually in younger patients, impotency rare
- commonly with features of the malaise complex

Gastrointestial

Nausea, dyspepsia, pain. Reaction volunteered frequently, variable relief with meals and/or bicarbonate

Metallic taste to foods, carbonate beverages lose flavor. Well tolerated reaction

Loss of appetite. Rare for reaction to occur alone: Consider malaise complex, altered taste of food

Chronic diarrhea: Reaction uncommon but debilitating, association with CAI overlooked frequently

Uncommon Side Effects

Renal/Urological

Frequency, nocturia: Reaction frequent but transient, typically occurs when drug is initiated

Urolithiasis: Reaction serious, requires prompt attention
- risk of a stone is 10 to 15 × age-matched controls
- presents with hematuria, renal colic

Metabolic acidosis: Mild disturbance, expected reaction, pre-existing disturbance can be increased significantly

Hypokalemia: Reaction transient on initiation of therapy
- initial loss may effect patients on cardiac glycosides
- chronic supplements required only in high risk patients

Hyperuricemia: Reaction normally not significant
- potentiated by thiazide diuretics and other drugs
- provoke acute gouty attack in predisposed patients

Anuria.* Reaction rare but medical emergency: Can occur with or without obstruction by stone

Rare Side Effects

Hematological

Bone marrow depression: Reaction life-threatening
- idiosyncratic reaction, not dose related
- usually presents 60-90 days after CAI initiated
- subtle symptoms; sore throat, fever, easy bruisability
- obvious symptoms; purpura, epitaxis, pallor, jaundice

Hemolytic anemia: Reaction may be dose/time-related, incentive for early recognition and treatment

Allergic and hypersensitivity reactions

Dermatologic response: Some reactions dose related
- erythema, papular rash, hives, facial edema
- erythema multiforme,* exfoliative dermatitis*

Table 5-1. (cont)

Liver failure*
Febrile response*

Ocular
Transient bilateral myopia
Delayed hypotony following filtering surgery
IOP problems in hyphema patients with sickle cell

Miscellaneous
Alopecia, infantile hirsuitism*
Tinnitus, hearing loss*

*Isolated reports only

Table 5-2. Drug Interactions with Carbonic Anhydrase Inhibitors

Adverse effect enhanced
Thiazide diuretics: Hypokalemia, hyperuricemia
Corticosteroids: Hypokalemia

Desired effect potentiated
Oral hypoglycemics
Oral anticoagulants

Desired effect antagonized
Anticholinesterase at neuromuscular junction
Bronchodilators in presence of bronchospasm

Toxic effect precipitated
High-dose salicylates
Cardiac glycosides
Quinidine

Table 5-3. Disease Interactions with Carbonic Anhydrase Inhibitors*

Pre-existing Disease	Potential Adverse Interaction
Hepatic insufficiency/cirrhosis	Hepatic encephalopathy
Severe COPD	Carbon dioxide narcosis
Diabetes mellitus with ketoacidosis	Hypotension, coma
Adrenocortical/renal insufficiency	Marked metabolic acidosis
Idiopathic/secondary hypercalciuria	Increased risk of renal stones
Primary hyperparathyroidism	Increased risk of renal stones
Primary/secondary gout	Precipitate acute gouty attack
Idiopathic orthostatic hypotension	Fall in upright systolic pressure
Sickle cell anemia	Precipitate sickle cell crisis

*CAI contraindicated if previous hemopoietic toxicity to any sulfonamide derivative is suspected

A new syndrome of delayed hypotomy and ciliochoroidal detachment following pharmacologic aqueous suppressant therapy in previously filtered eyes has been suggested. It is believed that eyes exposed to a CAI that undergo glaucoma filtering surgery can develop a hypersensitivity reaction to these drugs when used alone or in combination with β-blockers. Typically, the patient has undergone a filtering procedure months earlier and a CAI is reinstituted because of a failing bleb or uncontrolled IOP in the fellow eye. Within weeks, the patient presents with a red, irritated eye; examination reveals hypotony and a ciliochoroidal detachment in the operated eye. Resolution can occur spontaneously or on discontinuation of aqueous suppressants and can reoccur with a second challenge.[22] This syndrome has been reported in the absence of aqueous suppressants. Adjunct therapy consists of cycloplegic eyedrops and coricosteroids. In resistant cases, surgical intervention might be required.[23]

The effectiveness of CAI to control elevated IOP following cataract surgery is variable, depending on the mechanisms.[24,25] In otherwise normal, cataractous eyes adverse ocular effects would not be expected and a therapeutic trial is appropriate. However, in the presence of central corneal guttae (Fuchs' endothelial dystrophy), fluid transport across the corneal endothelium might be altered by a CAI. Following cataract surgery corneal swelling, measured by central corneal thickness, might be significantly increased when a CAI is administered in the immediate postoperative period.[26]

Another situation where a CAI can induce an undesirable ocular effect is in the management of increased IOP secondary to hyphema in patients with sickle cell hemoglobinopathy or sickle cell trait.[27] Sickled erythrocytes in the anterior chamber have a greater propensity for obstructing outflow channels.[28] Acetazolamide encourages the formation of sickled erythrocytes in the anterior chamber by lowering aqueous humor pH, increasing aqueous humor pCO_2, and increasing aqueous concentration of ascorbic acid.[29,30,31] These properties make it a poor choice for hyphema management in patients with sickle cell tendencies. If a CAI must be used, methazolamide might be more desirable, but not free of the same problems.[31]

A CAI can alter the results of certain ophthalmic tests. An increase in the amplitude of the b-wave on a electroetinogram occurs.[32] Differential light threshold might be improved in patients with glaucomatous visual field loss following short-term use.[33] These effects do not represent adverse reactions but rather reflect poorly understood physiologic mechanisms.

Systemic Effects

Unlike the adverse ocular effects, undesired systemic effects are common (Table 5-1). They are of sufficient severity to cause discontinuation of the drug in 30 to 50% of properly monitored patients.[34,35] The ability to tolerate a CAI seems to be greater in patients under the age of 40.[35,36] The majority of systemic side effects are dose-related;[37,38,39,40] an exception worth noting is that on the hemopoietic system. Most symptoms appear within the first few weeks of therapy. Even if a CAI is well tolerated for a long period of time, adverse systemic reactions can surprise the practitioner. Decompensation might occur because of worsening of a preexisting systemic disease or the development of a new one, increasing the dose of a CAI or the addition of a new systemic drug, or sudden appearance of a catastrophic adverse effect such as urolithiasis or hemopoietic toxicity. The search for debilitating side effects must continue as long as the patient is taking a CAI. It is prudent to alert the patient's general medical physician to the intended use of this drug and solicit the physician's advice and help in following the patient long term.

The most commonly recognized systemic side effect from a CAI is paresthesia.[41] Within a short period of time the patient notices a tingling sensation or numbness over the hands and feet. Typically, it is a minor problem that spontaneously resolves or improves over time. It is best handled by preparing the patient for its occurrence and assuring the patient that it is reversible on stopping the medication. It has not been associated with any long-term disability. This side effect does not correlate with any serum chemical change although uncontrolled studies have reported relief with potassium supplements.[41,42,43] Rarely, the patient will find this symptom intolerable and the CAI will have to be reduced, changed, or discontinued.[35] In a similar vein, initiation of therapy might be met with complaints of urinary frequency and nocturia.[37] Because of renal adaptation, these problems are usually temporary and can be handled as described.

Another commonly recognized systemic side effect from CAI is gastrointestinal dysfunction.[38,41,42,43] It is well known that a CAI changes the chemical composition of gastric, pancreatic, hepatic, and bile secretions.[1,44,45] It is not known whether the occurrence of gastrointestinal problems are because of systemic absorption and/or local irritation. Typically, the patient complains of nausea, burning (dyspepsia), and/or abdominal cramps. Less common but more debilitating is the development of chronic diarrhea.[37] Some of these complaints might not be volunteered by the patient or recognized by the medical physician as secondary to an oral CAI. If this symptom complex is not identified, a complete gastrointestinal work up might be performed before the connection is made. Again, these problems can be handled by changing the type or dose of the CAI.[35,42,43] A simple measure to help alleviate symptoms is to have the patient take the drug with meals.[42,43] Although the palliative effect may be due only because of reduced absorption,[35] it is worth trying. The use of concurrent bicarbonate has been suggested,[42,43] but remains controversial. The presence of these symptoms do not correlate with any serum chemical change.[43] Finally, patients might complain of a metallic taste to foods and a loss of taste for carbonated beverages.[35,38] Rarely does the patient find this intolerable and merely an explanation is required.

The most common systemic side effect from a CAI leading to intolerance is the so-called malaise complex.[42,43] Its onset is insidious and can gradually build with time. It can be missed by the patient, family, and physician. Typically, the patient's symptoms are fatigue, depression, anorexia, and/or weight loss. Its presentation can be as dramatic as a suicide attempt or as subtle as a presumed increase in the severity of an underlying dementia. The hallmark of this complex seems to be an indifference to life. The etiology of this complex is poorly understood. Its management is straightforward: reduce, change or stop the drug. Potassium and bicarbonate supplements have been reported to be beneficial in some cases, but controlled studies have not been conducted.[42,43] The problem is recognition of a change in the patient's quality of life and to intervene appropriately. Information might be required from family, friends, and other physicians before a decision is made. Sometimes the only way to decide definitely if the drug is causing a problem is to discontinue it for weeks to months. It might be only then that the patient appreciates the detrimental effect of the drug on his or her life-style.

Similar difficulties occur when identifying the adverse reaction of decreased or absent sexual libido. Commonly, it occurs in younger patients and, in some degree, with the malaise complex just described.[42,43,46] Typically the patient, male or female, does not make the association and does not complain. With tactful prodding, however, the problem can be identified and managed. In more severe cases, impotency can develop.[46,47] Recently because of increased awareness, this problem is being appreciated with increased frequency.

Renal stones or urolithiasis is a frequent finding in an adult population with an incidence of 2 to 3%. The chronic use of a CAI increases the risk of stone formation 10 to 15 times over the expected rate.[48] The kidney, under the influence of a CAI, excretes less citrate and magnesium while producing an alkaline urine.[49,50] These factors encourage the precipitation of certain insoluble inorganic salts such as calcium oxalate and calcium phosphate, which can lead to calcareous stones. Noncalcareous stones are less of a problem. Typically, the patient will present with symptoms of hematuria or renal colic secondary to a stone within the first year of treatment. If therapy is continued despite the first stone, there is a 50% chance of recurrence.[48] In the ophthalmic literature, concurrent medical treatment with a variety of agents has been suggested to try and prevent stone formation. The reports are inconclusive and often fail to appreciate potential complications. In the urologic literature, the use of potassium and sodium citrate shows promise and both have been shown to reduce significantly the incidence of stone formation in glaucoma patients taking acetazolamide.[51]

An attractive alternative is low dose methazolamide because metabolic acidosis is minimized and urinary citrate concentrations are maintained.[17,38] Because of the complexity of the problem, patients who develop a stone or who are at increased risk for urolithiasis should be handled in conjunction with an appropriate specialist. Hypercalciuria, either idiopathic or associated with a systemic disease such as primary hyperparathyroidism or Paget's diseases,[52] is a relative contraindication to the use of a CAI. The risk of stone formation might be increased by previous bladder surgery or trauma[53] and diets high in vitamin D, calcium, and phosphate. Anuria has been report both in the presence and absence of demonstrable crystalluira.[54,55] This is an extremely rare complication of CAI therapy.

The importance of potassium depletion in patients receiving CAI is controversial. When therapy is initiated, serum potassium levels reflecting extracellular concentration can be acutely lowered during the early diuretic phase. With chronic therapy, however, total body potassium—the bulk being intracellular—is usually normal and supplemental potassium is not required.[56] Potassium replacement is recommended under the following circumstances: concurrent use of potassium depleting drugs such as thiazide diuretics, corticosteroids, and/or hyperosmotic agents; excessive loss of potassium through the gastrointestinal tract as with vomiting and/or diarrhea; and preexisting hypokalemia secondary to inadequate dietary intake and/or a potassium depleting systemic disease. Supplemental potassium is administered best by dietary means. Fruits, freshly squeezed juices, nuts, and vegetables provide an adequate source in most cases. Enteric-coated potassium tablets should be avoided because of possible small bowel ulceration.[56] Extra care must be taken to monitor potassium stores when a cardiac glycoside is being used concurrently. Potassium depletion is the most common precipitating cause of digitalis intoxication. It must be emphasized that potassium supplements are not required in the normal population and have not been shown to alter CAI side effects reliably.[43] However, replacement therapy in the presence of known or anticipated hypokalemia secondary to any of the above problems might improve symptomology.[35]

The most feared complication of CAI therapy is a secondary blood dyscrasia leading to death. Considering the large number of new prescriptions written for CAI yearly and the number of case reports of hemopoietic depression, the risk is low. It is on the order of 0.01% and is less than those because of chloramphenicol or phenylbutazone. Drug-induced bone marrow depression can be of two types. The first type is an idiosyncratic reaction that is not dose-related and is not aborted by stopping the drug. This mechanism is accepted widely for the more commonly reported severe CAI-induced hemopoietic toxicities and helps explain the 50% mortality rate of drug-induced aplastic anemia. The second type is dose-related and time dependent with reversibility or cessation of therapy. At the present time this mechanism is speculative, but might be responsible for CAI-induced hemolytic anemia and might play some role in other blood dyscrasias as well. Clearly, this provides an additional incentive for early recognition and treatment.

Typically, the patient presents within 60 to 90 days after starting a CAI with a variety of different symptoms. Possible complaints are: persistent sore throat, fever, pallor, easy bruisability, epitaxis, purpura, or jaundice. It is a medical emergency if the work up reveals aplastic anemia, pancytopenia, leukopenia, agranulocytosis, or thrombocytopenia. The CAI should be discontinued immediately and the patient admitted for appropriate therapy. Rarely, symptoms can occur as early as 2 weeks or as late as 6 months after treatment. Additional reported toxicities are hypochromic anemia, neutropenia, thrombocytopenic purpura, eosinophilia, and red blood cell aplasia.[57,58,59,60] Rarely, a blood dyscrasia has presented in combination with another hypersensitivity reaction such as hepatitis, interstitial renal disease, or exfoliative dermatitis.[61,62,63] Although controversial,[59,60] present recommendations concerning the use of a CAI are: complete blood count, including platelets initially and at regular intervals; education of the patient to report new symptoms, and cessation of therapy if there is a signification fall in any formed blood element.[57] These recommendations should be considered carefully before chronic care is initiated. The risk of a rare but serious drug reaction should be discussed. Alternate treatment modalities should be explained and offered to the patient. An informed patient placed on a CAI is more likely to report new symptoms. The patient should be seen or contacted regularly and questioned specifically for adverse reactions. Most ophthalmologists prefer to follow patients on a CAI with their general medical physician, making all decisions jointly on a case by case basis.

It is not surprising that a CAI can produce allergic manifestations. Although rare, the most typical is a skin eruption. Erythema of the extremities, facial edema, hives, papular rash, erythema multiform bullosum, and exfoliative dermatitis have all been reported.[63,64] If an allergic response is suspected, it is recommended the drug be discontinued. It is of interest that some skin reactions are dose-related, disappearing only at lower drug levels. Other hypersensitivity reactions can occur. They range from a febrile response[65] to liver failure.[61,66]

In isolated case reports a CAI has been associated with alopecia in adults,[67] hirsutism in infants,[68] tinnitus,[56] and hearing loss.[13,41] Teratogenesis has been shown only in animals, but CAI use should be avoided during pregnancy.[69]

Drug Interactions

It is agreed that CAI are additive in lowering ocular pressure when used in combination with other medications for the treatment of glaucoma. The interaction of a CAI with other systemic drugs for a preexisting disorder might be detrimental (Table 5-2). The most common problem is that an undesired effect is potentiated. For example, a CAI produces a relative hyperuricemia that increases by the concurrent use of a hydrochlorothiazide.[70] Clinically, this is not important unless there is a known or suspected history of gout. More importantly, the early transient hypokalemia induced by the sole use of a CAI can become chronic when combined with other potassium depleting drugs. Urinary potassium loss can be increased dramatically by the concurrent use of thiazide diuretics and/or systemic corticosteroids.[71] Symptoms of potassium depletion, such as mental aberration, fatigue, nocturia, and impaired neuromuscular function might develop and mimic the known side effects of a CAI. An electrocardiogram demonstrating conduction defects, flattened T waves, and/or abnormal U waves confirms marked intracellular depletion of potassium. In addition, even a mild to moderate potassium deficiency enhances the cardiac toxicity of digitalis preparations. A patient on a cardiac glycoside who complains of anorexia, nausea, and/or vomiting following the use of a CAI could be developing the early signs of digitalis intoxication. If unrecognized, continued potassium loss could lead to cardiac arrythmias and atrioventricular block.

A CAI increases the risk of developing salicylate intoxication in patients receiving high dose aspirin. The metabolic acidosis caused by the CAI increases the proportion of the nonionized form of salicylic acid that enhances penetration into the central nervous system and other tissues. Symptoms such as tinnitus, tachypnea, and/or mental confusion should suggest salicylate intoxication. In severe cases coma can result.[72]

Sulfonamide binds significantly to plasma proteins. For CAI, a sulfonamide derivative, binding is as high as 95% with acetazolamide and 55% with methazolamide.[3] Oral anticoagulants and oral antidiabetic agents are plasma protein bound and can be displaced when a CAI is introduced. Competitive binding by CAIs increases bioavailability and enhances the action of these two groups of oral agents.[73] In patients receiving these oral agents who require CAI, methazolamide would seem to be the more desirable choice.

Two other interactions should be considered, but reports are rare. Alkalinization of the urine by CAI can enhance renal tubular reabsorption of quinidine. This leads to increased serum levels of this antiarrhythmic agent and potential toxicity.[73] A CAI might antagonize the effect of an anticholinesterase drug at the neuromuscular junction in myasthenia gravis causing an exacerbation in symptoms.[74]

The lesson to be learned is that a well-compensated patient can develop signs of drug toxicity at the same dosage level only when challenged by the addition of a CAI. The intoxication to a preexisting drug can be overlooked and misinterpreted as a new side effect attributable only to the recently started CAI. This can be a costly mistake for the patient.

A previous reaction to an antibacterial sulfonamide is not a contraindication to the use of a CAI. Their chemical structures are not closely related and there is no evidence to support overlapping sensitivities between the two classes of drugs.[3] Prior hemopoietic toxicity or anaphylactic reaction to any sulfonamide derivative should strongly discourage the use of any CAI.[58]

Disease interactions

A CAI has been used as adjunctive treatment in nearly all forms of glaucoma. A reduction in IOP is interpreted as a positive therapeutic response and long-term therapy is considered. Caution must be taken to rule out treatable causes of progressive angle closure disease that might be missed if only ocular pressure response is considered. Clinically, the most commonly missed diagnoses are chronic angle closure glaucoma and early neovascular glaucoma. Iridectomy for pupillary block and panretinal photocoagulation for ischemia can halt synechial closure that might otherwise lead to intractable disease. An active, underlying mechanism must be ruled out before a chronic CAI is recommended.

Before a CAI is administered possible adverse interactions with any preexisting disease state should be considered (Table 5-3). A CAI should not be used in patients with cirrhosis of the liver, severe chronic obstructive pulmonary disease (COPD), or diabetes mellitus with ketoacidosis. In hepatic cirrhosis, an alkaline urine leads to decreased urinary excretion of ammonia and increased plasma levels. Hyperammonemia causes impaired glucose metabolism and decreased oxygen uptake in the brain. Both factors contribute to hepatic encephalopathy.[75] Similar problems can occur in hepatic insufficiency. In severe COPD, inhibition of red blood cell carbonic anhydrase leads to carbon dioxide retention. Alveolar ventilation cannot be increased and carbon dioxide narcosis can result.[76] Caution must be exercised whenever bronchospasm is present, whether because of COPD or asthma.[77]

Induced acidosis decreases the effectiveness of bronchodilator therapy. In diabetic ketoacidosis, dehydration coupled with potassium and sodium depletion are potentiated leading to a more severe metabolic acidosis. Vomiting, abdominal pain, and "air hunger" might develop, followed by hypotension and coma in severe cases.

A CAI should be used cautiously in patients with preexisting metabolic acidosis and/or electrolyte imbalance. Adrenocortical and renal insufficiency are associated commonly with a secondary metabolic acidosis, hyperkalemia, and hyponatremia. Clinically, these patients present with symptoms identical to the malaise complex combined with nausea and vomiting in more severe cases. It is easy to see that these symptoms can be made worse with a CAI. In addition, the metabolic acidosis and hyponatremia are exacerbated. The postural hypotension that occurs in adrenocortical insufficiency can be increased. With renal insufficiency, there is a further decrease in renal concentrating ability adding to fluid loss. Hypokalemia is not a problem unless renal tubular acidosis is present.

Because it is known that a CAI encourages the precipitation of insoluble calcium salts in urine, patients with increased calcium excretion are at a higher risk of urolithiasis. Idiopathic hypercalciuria and primary hyperparathyroidism are the diseases most frequently linked to calcium stone formation. Other disorders that have been recognized to cause calcareous stones include metastatic cancer, multiple myeloma, osteoporosis, sarcoid, vitamin D intoxication, and Paget's disease. In the presence of these conditions consultation concerning prophylaxis and follow up is advisable.

Although documented, the ability of a CAI to provoke an acute attack of gouty arthritis is not appreciated as a possible disease interaction.[78] Decreased renal excretion and clearance of uric acid produce a relative hyperuricemia. With proper medical therapy as prophylaxis a CAI can be administered safely. If a gouty attack occurs certain other factors should be considered. A CAI induced hyperuricemia can be potentiated by thiazide diuretic[70] and other drugs such as ethacrynic acid, furosemide, and some antineoplastic agents. Secondary forms of gout because of underlying systemic disease such as leukemic and polycythemia might be active.

Other disease where a CAI might not be desirable are: idiopathic orthostatic hypotension where symptoms can be excerbated because of decrease in standing systolic blood pressure, sickle cell anemias where a metabolic acidosis favors erythrocytic sickling and can precipitate a painful crisis,[79] and carbonic anhydrase II deficiency where no effect on IOP is obtained.[80]

Recommendations

The decision to start a patient on chronic CAI therapy requires a thoughtful analysis. The high incidence of side effects and low rate of compliance[81,82] must be weighed carefully against the risk of alternative therapeutic intervention and progressive glaucomatous damage. The presence and severity of preexisting systemic disease, the type and amount of concurrent medications, as well as the personality and the mental condition of the patient are all factors that influence the physician's final judgment. In difficult cases, the ophthalmologist should consider consultation with the patient's general medical doctor. Once it is decided to initiate a CAI, the patient and/or family members must be educated in an appropriate and timely manner to potential adverse reactions. The ophthalmologist, preferably in conjunction with the patient's general physician, must decide if a baseline CBC with platelets[57,60] and/or other tests are indicated. The type and dose of a CAI is chosen. Methazolamide, given at 25 mg twice a day, is a reasonable start. Reduction in IOP can be expected without significant metabolic acidosis.[17,38] If IOP is not reduced or a larger reduction is required, the drug can be increased to 50 or 100 mg per dose.[40] If this is unsuccessful, poorly tolerated, or too expensive, acetazolamide can be tried. A sustained-release capsule should be given once a day and increased to twice a day only if needed.[37,38] An alternate choice is a tablet, broken appropriately to give 62.5 mg four times a day.[39] Each dose can be adjusted in increments up to 250 mg. The goal is to achieve the maximum pressure lowering effect with the minimum amount of CAI, since almost all side effects are dose-related. Dosage schedules should be as simple as possible to try and improve compliance. Patients should immediately report persistent infections, easy bruisability, bleeding tendencies, rashes, and/or change in skin color (pallor/jaundice). Initially, the patient should be scheduled in at least 10 to 14 days since most side effects begin to appear by this time. At each visit the patient should be interviewed for the presence of side effects and any significant change in his/her medical condition. This should be done on a regular basis, especially during the first six months of therapy.

Despite IOP control in the office, the ophthalmologist must continue to reevaluate the patient with a suspicious eye. Underlying angle closure problems and unsuspected poor compliance[80,81] might be missed. Successful glaucoma treatment must be based on stabilization of visual function, disc integrity, and gonioscopic anatomy. Successful patient management becomes more complicated because their quality of life must be maintained as well. The patient and others might fail to recognize an insidious, progressive, detrimental change in life-style. If this is suspected by the alert physician, a trial off CAI is indicated.

Although this chapter has emphasized the complications of CAI treatment, these substances are a powerful tool in the armamentarium of the glaucomatologist. Rational use of these agents has saved the sight of multitudes of patients who would have otherwise gone blind. It is through the cooperation and communication of physicians and patients that adverse effects can be identified and dealt with appropriately. The CAI can be changed, the dose reduced, or discontinued. Risk factors can be identified, drug interactions anticipated, and disease relationships understood. The informed physician can meet the challenge offered by chronic CAI treatment with confidence knowing that ultimately it is the patient who benefits from his or her expertise.

References

1. Maren TH. Carbonic anhydrase: chemistry, physiology, and inhibition. Physiol Rev 47:595-766, 1967.

2. Maren TH. The development of ideas concerning the role of carbonic anhydrase in the secretion of aqueous humor: relation to the treatment of glaucoma. In Drance SM, Neufeld AH (eds.): Glaucoma: applied pharmacology in medical treatment. Orlando, Florida: Grune and Stratton, 1984, pp. 331-340.
3. Friedland BR, Maren TH. Carbonic anhydrase: pharmacology of inhibitors and treatment of glaucoma. In Sears ML (ed.): Pharmacology of the eye. New York: Springer-Verlag, 281-288, 1984.
4. Friedenwald JS. The formation of intraocular fluid. Am J Ophthalmol 1942; 32:9-27.
5. Kinsey VE. A unified concept of aqueous humor dynamics and the maintenance of intraocular pressure. Arch Ophthalmol 1950; 44: 215-235.
6. Wistrand PJ. Carbonic anhydrase in the anterior uvea of the rabbit. Acta Physiol Scand 1951; 24:144-148.
7. Kinsey VE. Comparative chemistry of aqueous humor in posterior and anterior chambers of rabbit eye. Arch Ophthalmol 1953; 50:401-417.
8. Becker B. Decrease in intraocular pressure in man by a carbonic anhydrase inhibitor, Diamox. Am J Ophthalmol 1954; 37:13-15.
9. Becker B. The mechanism of the fall in intraocular pressure induced by the carbonic anhydrase inhibitor, Diamox. Am J Ophthalmol 1955; 39:177-183.
10. Wistrand PJ, Garg LC. Evidence of a high-activity C type of carbonic anhydrase in human ciliary processes. Invest Ophthalmol 1979; 18: 802-806.
11. Dobbs PC, Epstein DL, Anderson PJ. Identification of isoenzyme C as the principal carbonic anhydrase in human ciliary processes. Invest Ophthalmol 1979; 18:867-870.
12. Maren TH. The rates of movement of Na^+, Cl^-, and HCO^{3-} from plasma to posterior chamber: effect of acetazplamide and relation to the treatment of glaucoma. Invest Ophthalmol 1976; 15:356-364.
13. Becker B. Use of methazolamide (Neptazane) in the therapy of glaucoma: comparison with acetazolamide (Diamox). Am J Ophthalmol 1960; 49:1307-1311.
14. Kass MA, Gordon M. The effect of a generic drug law on the retail cost of antiglaucoma medications. Am J Ophthalmol 1981; 92:273-278.
15. Kooner KS, Zimmerman TJ. The cost of antiglaucoma medications. Ann Ophthalmol 1987; 19:327-328.
16. Shields MB. Carbonic anhydrase inhibitors. In: Shields MB. A study guide for glaucoma. Baltimore: Williams and Wilkins, 1982: 431-432.
17. Maren TH, Haywood JR, Chapman SK, et al. The pharmacology of methazolamide in relation to the treatment of glaucoma. Invest Ophthalmol 1977; 16:730-742.
18. Galen MA, Baras I, Zweifach P. Diamox-induced myopia. Am J Ophthalmol 1962; 54:237-240.
19. Muirhead JF, Scheie HG. Transient myopia after acetazolamide. Arch Ophthalmol 1960; 63:143-146.

20. Hook SR, Holladay JT, Prager TC, et al. Transient myopia induced by sulfonamides. Am J Ophthalmol 1986; 101:495-496.
21. Chandler PA, Grant WM. Angle-closure glaucoma secondary to bilateral transitory myopia. In: Chandler PA, Grant WM. Glaucoma, 2nd edition. Philadelphia. Lea and Febiger, 1979, pp. 192-193.
22. Vela MA, Campbell DG. Hypotony and ciliochoroidal detachment following pharmacologic aqueous suppressant therapy in previously filtered patients. Ophthalmology 1985; 92:50-57.
23. Burney EN, Quigley HA, Robin AL. Hypotony and choroidal detachment as late complications of trabeculectomy. Am J Ophthalmol 1987; 103:685-688.
24. Beidner B. Rothkoff L, Blumenthal M. The effect of acetazolamide on early increased intraocular pressure after cataract extraction. Am J Ophthalmol 1977; 83:565-568.
25. Lewen R, Insler MS. The effect of prophylactic acetazolamide on the intraocular pressure rise associated with Healon-aided intraocular lens surgery. Ann Ophthalmol 1985; 17:315-318.
26. Nielsen CB. The effect of carbonic anhydrase inhibition on central corneal thickness after cataract extraction. Acta Ophthalmol 1980; 58: 985-990.
27. Goldberg MF. Sickled erythrocytes, hyphema, and secondary glaucoma: I. The diagnosis and treatment of sickled erythrocytes in human hyphemas. Ophthalmic Surg 1979; 10(4):17-31.
28. Goldberg MF, Tso MOM. Sickled erythrocytes, hyphema, and secondary glaucoma: VII. The passage of sickled erythrocytes out of the anterior chamber of the human and monkey eye: light and electron microscopic studies. Ophthalmic Surg 1979; 10(4):89-123.
29. Gamm E. Effect of certain hypotensive drug on pH, PCO_2, PO_2, and bicarbonate content of aqueous humor. Glaucoma 1982; 4:249-252.
30. Goldberg MF, Dizon R, Moses VK. Sickled erythrocytes, hyphema, and secondary glaucoma: VI. The relationship between intracameral blood cells and aqueous humor pH, PO_2, and PCO_2. Ophthalmic Surg 1979; 10(4):78-88.
31. Goldberg MF. Sickled erythrocytes, hyphema, and secondary glaucoma: V. The effect of vitamin C on erythrocyte sickling in aqueous humor. Ophthalmol Surg 1979; 10(4):70-77.
32. Stanescu B, Michiels J. The effects of acetazolamide on the human electroretinogram. Invest Ophthalmol 1975; 14:935-937.
33. Flammer J, Drance SM. Effect of acetazolamide on the differential threshold. Arch Ophthalmol 1983; 101:1378-1380.
34. Lichter PR, Newman LP, Wheeler NC, et al. Patient tolerance to carbonic anhydrase inhibitors. Am J Ophthalmol 1978; 85:495-502.
35. Lichter PR. Reducing side effects of carbonic anhydrase inhibitors. Ophthalmology 1981; 88:266-269.
36. Shrader CE, Thomas JV, Simmons RJ. Relationship of patient age and tolerance to carbonic anhydrase inhibitors. Am J Ophthalmol 1983; 96:730-733.

37. Garner LL, Carl EF, Ferwerda JR. Advantages of sustained-release therapy with acetazolamide in glaucoma. Am J Ophthalmol 1963; 55: 323-327.
38. Stone RA, Zimmerman TJ, Shin DH, et al. Low dose methazolamide and intraocular pressure. 1977; 83:674-679.
39. Friedland BR, Mallonee J, Anderson DR. The short-term dose response characteristics of acetazolamide in man. Arch Ophthalmol 1977; 95:1809-1812.
40. Dahlen K, Epstein DL, Grant WM, et al. A repeated dose-response study of methazolamide in glaucoma. Arch Ophthalmol 1978; 96: 2214-2218.
41. Becker B, Middleton WH. Long-term acetazolamide (Diamox) administration in therapy of glaucomas. Arch Ophthalmol 1955; 54:187-192.
42. Epstein DL, Grant WM. Management of carbonic anhydrase inhibitor side effects. In: Leopold IH, Burns RP, eds. Symposium on ocular therapy, vol. 2. New York: John Wiley and Sons, 1979, pp. 51-64.
43. Epstein DL, Grant MW. Carbonic anhydrase inhibitor side effects: A chemical analysis. Arch Ophthalmol 1977; 95:1378-1382.
44. Banks PA, Sum PT. Mode of action of acetazolamide on pancreatic exocrine secretion. Arch Surg 1971; 102:505-508.
45. Waitman AM, Dyck WP, Janowitz HD. Effect of secretin and acetazolamide on the volume and electrolyte composition of hepatic bile in man. Gastroenterology 1969; 56:286-294.
46. Wallace TR, Fraunfelder FT, Petursson GJ, et al. Decreased libido – a side effect of carbonic anhydrase inhibitor. Ann Ophthalmol 1979; 11:1563-1566.
47. Epstein RJ, Allen RC, Lunde MW. Organic impotence associated with carbonic anhydrase inhibitor therapy for glaucoma. Ann Ophthalmol 1987; 19:48-50.
48. Kass MA, Kolker AE, Gordon M, et al. Acetazolamide and urolithiasis. Ophthalmology 1981; 88:261-265.
49. Constant MA, Becker B. The effect of carbonic anhydrase inhibitors on urinary execution of citrate by humans. Am J Ophthalmol 1960; 49: 929-934.
50. Gyory AZ, Edwards KDG, Robinson J, et al. The relative importance of urinary pH and urinary content of citrate, magnesium and calcium in the production of nephrocalcinosis by diet and acetazolamide in the rat. Clin Sci 1970; 39:605-623.
51. Takemoto M. Prophylaxis for acetazolamide induced urolithiasis: Clinical study. Jpn J Urol 1978; 69:963-987.
52. Shields MB, Simmons RJ. Urinary calculus during methazolamide therapy. Am J Ophthalmol 1976; 81:622-624.
53. Gill WB, Vermeulen CW. Causation of stones by 2 co-acting agents — Diamox and operative insult upon the tract. J Urol 1962; 88:103-109.
54. Charron RC, Feldman F. Acetazolamide therapy with renal complications. Can J Ophthalmol 1974; 9:282-284.
55. Yates-Bell JG. Renal colic and anuria from acetazolamide. Brit Med J 1958; 2:1392-1393.

56. Spaeth GL. Potassium, acetazolamide and intraocular pressure. Arch Ophthalmol 1967; 78:578-582.
57. Fraunfelder FT, Meyer M, Bagby GC, et al. Hematologic reations to carbonic anhydrase inhibitors. Am J Ophthalmol 1985:100:79-81.
58. Weblin TP, Pollack IP, Liss RA. Blood dyscrasias in patients using methazolamide (Neptazane) for glaucoma. Opthalmology 1980; 87:350-354.
59. Johnson T, Kass MA. Hematologic reactions to carbonic anhydrase inhibitors. (correspond.) Am J Ophthalmol 1986; 101:128-129.
60. Zimran A, Beutler E. Can the risk of acetazolamide-induced aplastic anemia be decreased by periodic monitoring of blood cell counts? Am J Ophthalmol 1987; 104:654-658.
61. Krivoy N, Ben-Arieh Y, Carter A, et al. Methazolamide-induced hepatitis and pure RBC aplasia. Arch Intern Md 1981; 141:1229-1230.
62. Bertino JR, Rodman T, Myerson RM. Thrombocytopenia and renal lesions associated with acetazolamide (Diamox) therapy. Arch Int Med 1957; 99:1006-1008.
63. Turtz CA, Turtz AI. Toxicity due to acetazolamide (Diamox). Arch Ophthalmol 1958; 60:130-131.
64. Spring M. Skin eruptions following the use of Diamox. Ann Allergy 1956; 14:41-43.
65. Schwimmer J, Schaffer AI, Guido J. Febrile reaction to acetazolamide (Diamox). NY State J Med 1954; 54:692-693.
66. Kristinsson A. Fatal reaction to acetazolamide. Br J Ophthalmol 1967; 51:348-349.
67. Aminlari A. Falling scalp hairs: A side effect of the carbonic anhydrase inhibitor, acetazolamide. Glaucoma 1984; 6:41-42.
68. Weiss IS. Hirsutism after chronic administration of acetazolamide. Am J Ophthalmol 1974; 78:327-328.
69. Maren TH. Teratology and carbonic anhydrase inhibitation. Arch Ophthalmol 1971; 85:1-2.
70. Ayvazian JII, Ayvazian LF. A study of the hyperuricemia induced by hydrochlorothiazide and acetazolamide separately and in combination. J Clin Invest 1961; 40:1961-1966.
71. Bateson ML, Lant AF. Dietary potassium and diuretic therapy. Surv Ophthalmol 1974; 19: 193-195.
72. Anderson CJ. Kaufman PL, Sturm RJ. Toxicity of combined therapy with carbonic anhydrase inhibitors and aspirin. Am J Ophthalmol 1978; 86:516-519.
73. Boyd JR, ed. Drug facts and comparisons, 1983 ed. St. Louis, MI: J.B. Lippincott Co., 1983; 179, 344, 444.
74. Carmignani M, Scoppetta C, Ranelletti FD, Tonali P. Adverse interaction between acetazolamide and anticholinesterase drugs at the normal and myasthenic neuromusclar junction level. Int J Clin Pharmacol Ther Toxicol 1984; 22:140-144.
75. Posner JB, Plum F. The toxic effects of carbon dioxide and acetazolamide in hepatic encephalopathy. J Clin Invest 1960; 39:1246-1258.

76. Block ER, Rostand RA. Carbonic anhydrase inhibition in glaucoma: Hazard or benefits for the chronic lunger? Surv Ophthalmol 1978; 23: 169-172.
77. Coudon WL, Block AJ. Acute respiratory failure precipitated by a carbonic anhydrase inhibitor. Chest 1976; 69:112-113.
78. Ferry AP, Lichtig M. Gouty arthritis as a complication of acetazolamide (Diamox) therapy for glaucoma. Can J Ophthalmol 1969; 4:145-147.
79. Finney RA, Hatch FE. Effect of a carbonic anhydrase inhibitor (Dichlorphenamide) on sickle cell anemia. Am J MEd Sci 1965; 250:154-160.
80. Krupin T, Williams SS, Whyte MP, et al. Failure of acetazolamide to decrease intraocular pressure in patients with carbonic anhydrase II deficiency. Am J Ophthalmol 1985; 99:396-399.
81. Davidson SI, Akingbehim T. Compliance in ophthalmology. Trans Ophthalmol Soc UK 1980; 100:286-290.
82. Alward PD, Wilensky JT. Determination of acetazolamide compliance in patients with glaucoma. Arch Ophthalmol 1981; 99:1973-1976.

CHAPTER 6

Potential New Drugs For Glaucoma

Joseph Caprioli, MD

Introduction

Surgery for glaucoma can be associated with significant morbidity, and can lead to potentially disastrous complications such as endophthalmitis, suprachoroidal hemorrhage, and malignant glaucoma. The introduction of laser surgery for the treatment of glaucoma was initially widely met with great enthusiasm. However, the modest pressure reductions and the relatively short-term effects that are often realized after such procedures might fall short of the appropriate therapeutic goals. The search for additional medical modalities for the treatment of glaucoma has been fueled by these realizations. This chapter will summarize current work on new, potentially useful classes of topical agents for the treatment of glaucoma.

Topical Carbonic Anhydrase Inhibitors

The effects of systemically administered CAIs on intraocular pressure are well known. Acetazolamide was reported to lower human IOP in 1954[1] and has since found a secure place in the treatment of glaucoma patients. Inhibition of ciliary carbonic anhydrase predictably causes a 40 to 50% decrease in aqueous humor production, probably by reducing solute transfer to the posterior chamber.[2] Unfortunately, dosage levels of CAIs required to lower IOP adequately are often accompanied by frequently bothersome and sometimes serious systemic side effects that limit their clinical usefulness. These untoward effects can severely limit patient compliance, and are reviewed in Chapter 5. The availability of an effective topical CAI would increase the success rate of medical treatment.

Early attempts at local ocular application of acetazolamide did not result in IOP reduction, since the drug penetrates the cornea poorly.[3-5] Interest in this approach has recently been renewed, sparked by reports that some agents cause modest reductions of IOP. Maren and Edelhauser's group studied 11 sulfonamides for transcorneal permeability and reduction of intraocular flow and pressure.[6] One of these, trifluoromethazolamide, entered the rabbit eye in sufficient concentration after prolonged corneal exposure to modestly lower the IOP. Aqueous flow, measured by fluorophotometry, was decreased in rabbit eye by 29% after topical delivery of this drug.[7] Although the drug could not be clinically tested because of its chemical instability and the long corneal contact time required for penetration, the feasibility of treating glaucoma with topical CAIs was demonstrated.

Flach and coworkers[8] demonstrated that topical acetazolamide blunted the IOP rise of water-loaded pigmented rabbits, and that a 10% topical solution potentiated the ocular hypotensive effect of systemically administered acetazolamide. Sugrue and others showed that a potent carbonic anhydrase inhibitor, a pivaloyl ester of 6-hydroxybenzothiazole-2-sulfonamide, lowers the elevated intraocular pressure of alpha-chymotrypsinized rabbit eyes.[9] Acetazolamide and methazolamide delivered by soft contact lenses saturated with these drugs caused significant unilateral reductions of IOP in rabbits.[10]

Ethoxzolamide is a relatively lipophilic carbonic anhydrase inhibitor with high activity. Corneal penetration was enhanced by adding a hydrophilic moiety to the molecule, producing the active compound 6-hydroxyethoxzolamide.[11] As a 1% topical suspension, this compound causes a small reduction of IOP (1 to 2 mm Hg) in albino rabbits which lasted approximately 2 hours. When used in a gel vehicle to increase corneal contact time, slightly larger and longer reductions of IOP were achieved. Another analog of ethoxzolamide, 6-amino-2-benzothiazolesulfonamide (aminozolamide), was tested in 18 patients with ocular hypertension.[12] A 50 μl application of a 3% aminozolamide gel produced a substantial (6 to 8 mm Hg) unilateral decrease of IOP lasting 8 hours. The lack of a significant contralateral response suggested a local mechanism of action. Local side effects included mild stinging and conjunctival hyperemia.

A recently introduced CAI shows good corneal penetration and appears to be topically active: 4-alkylaminothienothiopyran-2-sulfonanide (Merck Sharp & Dohme, MK.927). It produces a clinically significant reduction of IOP in glaucomatous monkey eyes[14] and in humans with primary open angle glaucoma or ocular hypertension.[15] This compound holds the greatest promise for clinical utility of the topical agents tested thus far.

Topically applied CAIs might produce clinically useful reductions of IOP if they can be delivered to the ciliary processes in sufficient concentrations. Corneal penetration can be increased by developing congeners with suitable lipophilic/hydrophilic properties, and by increasing corneal contact time. It is likely that a suitable preparation will be found that satisfies the criteria of high CAI activity and good corneal penetration. Inhibition of corneal endothelial carbonic anhydrase by the topical agents raises some concern regarding possible effects on corneal clarity with prolonged administration.

This complication has not been encountered in animals (Maren, personal communication). The efficacy and side effects of such drugs will ultimately determine their clinical utility, and must await careful evaluation of prolonged human use.

Forskolin and its Analogs

It seems paradoxical, in view of the action of the beta-adrenergic blockers, that stimulation of ciliary adenylate cyclase could lower IOP by reducing aqueous production.[16,17] The uncertain results and complex physiologic effects of the adrenergic agonists led to studies with potent, non-adrenergic cyclase activators. Cholera toxin, a potent irreversible cyclase stimulator, given intravitreally or as a local arterial injection in rabbits causes a large reduction of IOP accounted for entirely by a decrease of aqueous humor formation.[18] Forskolin, a diterpene derivative of the plant *Coleus forskolhii*, increases intracellular cyclic AMP by stimulating the enzymatic subunit of the adenylate cyclase complex in diverse cellular systems.[19] A topical 1% suspension of forskolin lowers IOP in rabbits, monkeys, and normal humans.[20] Subsequent work demonstrated increased ciliary body blood flow and decreased aqueous production in rabbits after topical administration.[21] Fluorophotometric measurements demonstrated that the ocular hypotensive effect in monkeys was secondary to decreased aqueous formation.[22] In eight normal human volunteers in whom a reduction of IOP after topical forskolin occurred, aqueous humor formation was 34% lower in the treated eye compared to the contralateral control eye.[23] Tonographic outflow facility was unaltered. In young human eyes not selected for an IOP response, topical forskolin did not produce a significant effect on aqueous humor formation.[24] Indeed, forskolin failed to lower IOP in this group from a pretreatment level of 12.3 mm Hg. Poor corneal penetration or a low baseline pressure could explain the lack of an effect. Recently, topical forskolin was reported to cause a 13% reduction of aqueous flow in 10 normal Japanese volunteers compared to contralateral control eyes, associated with small but statistically significant IOP reductions.[25] Sympathetic innervation might play a role in forskolin-induced ocular hypotension because in one study with rabbits, control eyes but not sympathectomized eyes responded with IOP reduction.[26]

The results of initial multiple dose human studies were mixed.[27] Bilateral topical administration of 0.5% or 1.0% forskolin suspensions to 12 glaucoma patients resulted in small, nonstatistically significant reductions of IOP compared to 6 glaucoma patients treated with placebo. Transient conjunctival hyperemia that lasted 15 to 30 minutes was a constant finding in the treated group. Although there was no statistically significant change of average IOP in the treated group, several patients displayed large significant reductions (4 to 7 mm Hg) of IOP. Variability of the response to treatment might be related to poor corneal penetration, binding by pigment, the prevailing level of adrenergic tone, or other factors. Water soluble chemical analogs of forskolin might enhance corneal penetration and might be worthy of a more extensive clinical trial. Twenty-three compounds with chemical structures similar to forskolin were assayed for adenylate cyclase activation in vitro and IOP lowering effect in rabbits.[28] Each compound was applied topically as a 1% suspension. Compounds with potent cyclase stimulatory activity lowered IOP significantly, while those with little or no cyclase effect did not lower IOP. These findings provided further evidence of the link between the cyclase stimulatory properties of these agents and their ability to lower IOP.

Forskolin has facilitated the study in the human eye of the effects of potent adenylate cyclase activation on aqueous humor dynamics. The role of forskolin and related compounds in the treatment of elevated pressure in human glaucoma needs further evaluation.

Prostaglandins

Prostaglandins, products of the cyclooxygenase pathway of arachidonic acid metabolism, are mediators of the ocular irritative response. This response consists of hyperemia, miosis, breakdown of the blood aqueous barrier, and ocular hypertension.[29] Prostaglandins are found in increased amounts in inflamed eyes; the signs of acute inflammation can be reproduced by topical or intracameral application of prostaglandins and hyperemia can be prevented by inhibitors of their synthesis such as aspirin, indomethacin, and related anti-inflammatory agents.[30] The situation is complicated since lipoxygenase products of arachidonic acid metabolism, such as the leukotrienes, have been implicated as mediators of chemotaxis and increased vascular permeability.

Topical application of a small dose (5 μg) of prostaglandin $F_2\alpha$ reduces IOP in rabbits.[31] This species has a notoriously labile blood aqueous barrier and a narrow limit exists between concentrations of prostaglandins that cause hypotensive and hypertensive effects. The rabbit is therefore probably not a suitable model for these studies. Higher topical doses (100 μg) were required to lower IOP in normal owl monkeys.[32] Applications of 50 to 100 μg of prostaglandins caused intraocular pressure reduction in rhesus monkey and cat eyes.[33]

Bito and coworkers investigated repeated topical applications of prostaglandins in rabbits, cats, and rhesus monkeys.[34] While tachyphylaxis developed in rabbits after 1 or 2 days, reduced IOP was maintained in cats for up to 9 months with daily applications of PGE_2. Treatment of two rhesus monkeys demonstrated lowering of intraocular pressure for 29 days. Marked pupillary constriction occurred after $PGF_2\alpha$ administration in cats but only a light miosis occurred with PGE_2, or with $PGF_2\alpha$ in monkey eyes. Prostaglandin-treated eyes frequently demonstrated mild degrees of flare and cell. Conjunctival hyperemia was not noted in cat and monkey eyes.[35] Recent work by Bito and coworkers in cat eyes suggests that the chemically derived prostaglandins of the A and B types might more effectively reduce IOP and cause less miosis than the classic primary prostaglandins of the E, F, and D types.[36]

Giuffre investigated the effects of topical $PGF_2\alpha$ (200 μg) in 18 normal human volunteers.[37] Reductions of IOP occurred in the prostaglandin-treated eyes compared to control eyes, and were maximum at 7 hours and lasted 24 hours. Miosis did not occur, and biomicroscopic examination did not reveal cell or flare. Conjunctival hyperemia, however, always occurred and patients frequently complained of severe stinging and headache. Preliminary reports indicate that the isopropyl ester prodrug of $PGF_2\alpha$ delivered topically in humans also significantly lowers IOP.[38,39]

Topically applied prostaglandins were initially reported to increase the tonographic outflow facility in rabbits.[31,40,41] Lee and colleagues studied aqueous humor dynamics in cats and monkeys treated with topical $PGF_2\alpha$. Only small increases of outflow facility were observed, and no measurable changes of aqueous humor flow were found with fluorophotometry.[42] In the same study, increased levels of aqueous humor protein were found in cats treated topically with 750 μg of $PGF_2\alpha$. In cats, PGA_2 and $PGF_2\alpha$-1-isopropylester lowered IOP but produced no significant changes in either aqueous flow or outflow facility.[43] The mechanism of pressure lowering with in the $PGF_2\alpha$-1-isopropylester was investigated with fluorophotometry in human subjects, and no effect was found on the rate of aqueous flow.[38] Animal and human studies have shown that the changes in aqueous production, episcleral venous pressure, and outflow facility are insufficient to explain the magnitude of IOP reduction after the application of topical prostaglandins. This suggests that uveoscleral flow might be somehow increased by these agents, a notion that has been supported recently by the work of Crawford and Kaufman.[44] They have shown that pilocarpine blocks the hypotensive effect of topical prostaglandins in monkeys. Although prostaglandins might therefore not be useful in combination with the classical miotics, the finding that they increase uveoscleral flow might make these drugs especially helpful in patients whose conventional outflow pathways are so compromised that miotics are not effective.

The prostaglandins and related compounds represent a potential class of agents for the treatment of glaucoma. The side effects of burning, conjunctival hyperemia, and destabilization of the blood-aqueous barrier remain a concern in human eyes. Long-term clinical safety and efficacy and the differential effects of the various primary and derived prostaglandins require further evaluation if these compounds are to achieve clinical usefulness.

Alpha Adrenergic Agents

Alpha receptors are present at adrenergic junctions on the surfaces of prejunctional neurons and postjunctional cells. Prejunctional alpha receptors differ in their pharmacologic properties from postjunctional alpha receptors.[45] $Alpha_1$ receptors include typical postjunctional receptors and classically mediate smooth muscle contraction. $Alpha_2$ receptors include presynaptic autoregulatory receptors as well as some atypical receptors such as those on human platelets. The α_2 (prejunctional) receptors regulate the amount of neurotransmitter (norepinephine) released from the nerve terminal by negative feedback inhibition. Thus, stimulation of α_2 receptors decreases the amount of norepinephine released from the nerve terminal during nerve stimulation. Blockade of α_2 receptors causes increased release of norepinephine from the nerve terminal during stimulation.

Thymoxamine is a non-selective alpha adrenergic blocker, and is the only alpha adrenergic agent in clinical use as an ophthalmic preparation. Commercially available in Europe, it is not currently approved for general use in the United States.[46] Thymoxamine has little or no effect on IOP, but causes pupillary constriction by competitive inhibition of norepinephine at the pupillary dilator muscle. The miosis is not accompanied by shallowing of the anterior chamber,[47] as opposed to the miosis induced by cholinergic agents. This property represents a theoretical advantage in the treatment of angle closure glaucoma. Thymoxamine has been used to reverse mydriasis induced with adrenergic agents,[48,49] to differentiate angle closure glaucoma from open angle glaucoma associated with narrow angles,[50] and has potential for the treatment of pigmentary glaucoma to prevent further pigment dispersion.[51]

Prazosin is an α_1 adrenergic antagonist used for its peripheral vasodilatory properties to treat systemic hypertension. Applied topically, it lowers IOP in normal rabbits.[52,53] Tonographic outflow facility remains unchanged after topical administration of the drug, and posterior chamber ascorbate concentrations increase.[53] These findings are compatible with decreased aqueous production. Topical administration has not been reported to lower IOP in humans.

Corynanthine, an α_1 antagonist, lowered IOP in rabbits, monkeys, and humans in single-dose studies.[62] Topical corynanthine did not alter tonographic outflow facility or aqueous flow rate, and was thought to act by increasing uveoscleral outflow, though solid evidence for this mechanism is lacking. In multiple dose studies in ocular hypertensive patients, topical administration of 2% corynanthine two or three times daily failed to produce a lasting effect on IOP.[63]

Clonidine is a partial alpha (nonselective) agonist used orally to lower blood pressure. Although the exact mechanism(s) of blood pressure reduction are unknown, the drug's interaction with alpha receptors in the central nervous system is likely involved. Topical administration of clonidine lowered IOP in laboratory animals[54] and in humans.[55,56] Topical human use was associated with large reductions of blood pressure that prevented clinical use.[56] Smaller topical doses (15 μl of a 0.25% or 0.50% solution) lowered IOP without causing significant systemic hypotension,[57] and might have proved a useful approach had it not been for the introduction of a para-amino derivative. This derivative, apraclonidine (Iopidine, Alcon), 2-(4-amino-2,6-dichloro)-phenylimino-imidazolidine), does not cross the blood brain barrier and has little or no effect on blood pressure or heart rate.[58] It significantly blunts the IOP rise after anterior segment laser surgery[59,60,61] and reduces by approximately 25% the IOP of normal volunteers.[58] While it has been approved in this country for use in conjunction with laser surgery for glaucoma, chronic studies in glaucoma patients are awaited to establish its long-term safety and efficacy.

Alpha adrenergic agents might be useful to treat glaucoma if compounds with sustained effectiveness can be found. The down-regulation of cell surface receptors with prolonged treatment could represent a problem.

Other Agents

Vanadate

Vanadium is a ubiquitous element normally consumed by humans at the rate of 1 to 4 mg per day.[64] Vanadate displays diverse pharmacologic actions in vitro, including inhibition of Na^+ K^+-ATPase[65,66] and stimulation of adenylate cyclase.[67] Vanadate might inhibit the removal of epinephrine or norepinephrine from their active sites.[68] Topical administration of 1% vanadate (as $NaVO_3$ or Na_3VO_4) lowers IOP in rabbits and monkeys.[69,70] Tonographic outflow facility is not altered by the drug,[69] and fluorophotometric measurements reveal decreased aqueous production.[70] The decreased aqueous flow rate was initially ascribed to inhibition of the ciliary Na^+K^+ pump.[71] Mittag and coworkers found the ciliary body content of vanadate after topical administration insufficient to inhibit a significant fraction of Na^+K^+-ATPase or to significantly stimulate adenylate cyclase.[72] The IOP lowering effect of intravenous vanadate was effectively blocked, however, by propranolol, a beta adrenergic blocker.[73] The pharmacologic basis for reduced aqueous production remains unclear. Topical vanadate appears to have little or no effect on human intraocular pressure when delivered as an aqueous solution. Formulations to enhance corneal penetration might produce more encouraging results. Consideration of vanadate in the treatment of glaucoma must take into account the possible effects of ATPase inhibition on the Na^+K^+ pump of the lens and cornea, which could lead to cataract and corneal edema.

Angiotensin Converting Enzyme Inhibitor

Angiotensin converting enzyme is normally present in aqueous humor, although the mechanism by which it is produced and its physiologic role in the eye, if any, are unknown. It has recently been reported by Constad and coworkers[74] that an angiotensin converting enzyme inhibitor (Schering 33861) lowered IOP in patients with ocular hypertension and primary open angle glaucoma. In a double-masked cross-over study with placebo and timolol, the drug significantly reduced IOP, though the magnitude of the effect was less than that with timolol 0.5%. Investigation into the mechanism of action of this unique drug might provide insight into the possible role of angiotensin converting enzyme in the control of aqueous humor dynamics, and provide a rationale for further studies on the use of this drug to treat glaucoma.

Calcium Channel Blockers

Flammer and coworkers have suggested that vasospasm might be a factor in the genesis of some cases of low tension glaucoma.[75,76] The vasospastic syndrome can be uncovered in susceptible patients by examining the nailfold capillaries after exposure of the fingers to cold. Fifteen patients with visual field defects and vasospastic syndrome showed a marked improvement of their visual fields after treatment with nifedipine, a calcium channel blocker used for the treatment of angina.[77] Identification of a subset of patients with low-tension glaucoma who might benefit from such treatment is required, and further prospective study should be undertaken to establish the safety and efficacy of this approach.

Pentoxifylline

The treatment of glaucoma is currently limited to lowering IOP. A considerable mass of clinical evidence indicates that lowering IOP, at least in some patients, will improve visual prognosis. Other patients, particularly those with advanced primary open angle glaucoma or low tension glaucoma, will lose additional visual function despite reduction of IOP to the lowest possible levels. This latter group of patients might require alternative forms of treatment. If some forms of glaucoma are secondary to microvascular disease of the optic nerve head, then treatment of the underlying circulatory disorder should be sought.

Pentoxifylline is a xanthine derivative with unique hemorheologic effects. Prolonged oral administration reduces blood viscosity by improving impaired red blood cell flexibility and increases perfusion of microcirculatory beds.[78,79] Pentoxifylline is well tolerated and effective for the symptomatic treatment of intermittent claudication.[80] A single report suggested that the drug may be beneficial in the treatment of acute retinal circulatory disorders.[81] Its use to increase microcirculation in the optic nerve of glaucoma patients with vascular disease for now remains speculative.

References

1. Becker B. Decrease in intraocular pressure in man by a carbonic anhydrase inhibitor. Diamox. Am J Ophthalmol 37:13, 1954.
2. Maren TH. The rates of movement of Na^+, Cl^-, and HCO_3 from plasma to posterior chamber: effect of acetazolamide and relation to the treatment of glaucoma. Invest Ophthalmol Vis Sci 15:356, 364, 1976.
3. Foss RH. Local application of Diamox: An experimental study of its effect on the intraocular pressure. Am J Ophthalmol 36:336, 339, 1955.
4. Green H, Leopold IH. Effects of locally administered Diamox. Am J Ophthalmol 40(suppl):137, 1955.
5. Gloster J, Perkins ES. Effect of a carbonic anhydrase inhibitor (Diamox) on intraocular pressure of rabbits and cats. Br J Ophthalmol 39:647-658, 1955.
6. Maren TH, Jankowska L, Sanyal G, Edelhauser HF. The transcorneal permeability of sulfonamide carbonic anhydrase inhibitors and their effect on aqueous humor secretion. Exp Eye Res 36:457-480, 1983.
7. Stein A, Pinke R, Krupin T, et al. The effect of topically administered carbonic anhydrase inhibitors on aqueous dynamics in rabbits. Am J Ophthalmol 95:222, 238, 1983.
8. Flach AJ, Peterson JS, Seligmann KA. Local ocular hypotensive effect of topically applied acetazolamide. Am J Ophthalmol 98:66-72, 1984.
9. Sugrue MF, Gautheron P, Schmitt C, et al. On the pharmacology of L.645,151: A topically effective ocular hypotensive carbonic anhydrase inhibitor. J Pharm Exp Ther 232:534-540, 1985.

10. Friedman Z, Allen RC, Raph SM. Topical acetazolamide and methazolamide delivered by contact lenses. Arch Ophthalmol 103:963-966, 1985.
11. Lewis RA, Schoewald RD, Eller MG, Barfknecht CF, Phelps CD. Ethoxzolamide analogue gel: a topical carbonic anhydrase inhibitor. Arch Ophthalmol 102:1821-1824, 1984.
12. Lewis RA, Schoewald RD, Barfknecht CF, Phelps CD. Aminozolamide gel. Arch Ophthamol 104:842-844, 1986.
13. Maren TH, Bar-Ilan A. Ocular pharmacology and hypotensive activity of a topically active carbonic anhydrase (CA) inhibitor, a 4-alkylaminothienothiopyran-2-sulfonamide, MK-927. Invest Ophthalmol Vis Sci Suppl 29:16, 1988.
14. Wang RF, Serle JB, Podos SM, Sugrue MF. The ocular hypotensive effect of the topical carbonic anhydrase inhibitor MK-927 in glaucomatous monkeys. Invest Ophthalmol Vis Sci Suppl 29:16, 1988.
15. Hennekes R, Pfeiffer N, Lippa E, et al. MK-927: An active topical carbonic anhydrase inhibitor in patients. Invest Ophthalmol Vis Sci Suppl 29:82, 1988.
16. Caprioli J, Sears M. The adenylate cyclase receptor complex and aqueous humor formation. Yale J Biol Med 57:283-300, 1984.
17. Sears ML. Regulation of aqueous flow by the adenylate cyclase receptor complex in the ciliary epithelium. Am J Ophthalmol 100:194-198, 1985.
18. Gregory D, Sears M, Bausher L, Mishima H, Mead A. Intraocular pressure and aqueous flow are decreased by cholera toxin. Invest Ophthalmol Vis Sci 20:371-381, 1981.
19. Seamon KB, Daly JW. Forskolin: A unique diterpene activator of cyclic AMP-generating systems. J Cyclic Nucleotide Res 7(4):201-224, 1981.
20. Caprioli J, Sears M. Forskolin lowers intraocular pressure in rabbits, monkeys, and man. Lancet 30:958-960, 1983.
21. Caprioli J, Sears M, Bausher L, Gregory D, Mead A. Forskolin lowers intraocular pressure by reducing aqueous inflow. Invest Ophthalmol Vis Sci 25:268-277, 1984.
22. Lee PY, Podos SM, Mittag T, Severin C. Effect of topically applied forskolin on aqueous humor dynamics in cynomolgus monkey. Invest Ophthalmol Vis Sci 25:1206-1209, 1984.
23. Burstein NL, Sears ML, Mead A. Aqueous flow in human eyes is reduced by forskolin a potent adenylate cyclase activator. Exp Eye Res 79:745-749, 1984.
24. Brubaker RF, Carlson KH, Kullerstrand LJ, McLaren JW. Topical forskolin (Colforsin) and aqueous flow in humans. Arch Ophthalmol 105:637-641, 1987.
25. Seto C, Eguchi S, Araie M, Matsumoto S, Takase M. Acute effects of topical forskolin on aqueous humor dynamics in man. Jpn J Ophthalmol 30:238-244, 1986.
26. Potter DE, Burke JA, Temple JR. Forskolin suppresses sympathetic neuron function and causes ocular hypotension. Cur Eye Res 4:87-96, 1985.
27. Caprioli J, Sears M, Elman J. Clinical trial of topical forskolin in patients with glaucoma. J Ocular Pharm, in press.

28. Caprioli J, Sears M, Kosley R, Cherill R, Huger F. Cyclase activation and IOP reduction by forskolin analogs. Invest Ophthalmol Vis Sci 26(suppl):15, 1985.
29. Neufeld AH, Jampol LM, Sears ML. Aspirin prevents the disruption of the blood-aqueous barrier in the rabbit eye. Nature 238:158-159, 1972.
30. Eakins KE. Prostaglandin and non-prostaglandin mediated breakdown of the blood-aqueous barrier. Exp Eye Res 483-498, 1977.
31. Camras CB, Bito LZ, Eakins KE. Reduction of intraocular pressure by prostaglandins applied topically to the eyes of conscious rabbits. Invest Ophthamol Vis Sci 16:1125-1134, 1977.
32. Camras CB, Bito LZ. Reduction of intraocular pressure in normal and glaucomatous primate (Aotus trivirgaties) eyes by topically applied prostaglandin F2. Cur Eye Res 1:205, 1981.
33. Stern FA, Bito LZ: Comparison of the hypotensive and other ocular effects of prostaglandins E2 and F2 on cat and rhesus monkey eyes. Invest Ophthalmol Vis Sci 22:588-598, 1982.
34. Bito LZ, Draga A, Blanco J, Camras CB. Long-term maintenance of reduced intraocular pressure by daily or twice daily topical application of prostaglandins to cat or rhesus monkey eyes. Invest Ophthalmol Vis Sci 24:312-319, 1983.
35. Bito, LZ. Prostaglandins, other eicosanoids, and their derivatives as potential antiglaucoma agents. In Drance SM (ed): Medical Treatment of Glaucomas, Grune & Stratton, pp 477-505, 1984.
36. Bito LZ, Baroody RA, Miranda OC. Eicosanoids as a new class of ocular hypotensive agents. 1. The apparent therapeutic advantages of derived prostaglandins of the A and B type as compared with primary prostaglandins of the E, F, and D type. Exp Eye Res 44:825-837, 1987.
37. Giuffre G. The effects of prostaglandin $F_2\alpha$ in the human eye. Graefe's Arch Clin Exp Ophthalmol 222:139-141, 1985.
38. Kerstetter JR, Brubaker RF, Wilson SE, Kullerstrand L. Prostaglandin $F_2\alpha$-1-isopropylester effects on aqueous humor dynamics in human subjects. Invest Ophthalmol Vis Sci Suppl 28:266, 1987.
39. Villumsen J, Alm A. The effect of prostaglandin $F_2\alpha$ eye drops in open angle glaucoma. Invest Ophthalmol Vis Sci Suppl 28:378, 1987.
40. Casey WJ. Prostaglandin E2 and aqueous humor dynamics in the rhesus monkey eye. Prostaglandins 8:327-337, 1974.
41. Kass MA, Podos SM, Moses RA, Becker B. Prostaglandin El and aqueous humor dynamics. Invest Ophthalmol Vis Sci 11:1022-1027, 1972.
42. Lee PY, Podos SM, Severin C. Effect of prostaglandin $F_2\alpha$ on aqueous humor dynamics of rabbit, cat and monkey. Invest Ophthalmol Vis Sci 25:1087-1093, 1984.
43. Hayashi M, Yablonski ME, Bito LZ. Eicosanoids as a new class of ocular hypotensive agents. Invest Ophthalmol Vis Sci 28:1639-1643, 1987.
44. Crawford K, Kaufman PL. Pilocarpine antagonizes prostaglandin F2-induced ocular hypotension in monkeys. Arch Ophthalmol 105:1112-1116, 1987.
45. Hoffman BB, Lefkowitz RJ. Alpha-adrenergic receptor subtypes. N Engl J Med 302:1390-1396, 1980.

46. Wand M, Grant WM. Thymoxamine hydrochloride: An alpha-adrenergic blocker. Surv Ophthalmol 25:75-84, 1980.
47. Susanna R, Drance SM, Schulzer M, Douglas GR. The effects of thymoxamine on anterior chamber depth in human eyes. Can J Ophthalmol 13:250-251, 1978.
48. Turner P, Sneddon JM. Alpha receptor blockade by thymoxamine in the human eye. Clin Pharmacol Ther 9:45-49, 1967.
49. Mapstone R. Safe mydriasis. Br J Ophthalmol 54:690-692, 1970.
50. Wand M, Grant WM. Thymoxamine test: differentiating angle-closure glaucoma from open-angle glaucoma with narrow angles. Arch Ophthalmol 96:1009-1011, 1978.
51. Campbell DG. Pigmentary dispersion and glaucoma. Arch Ophthalmol 97:1667-1672, 1979.
52. Smith BR, Murray DL, Leopold IH. Influence of topically applied prazosin on the intraocular pressure of experimental animals. Arch Ophthalmol 97:1933-1936, 1979.
53. Krupin T, Feibl M, Becker B. Effect of prazosin on aqueous humor dynamics in rabbits. Arch Ophthalmol 98:1639-1642, 1980.
54. Bill A, Heilmann K. Ocular effects of clonidine in cats and monkeys (Macaca irus). Exp Eye Res 21:481-488, 1975.
55. Krieglstein GK, Langham ME, Leydhecker W: The peripheral and central neural actions of clonidine in normal and glaucomatous eyes. Invest Ophthalmol Vis Sci 17:149-158, 1978.
56. Hodapp E, Kolker AE, Kass MA, et al. The effect of topical clonidine on intraocular pressure. Arch Ophthalmol 99:1208-1211, 1981.
57. Peturssen G, Cole R, Hanna C. Treatment of glaucoma using minidrops of clonidine. Arch Ophthalmol 102:1180-1181, 1984.
58. Abrams DA, Robin AL, Pollack IP, deFaller JM, DeSantis L. The safety and efficacy of topical 1% ALO 2145 (p-aminoclonidine hydrochloride) in normal volunteers. Arch Ophthalmol 105:1205-1207, 1987.
59. Robin AL, Pollack IP, House B, Enger C. Effects of ALO 2145 on intraocular pressure following argon laser trabeculoplasty. Arch Ophthalmol 105:646-650, 1987.
60. Robin AL, Pollack IP, deFaller JM. Effects of topical ALO 2145 (p.aminoclonidine hydrochloride) on the acute intraocular pressure rise after argon laser iridotomy. Arch Ophthalmol 105:1208-1211, 1987.
61. Brown RH, Stewart RH, Lynch MG, et al. ALO 2145 reduces the intraocular pressure elevation after anterior segment laser surgery. Ophthalmol 95:378-384, 1988.
62. Serle JB, Stein AJ, Posos SM, Severen CH. Corynanthine and aqueous humor dynamics in rabbits and monkeys. Arch Ophthalmol 102:1385-1388, 1984.
63. Serle JB, Podos SM, Lustgarten JS, Teitelbaum C, Severin CH. The effect of corynanthine on intraocular pressure in clinical trials. Ophthalmol 92:977-980, 1985.
64. Schoeder HA, Bolassa JJ, Tipton IH. Abnormal trace metals in man-vanadium. J Chronic Dis 16:1047, 1963.

65. Cantley LC Jr, Josephson L, Warner R, et al. Vanadate is a potent (Na^+, $K^!+$)-ATPase inhibitor found in ATP derived from muscle. J Biol Chem 252:7421, 1977.
66. Bond GH, Hudgins PM. Kinetics of inhibition of Na^+, K^+ ATPase by $Mg^2{}_+$ K^+, and vanadate. Am Chem Soc 18:325, 1979.
67. Schwabe U, Puchstern C, Hannemann H, Sochtig E. Activation of adenylate cyclase by vanadate. Nature 277:143, 1979.
68. Delamere NA, Williams RN. Modulation by vanadate of the adrenergic characteristics of the iris, ileum. and vas deferens. Invest Ophthalmol Vis Sci 27:1336-1341, 1986.
69. Krupin T, Becker B, Podos SM. Topical vanadate lowers intraocular pressure in rabbits. Invest Ophthalmol Vis Sci 19:1360-1363, 1980.
70. Podos SM, Lee PY, Severin C, Mittag T. The effect of vanadate on aqueous humor dynamics in cynomolgus monkeys. Invest Ophthalmol Vis Sci 25:359-361, 1984.
71. Becker B. Vanadate and aqueous humor dynamics. Invest Ophthalmol Vis Sci 19:1156-1164, 1980.
72. Mittag TW, Serle JB, Podos SM, Cohen L, Liebowitz F. Vanadate effects on ocular pressure, (Na^+ K^+)-ATPase and adenylate cyclase in rabbit eyes. Invest Ophthalmol Vis Sci 25:1335-1338, 1984.
73. Delamere NA, Williams RN. The influence of reserpine and propranolol upon the IOP response to vanadate in the rabbit. Invest Ophthalmol Vis Sci 26:1442-1445, 1985.
74. Constad WH, Fiore P, Samson C, Cinotti AA. Use of an angiotensin converting enzyme inhibitor in ocular hypertension and primary open angle glaucoma. Am J Ophthalmol 105:674-677, 1988.
75. Flammer J, Guthauser U, Mahler F. Do ocular vasospasms help cause low tension glaucoma? E.L. Greve & A. Heyl (eds): Seventh International Visual Field Symposium, Amsterdam. 1986, Dr. W. Junk Publishers, Dordrecht. pp 397-399.
76. Gasser P, Flammer J. Influence of vasospasm on visual function. Doc Ophthalmol 66:3-18, 1987.
77. Flammer J, Guthauser U. Behandlung choroidaler vasospasmen mit, kalziumantagonisten. Klin Monastbl Augenheilkd 190:299-300, 1987.
78. Moller R, Tehrack F, Grigoleit HG. Fum Wirkingsmechanismus von pentoxifylline. Med Monatsschr Pharm 29:487, 1975.
79. Muller R. Pentoxifylline: a biomedical profile. J Med 10:307, 1979.
80. Porter JM, Cutler BS, Lee BY, et al. Pentoxifylline efficacy in the treatment of intermittent claudification: Multicenter controlled double-blind trial with objective assessment of chronic occlusive arterial disease patients. Am Heart J 104:66-72, 1982.
81. Flamm P. Pentoxifylline treatment of acute circulatory disturbances in the retina and optic nerve. Therapiewoche 33:2845-2853, 1983.

SECTION II

Complications of Surgical Laser Procedures — Their Prevention and Management

CHAPTER 7

Complications of Argon Laser Trabeculoplasty

Mark B. Sherwood, MD

Although argon laser trabeculoplasty (ALT) is a remarkably safe procedure, it can cause problems, some of marked clinical significance. The possible complications following ALT are listed in Table 7-1.

A sharp rise in IOP in the hours immediately following argon laser trabeculoplasty is one of the most common complications and potentially the most serious. It can lead to further visual field loss and even, in cases with far advanced glaucomatous cupping, to decreased visual acuity from "snuff-out" of a small residual central island of field. This latter is rare but has been reported.[1,2]

In most cases, the pressure rise, if it occurs, is small; less than 10 mm Hg above prelaser IOP. The reported incidence varies widely, but approximately 25 to 35% of patients can expect a pressure spike of greater than 5 mm Hg[1,3,4] and about 5 to 20% an elevation of 10 mm Hg or more following ALT.[1-7] Occasionally the pressure can abruptly rise to levels approaching 60 mm Hg or greater, and it is in these cases that further damage to the optic nerve and field loss is most likely if urgent medical therapy (usually including an oral or intravenous osmotic agent) is not provided.

As it is hard to know which patient will develop a pressure rise after ALT, it is important to measure the postlaser pressures of all patients hourly for the first two to three hours. Certain patient factors, listed in Table 7-2, make pressure spikes more common or potentially more hazardous, and in these cases close monitoring over a longer period is advisable.

Preexisting advanced glaucomatous nerve damage is the major factor determining the susceptibility of a patient to significant visual damage from a transient pressure spike. Included are patients whose visual field loss is within 5° of fixation and especially those whose field loss splits fixation. Another important determinant of susceptibility to damage is the starting IOP. A pressure rise of 20 mm Hg in a patient whose initial pressure is 45 mm Hg is more likely to lead to field loss than a similar pressure rise in a patient with an initial pressure of 20 mm Hg. Significant postlaser pressure elevation is more common in patients with exfoliation syndrome glaucoma[8] than in primary open angle glaucoma and patients with a poor outflow facility are also at higher risk.[9]

Table 7-1. Complications of Argon Laser Trabeculoplasty
Elevation of IOP
Early and transient pressure "spike"
Early and sustained pressure increase
Late pressure rise—loss of laser effect
Visual field loss
Secondary to increased IOP
Despite lowered IOP
Visual acuity decrease
Transient—associated with gonisol, SPK, or bright light
Permanent—associated with field loss
Iridocyclitis
Transient (1 week or less)
Sustained
Peripheral anterior synichiae
Hyphema (usually microscopic)
Cornea—Epithelial burns
—Endothelial burns
Corneal edema
Syncope
Cystoid macular edema
Cataract

Table 7-2. Patient Factors Calling for Close Monitoring for Pressure Spikes
Advanced glaucomatous nerve damage and field loss
High prelaser IOP
Patient diagnosis: exfoliation syndrome glaucoma, secondary glaucomas
Low outflow facility
Previous 360° laser trabeculoplasty

Patients undergoing repeat laser trabeculoplasty, following previous 360° angle treatment, have an increased risk of pressure elevation that might necessitate urgent surgical intervention. The incidence of this was 12% in one study,[10] although other studies, in which only 180° of angle meshwork was retreated[11] or where only 50 to 60 burns were applied to the entire circumference,[12] found no cases requiring urgent surgery. All studies agree, however, that the long-term success rate of laser trabeculoplasty retreatment is poor.

The need medically to treat an early postlaser spike in pressure depends on the individual patient. Where there is minimal disc or field damage, a small pressure rise from an initial moderate level might require only observation. In patients with little residual field, pretreatment with an osmotic agent prior to laser therapy might be advisable as a prophylaxis against even a small pressure spike.[13] Administration of 500 mg of acetazolamide 30 to 60 minutes before laser treatment is of questionable benefit in reducing the occurrence of early pressure spikes.[7] Any treatment administered will partly depend on the patient's previous history of intolerances and allergic reactions. In general, oral osmotic agents such as isosorbide, or in nondiabetics, glycerin, are particularly effective in cutting short an early pressure spike. Topical pilocarpine is also helpful and some recommend its prophylactic use.[14,15] Additional aqueous suppression from CAIs or beta blockers can be useful, post laser especially in maintaining a pressure reduction obtained from the osmotic agents.

More recently, trials of a new topical drug, apraclonidine hydrochloride 1% (Iopidine, Alcon) an α_2 agonist, have shown a reduction both in the incidence and in the magnitude of pressure spikes following laser trabeculoplasty.[4,16] A single drop is administered one hour prior to ALT and a second drop immediately after treatment. To date, in short-term use, there have been no significant side effects reported, although eyelid retraction, conjunctival blanching, and mydriasis have been noted.[17] Despite the decrease in pressure elevation using apraclonidine, IOP rises of 10 mm Hg or greater might still occur in a small number of cases (4% in one study[4]) and close monitoring of postlaser IOP remains advisable.

Several modifications of the laser technique initially described by Wise[18] have been suggested to help reduce the incidence or height of early pressure rise. These are listed in Table 7-3.

Table 7-3. Suggested Modifications to Reduce Pressure Spike
Reduction of number of burns and area lasered per session
Placing burns anteriorly on pigmented trabecular meshwork
Accurate control of spot size
Pretreatment with apraclonidine hydrochloride or osmotic agents

Decreasing the area of meshwork lasered and the number of spots applied is associated with a decrease in the magnitude of — but not in the incidence of — early pressure spikes.[2,7] The pressure rise also occurs earlier and does not last so long.[2] Some authors recommend treating 180° of the angle with approximately 50 burns at a single sitting and to later treat the remaining 180° if pressure-lowering is inadequate. Initial studies suggested that treating only half the angle is as effective as treating the full 360° at one session.[1,19,20] Treatment of only 90 with 25 burns has been reported but this produces a smaller pressure reduction than 180° or 360° protocols.[20,21] Pressure is further lowered at the second laser treatment in the majority of these cases; however, in patients with "fragile" optic nerves, divided sessions might be preferable. Since pressure rises of 10 mm Hg or more can still be seen even when laser is applied to only 90° of the meshwork, postlaser monitoring of IOP remains essential.

The positioning of the laser burns on the anterior part of the pigmented trabecular meshwork, rather than on the posterior part or scleral spur, greatly reduces the likelihood of early pressure rise.[13,20] This is demonstrated in Figs. 7-1 and 7-2. When anteriorly placed, most of the 50 μm laser spot lies on the pigmented meshwork band and the remainder of the spot extends just anterior to it. Following treatment, the blanching produced in the pigmented zone gives a saw-toothed appearance to the area lasered as shown in Fig. 7-3. The IOP reduction obtained from ALT is not lessened by anterior placement of the burns,[20] and in view of the reduction in the incidence of pressure spikes this location is recommended for all cases.

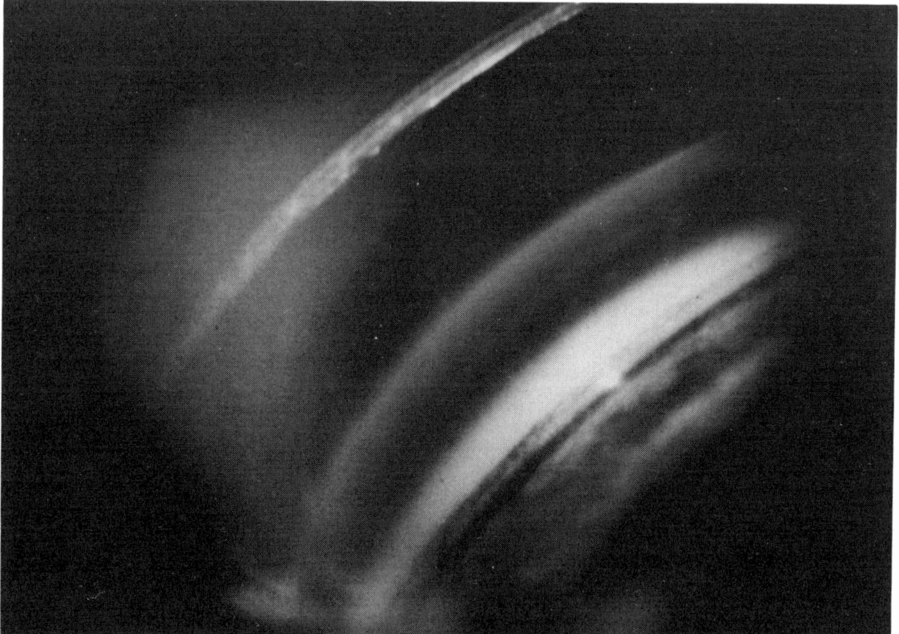

Figure 7-1. Argon laser aiming beam directed correctly on the anterior portion of the pigmented trabecular meshwork.

The laser itself has been evaluated as a factor in both final effectiveness of ALT and in complication rates. Analysis by microscopy has shown great variation between different makes of argon lasers in the size of lasers burn delivered. A 50 μm setting might produce a minimum spot diameter of 100 μm or more in some. It has been suggested that the larger spot sizes contribute to a higher incidence of iritis and early pressure spikes,[22] but this is not proven. Lasers of different wavelength, such as monochromatic green argon, krypton red, or krypton yellow, have been shown to produce essentially the same rate of early pressure rise and other complications as the standard blue/green argon laser.[23,24]

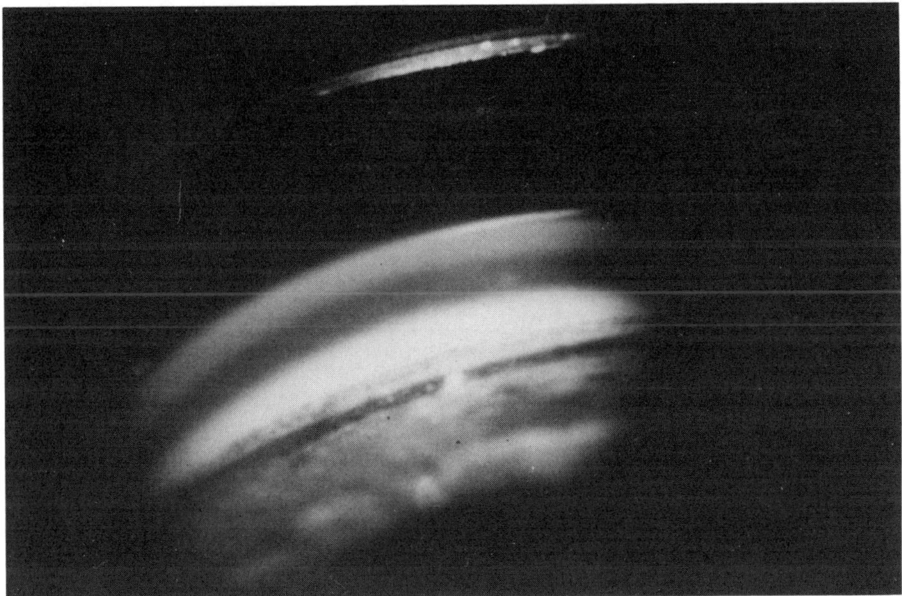

Figure 7-2. Argon laser aiming beam directed at the posterior part of the pigmented trabecular meshwork. There is a higher incidence of post ALT pressure spikes and PAS formation if the laser burn is placed this posteriorly.

Nonsteroidal anti-inflammatory topical agents such as indomethacin and flurbiprofen, administered prior to and for a short course following ALT, have been evaluated to determine if they can decrease early pressure rises. It has been suggested by some that there is increased anterior chamber inflammation in eyes exhibiting pressure spikes,[2] although others disagree.[25] On theoretical grounds, prostaglandin inhibition should be helpful in reducing this inflammation. In practice, however, no studies have demonstrated that these topical agents decrease early postlaser pressure rise.[25-28] Indeed, some have shown a decline in the longer-term pressure-lowering effect from ALT in patients given these drops.[27,28] They are therefore not recommended. Pretreatment with steroid drops has also been shown to be ineffective in preventing early pressure rises.[29] Topical steroids are routinely used for several days after laser surgery to reduce intraocular inflammation, although they have no effect on the final outcome of laser treatment.[1]

Although 80 to 90% of pressure rises occur within the initial three hours following ALT, a significant minority of patients spike later. Some patients with an early pressure elevation respond to additional medical therapy but

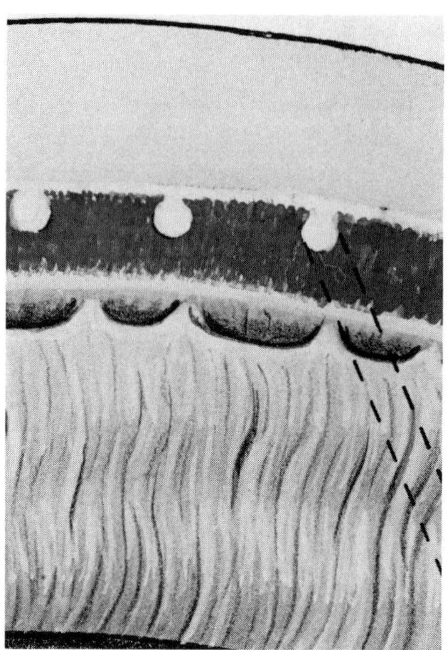

Figure 7-3. Saw-tooth appearance of pigmented trabecular meshwork produced by blanching following anteriorly placed laser burns.

then several hours later have a further rebound increase in pressure.[30] In about 5% of patients a persistent elevation of intraocular tension has been noted more than 24 hours after ALT.[1,7]

As laser trabeculoplasty is almost invariably an outpatient procedure, it is best performed in the morning so that adequate follow up for patients who do spike can be arranged. Further review should be tailored to the needs of the individual. If the disc and visual field are relatively healthy and there has been no evidence of pressure elevation, reevaluation in approximately one week is appropriate. In cases involving a high pressure spike, or especially where there is visual field loss close to fixation, reexamination at 24 hours might be required. The interval for further visits depends on the findings at these subsequent exams. In 1% or less of cases the pressure rise following ALT cannot be adequately controlled medically and in these cases it might be necessary to proceed promptly to filtration surgery. Patients should be informed of this remote but definite possibility prior to laser trabeculoplasty. In about 3% of cases glaucoma control can be worsened by laser therapy.[1,7] This has been particularly noted in certain forms or secondary glaucoma, such as uveitic[3] or juvenile glaucoma[31] and urgent surgery might be precipitated.

It is now generally believed that over several years there is a gradual decrease in the pressure-lowering effect achieved by an initially successful laser trabeculoplasty.[7,13] Some patients continue to maintain acceptable pressure levels even after 10 years, but the proportion of patients who remain controlled diminishes with time.[32] The failure rate is maximal in the first year following ALT and thereafter is approximately 7 to 10% per year.[33] Eyes with advanced glaucomatous optic nerve damage are much more likely to require subsequent filtration surgery, although for many elderly patients, ALT can provide IOP control for their remaining lifespan. [32] Fairly abrupt "late failure," many months or even years after laser trabeculoplasty, has been reported in 6 to 7% of exfoliation syndrome patients. [34,35] A further proportion of patients (approximately 10 to 15%) will continue to lose visual field despite a continued good response to laser therapy, with pressure reduction to a "normal" range. [3,7] These patients generally require filtering surgery to attempt to obtain still lower pressure. Prolonged follow up with review of intraocular pressures, visual fields, and disc appearances is essential.

Other Complications

Peripheral anterior synechiae (PAS) are not uncommon following ALT, occurring in 29 to 47% of eyes in early studies. [1,13,36] There is general agreement that PAS probably do not reduce the final pressure-lowering effect of laser trabeculoplasty, [1,13,36,37] although some disagree. [38] A higher incidence of early pressure spikes, however, has been reported in eyes that develop PAS. [37,39] No correlation has been found between the width of the chamber angle, the number of laser burns, or the amount of trabecular pigmentation, and the formation of PAS. [1,37] It is uncertain whether the laser energy level plays a role. [1,38] The major factor that does seem relevant in reducing the incidence of PAS is placement of the laser burns anteriorly on the trabecular meshwork. If the laser spots are directed anteriorly, the rate of occurrence of PAS falls to around 12%. [37] The PAS seen after laser treatment are in most cases small, peaked, and adherent at the level of the scleral spur. They form a total aggregate usually of less than two clock hours of angle circumference.

In one study 27% of eyes with PAS showed some attachment of iris further anteriorly, at the level of the posterior trabecular meshwork. [1] This again had no demonstrable effect on IOP reduction, presumably because of the small area of meshwork involved. Very rare cases with significant closure of greater than 180 have been reported. [7,14] This might be associated with a prolonged postlaser iritis. [7]

A mild **transient iritis** is seen almost universally following laser trabeculoplasty, but this normally settles within about a week. It is of no clinical significance and generally causes few symptoms. Topical steroids are prescribed routinely, often as a six hourly regimen, but even without these the inflammation will resolve spontaneously. A large number of the retrospective trials each detail one or two patients who developed a severe or persistent iritis. [5-7,40] Patients with uveitic glaucoma might develop a marked flare-up of their inflammation following ALT, along with an associated sustained pressure elevation. This might necessitate early filtration surgery. [3]

Hyphema occurs in 2 to 5% of eyes treated. [1,5,6,13,18,41] In most cases this is microscopic and rapidly clears. Rarely, a more significant hyphema occurs. The bleeding is usually from the trabecular meshwork and can be a sudden spurt or a slow ooze. [1] Bleeding has also been reported after delivery of inadvertent burns to the iris root [41] or circumferential ciliary vessel. [1] If bleeding is noted at the time of trabeculoplasty, it might be controlled by pressing more firmly on the eye with the goniolens or, if this is not sufficient, by directing a few laser burns at the site of the bleeding, using a larger spot and a lower power setting (for example: power, 200 mW; spot size 200 μm; duration, 0.2 sec). The occurrence of hyphema does not decrease the pressure reduction or the increase in outflow facility achieved by laser trabeculoplasty. [1,13]

Mild corneal epithelial abrasions or **superficial punctate erosions** can be seen following the use of the goniolens during the procedure. These resolve spontaneously, usually within hours, and generally cause only minor discomfort. In patients with "dry eyes" or other conditions predisposing to corneal erosions, special care must be taken to avoid traumatizing the cornea, causing more severe postoperative discomfort. Corneal burns, both epithelial and endothelial, have been reported but, again, are of little clinical importance. [41] Epithelial burns resolve within a few days without residual scarring. [42] Specular microscopy has shown that there is no significant decrease in endothelial cell count following laser trabeculoplasty. [43] Corneal edema can occur, either associated with underlying corneal disease (Fuchs' dystrophy and Chandler's syndrome have been described) or secondary to a major postlaser pressure spike. The edema clears in most cases within a few weeks. [41]

Cystoid macular edema has been reported in two aphakes following trabeculoplasty, [7] but no direct causal relationship has been proven. Likewise, there is no good evidence of cataract progression secondary to ALT.

Syncopal episodes, possibly related to either anxiety or to vasovagal effects from pushing on the eye with the goniolens, can occur while the patient is sitting at the laser. Beta blockers have been suggested as an additional factor. [7] The patient might be pale or perspiring on his forehead. This should alert the ophthalmologist to ask the patient whether he feels faint. The laser treatment, if underway, should be stopped and the patient reclined horizontally in an examination chair or on a couch.

In summary, the most serious complications of ALT are associated with a postlaser pressure rise. Particularly vulnerable are those patients with far advanced field loss. Pretreating with apraclonidine and directing the laser burns anteriorly and treatment of only 180° of the meshwork per sitting help to reduce the danger. The risk-to-benefit ratio is generally very favorable in laser trabeculoplasty, but this must be assessed for each case. The state of the optic disc, the starting IOP and the type of glaucoma are the important factors to consider. The likelihood of ALT giving a good result for a particular glaucoma diagnostic group is summarized in Table 7-4.

Table 7-4. Prognosis for ALT for Different Types of Glaucoma

Good Prognosis	Moderate Prognosis	Poor Prognosis
Exfoliation syndrome	Glaucoma in aphakia	Uveitic glaucoma
POAG	Previous trabecular surgery	Juvenile glaucoma
Pigmentary glaucoma	Combined mechanism glaucoma	Neovascular glaucoma
	Angle recession glaucoma	Angle anomaly syndromes

References

1. Thomas JV, Simmons RJ, Belcher CD. Argon laser trabeculoplasty in the presurgical glaucoma patient. Ophthalmology 89:187-197, 1982.
2. Weinreb RN, Ruderman J, Juster R, et al. Immediate intraocular pressure response to argon laser trabeculoplasty. Am J Ophthalmol 95:279-286, 1983.
3. Lieberman MF, Hoskins HD, Hetherington J. Laser trabeculoplasty and the glaucomas. Ophthalmology 90:790-795, 1983.
4. Brown RH, Stewart RH, Lynch MG, et al. ALO 2145 reduces the intraocular pressure elevation after anterior segment laser surgery. Ophthalmology 95:378-383, 1988.
5. Elsas T, Harstad HK. Laser trabeculoplasty in open angle glaucoma. Acta Ophthalmol 61:991-997, 1983.
6. Brooks AMV, Gillies WE. Do any factors predict a favorable response to laser trabeculoplasty? Aust J Ophthalmol 12:149-153, 1984.
7. Hoskins HD, Hetherington J, Minckler DS, et al. Complications of laser trabeculoplasty. Ophthalmology 90:796-799, 1983.
8. Svedbergh B, Sherwood MB. Argon laser trabeculoplasty in exfoliation glaucoma. A retrospective study. Dev Ophthalmol 11:116-123, 1985.
9. Keightley SJ, Khaw PT, Elkington AR. The prediction of intraocular pressure rise following argon laser trabeculoplasty. Eye 1:577-580, 1987.
10. Brown SVL, Thomas JV, Simmons RJ. Laser trabeculoplasty retreatment. Am J Ophthalmol 99:8-10, 1985.
11. Richter CU, Shingleton BJ, Bellows AR, et al. Retreatment with argon laser trabeculoplasty. Ophthalmology 94:1085-1088, 1987.
12. Messner D, Siegel LI, Kass MA, et al. Repeat argon laser trabeculoplasty. Am J Ophthalmol 103:113-115, 1987.
13. Schwartz AL, Kopelman J. Four-year experience with argon laser trabecular surgery in uncontrolled open-angle glaucoma. Ophthalmology 90:771-779, 1983.
14. Schwartz L, Spaeth GL, Brown GC. Laser therapy of the anterior segment, New Jersey: Charles B. Slack, 1984, Chapter 4.
15. Ofner S, Samples JR, Van Buskirk EM. Pilocarpine and the increase in intraocular pressure after laser trabeculoplasty. Am J Ophthalmol 97:647-649, 1984.
16. Robin AL, Pollack IP, House B, et al. Effects of ALO 2145 on intraocular pressure following argon laser trabeculoplaty. Arch Ophthalmol 105:646-650, 1987.
17. Robin AL. Short-term effects of unilateral 1% apraclonidine therapy. Arch Ophthalmol 106:912-915, 1988.
18. Wise J. Long-term control of adult open angle glaucoma by argon laser treatment. Ophthalmology 88:197-202, 1981.
19. Weinreb RN, Ruderman J, Juster R. Influence of the number of laser burns administered on the early results of argon laser trabeculoplasty. Am J Ophthalmol 95:287-292, 1983.
20. Schwartz LW, Spaeth GL, Traverso C, et al. Variations of techniques on the results of argon laser trabeculoplasty. Ophthalmology 90:781-784, 1983.

21. Wilensky JT, Weinreb RN. Low-dose trabeculoplasty. Am J Ophthalmol 95:423-426, 1983.
22. Wise JB. Errors in laser spot size in laser trabeculoplasty. Ophthalmology 91:186-190, 1984.
23. Smith J. Argon laser trabeculoplasty: Comparison of bichromatic and monochromatic wavelengths. Ophthalmology 91:355-360, 1984.
24. Spurny RC, Lederer CM. Krypton laser trabeculoplasty. Arch Ophthalmol 102:1626-1628, 1984.
25. Weinreb RN, Robin AL, Baerveldt G, et al. Flurbiprofen pretreatment in argon laser trabeculoplasty for primary open-angle glaucoma. Arch Ophthalmol 102:1629-1632, 1984.
26. Pappas HR, Berry DP, Partamian L, et al. Topical indomethacin therapy before argon laser trabeculoplasty. Am J Ophthalmol 99:571-575, 1985.
27. Gelfand Y, Wolpert M. Effects of topical indomethacin pretreatment on argon laser trabeculoplasty: a randomized, double-masked study on black South Africans. Br J Ophthalmol 69:668-672, 1985.
28. Hotchkiss ML, Robin AL, Pollack IP, et al. Nonsteroidal anti-inflammatory agents after argon laser trabeculoplasty. Ophthalmology 91:969-976, 1984.
29. Ruderman JM, Zweig KO, Wilensky JT, et al. Effects of corticosteroid pretreatment on argon laser trabeculoplasty. Am J Ophthalmol 96:84-89, 1983.
30. Krupin T, Kolker AE, Kass MA, et al. Intraocular pressure the day of argon laser trabeculoplasty in primary open angle glaucoma. Ophthalmology 91:361-365, 1984.
31. Wilensky JT, Weinreb RN. Early and late failures of argon laser trabeculoplasty. Arch Ophthalmol 101:895-897, 1983.
32. Wise JB. Ten year results of laser trabeculoplasty. Does the laser avoid glaucoma surgery or merely defer it? Eye 1:45-50, 1987.
33. Shingleton BJ, Richter CU, Bellows AR, et al. Long-term efficacy of argon laser trabeculoplasty. Ophthalmology 94:1513-1518, 1987.
34. Pohjanpelto P. Late results of laser trabeculoplasty for increased intraocular pressure. Acta Ophthalmol 61:998-1008, 1983.
35. Sherwood MB, and Svedburgh B. Argon laser trabeculoplasty in exfoliation syndrome. Br J Ophthalmol 69:886-890, 1985.
36. Schwartz AL, Whitten ME, Bleiman B, et al. Argon laser trabecular surgery in uncontrolled phakic open angle glaucoma. Ophthalmology 88:203-212, 1981.
37. Traverso CE, Greenidge KC, Spaeth GL. Formation of peripheral anterior synechiae following argon laser trabeculoplasty. Arch Ophthalmol 102:861-863, 1984.
38. Rouhiainen HJ, Terasvirta ME, Tuovinen EJ. Peripheral anterior synechiae formation after trabeculoplasty. Arch Ophthalmol 106:189-191, 1988.
39. Thomas JV. Laser Trabeculoplasty. In Belcher CD, Simmons RJ (eds): Photocoagulation in Glaucoma and Anterior Segment Disease. Baltimore, Williams & Wilkins, 61-86, 1984.

40. Horns DJ, Bellows AR, Hutchinson BT, et al. Argon laser trabeculoplasty for open angle glaucoma. A retrospective study of 380 eyes. Trans Ophthalmol Soc UK 103:288-295, 1983.
41. Weinreb RN, Wilensky JT. Clinical aspects of argon laser trabeculoplasty. Int Ophthalmol Clin 24:79-95, 1984.
42. Mandell AI, Terry SA. Manual of argon laser trabeculoplasty. Coherent Medical Publication, 1982.
43. Traverso CE, Cohen EJ, Groden LR, et al. Central corneal endothelial cell density after argon laser trabeculoplasty. Arch Ophthalmol 102:1322-1324, 1984.

CHAPTER 8

Argon and Nd:YAG Laser Peripheral Iridectomy

Louis W. Schwartz, MD

The first application of the laser in glaucoma was to perform iridectomies with the argon laser. At the present time, laser iridectomy has almost completely supplanted the use of surgical iridectomy because of its ease of use and safety. Many clinicians presently perform iridectomies with the argon laser, but more and more ophthalmologists are beginning to use the Q-switched Nd:YAG laser.

Indications

The indications for performing a laser iridectomy are exactly the same as for performing a surgical iridectomy and are listed in Table 8-1. However, one does not have the problems associated with an operating room and anesthesia. Therefore, some patients who might need an iridectomy, but because of medical reasons might not be able to lie flat on an operating room table or undergo anesthesia, could have a laser treatment sitting up as an outpatient.

Table 8-1. Indications for Laser Iridectomy
Acute primary angle closure
Chronic primary angle closure
Intermittent primary angle closure
Fellow eye of eye with above conditions
Incomplete surgical iridectomy
Occludable angle with historical or physical evidence of previous angle closure
Secondary angle closure

It has been documented that at least 50 to 75% of fellow eyes of individuals who develop acute angle closure glaucoma in one eye will develop an acute attack of glaucoma—despite miotics—within five to ten years. Prophylactic iridectomy in the fellow eye has been shown to be effective in preventing this acute attack. In some instances, however, even when the indications for a laser iridectomy are present, the media (cornea or anterior chamber) are not clear enough or the anterior chamber is too shallow to allow a laser iridectomy and thus one must resort to a surgical iridectomy.

Technique

The technique of laser iridectomy that has evolved over the years has been developed to facilitate penetration of the iris and to minimize complications. Preoperatively, pilocarpine 2% is given every 10 minutes for 3 doses starting 45 minutes before treatment. The media must be clear and the anterior chamber of adequate depth (1 mm for Nd:YAG, 0.5 mm for argon). If the cornea is edematous or cloudy, not enough of the laser energy will reach the iris because the cornea will absorb the energy. Topical glycerin or intravenous mannitol or oral hyperosmotic agents can be tried to clear the cornea. If the cornea is mildly edematous after these measures it is often possible to perform a Nd:YAG iridectomy successfully, but the cornea must be crystal clear to achieve a successful argon laser iridectomy. Often after an acute attack of glaucoma, the iris is inflamed and edematous. When this is present, it is easier to penetrate the iris by lowering the IOP, using steroid eyedrops to decrease the iris inflammation, and then perform the iridectomy a few days after the acute attack. If time is critical, one can usually achieve an iridectomy with the Nd:YAG, but not the argon laser, as the latter will just cause more inflammation. There is the added risk, however, of hemorrhage with a Nd:YAG iridectomy in the inflamed iris that has dilated vessels.

If the acute attack cannot be broken medically, and the cornea is clear enough, an argon laser iridoplasty (see Chapter 9) might be attempted to break the acute attack. When the inflammation subsides, a laser iridectomy can be performed. If the cornea remains cloudy, however, the distance between iris and cornea is not adequate, or the anterior chamber is not clear enough, then surgical iridectomy must be performed.

Local anesthetic drops are used; a retrobulbar anesthetic is needed only if nystagmus is present. An area is chosen in the superior iris (to prevent monocular diplopia), under the upper eyelid, preferably in the ten or two o'clock positions at least two thirds of the distance from the pupil margin in an argon laser iridectomy, and just inside the arcus as far in the periphery as possible for a Nd:YAG laser iridectomy. If an iris crypt is present in the proper zone, it is utilized because the iris is felt to be thinner in these crypts. An Abraham lens or any of the more recently designed iridectomy lenses should be utilized, because the lens facilitates focusing by magnification, widens the beam at the cornea to lessen the chance of corneal burns, decreases the spot size thus increasing the energy at the point of focus, and prevents the lids from closing during the procedure. Naturally, all efforts should be directed to aim the laser away from the macular area. The most important part of the technique, however, is proper focus!

Commonly used settings for the continuous wave argon, pulsed argon, and Nd:YAG lasers are listed in Table 8-2. Some authors have described "hump" or "drum" techniques to stretch the iris prior to argon iridectomy. Most clinicians, however, have found the technique of choosing a spot and just "firing away" until an adequate opening is formed to be most successful. Pretreating an area with argon prior to a YAG iridectomy also has been proven to be superfluous. After the iridectomy is performed, the patient is monitored for IOP spikes hourly for three hours. Posttreatment a drop of prednisilone acetate 1% and pilocarpine 2% are given immediately. Depending on the amount of inflammation, stronger or weaker steroid drops are continued for at least one week. Minimally, the patient should be seen in three days, one week, one month, and as needed thereafter.

Table 8-2. Laser Settings

Laser Type	Spot Size	Power	Pulse	Duration
Continuous wave argon	50 μm	700-1500 mW	1	0.2 sec.
Pulsed argon	50 μm	25 W	300/sec	0.2 sec.
Nd:YAG (Q-switched)	10-70 μm	6 mJ	3	12 nsec.

Complications

Although laser iridectomy seems relatively safe, numerous complications have been described (Table 8-3), including significant loss of vision. Thus, even though the procedure can be done in an office setting, one must be aware of the dangers and be careful to minimize the potential for serious ocular damage.

Table 8-3. Possible Complications of Argon and Nd: YAG Laser Iridectomy

Irritation (Pain)	Synechias
Blurred Vision	Lenticular Opacities
Pigment Dispersion	Closure of Iridectomy
Pupil Distortion	Retinal Burns
Elevation of IOP	Macular Burns
Hemorrhage	Monocular Diplopia
Corneal Endothelial Burns	Lens Dislocation
Corneal Epithelial Burns	Trabecular Meshwork Damage
Iritis	Failure of Patency

Irritation occurs in almost all patients and is because of the effect of the contact lens on the cornea. All patients are told of this effect. If iritis or significantly elevated IOP develops, "deep" pain can ensue, but is rare. All patients have markedly blurred vision for the first ten minutes because of the goniosol and dazzling effect of the bright light. By the next day, however, the vision returns to prelaser levels unless iritis occurs or corneal edema develops from high IOP or there is a corneal abrasion. If the IOP elevates enough to further damage the optic nerve, permanent visual loss might ensue, and can be documented in the visual field.

Pigment dispersion occurs in all cases and can be seen by particles in the anterior chamber immediately following the iridectomy. Within a few hours, the pigment precipitates into the inferior angle (Fig. 8-1). This has not been known to cause any long-term problem with pressure or outflow facility, except in the immediate postlaser period, and might contribute to the etiology of the transient rise in pressure that occurs within the first 24 hours in many patients.

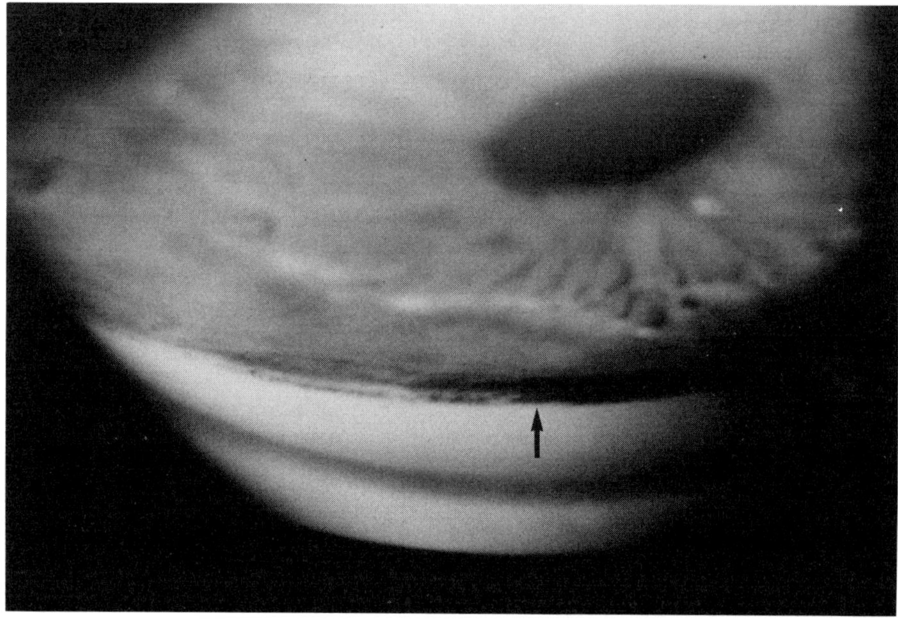

Figure 8-1. Marked trabecular pigmentation after laser iridectomy (arrow). This angle before treatment had little trabecular pigment. (Reprinted with permission from Schwartz L, Spaeth GL, Brown G. Laser Therapy of the Anterior Segment: A Practical Approach. Thorofare, N.J.: Slack, 1984.)

Pupil distortion rarely is seen with the Nd:YAG laser, but is noted in almost all argon laser iridectomies. It is caused by the shrinking effect of the heat on iris tissue pulling the pupil toward the site of treatment. It is transient and might even help to break an acute attack of pupil block glaucoma by allowing the aqueous to flow through the pupil before the iridectomy is completed.

Significant elevation of IOP greater than 10 mm Hg occurs in 20 to 30% of laser iridectomies within the first three hours for both argon and Nd:YAG. The reason for this is unclear, but might be because of the particulate matter released that clogs the trabecular meshwork or possibly because of inflammation in the trabecular meshwork caused by the shock wave of the laser bursts. If an individual already has a compromised optic nerve, even short but significant rises in pressure can further damage the nerve and lead to permanent visual loss. To dampen these potential rises in pressure, pretreating the patient with oral acetazolamide or oral or IV osmotic agents as well as giving pilocarpine 2% eye drops for several doses postlaser treatment has been shown to be beneficial. Recently, Robin and coworkers have shown that pretreatment with topical apraclonidine (Iopidine, Alcon) prevents this pressure rise. Pretreating the patient with prostaglandin inhibitors and/or steroid drops has not been helpful. Using steroid drops posttreatment might help however, because iritis can be a complication of the treatment. The steroid drops decrease the inflammatory cells and fibrin that can contribute to a decreased outflow facility. When performing an iridectomy on an eye greatly at risk, do not hesitate to hospitalize the patient, monitor the IOP frequently, and give intravenous mannitol as required, along with pilocarpine drops, timolol and carbonic anhydrase inhibitors.

Hemorrhage is a rare complication with argon laser iridectomy but has been seen in approximately 20 to 40% of Nd:YAG laser iridectomies. Most cases have just a small clot at the margin of the iridectomy but approximately 5% have a stream of blood (Fig. 8-2) and a few even have a layered hyphema. This bleeding usually stops within seconds, but a total hyphema has been reported. If hemorrhaging becomes significant, just pushing on the Abraham (or similar) lens increases the IOP and stops the flow of blood. If that does not stop the hemorrhage, coagulate the bleeding vessel by switching to free running Nd:YAG if it is available on your laser, or else switch the patient to an argon laser and coagulate the offending vessel. If an individual has a clotting disorder or cannot stop anticoagulant therapy for three days, an argon laser iridectomy is the treatment of choice. When hemorrhage does occur, the red cells in the anterior chamber might contribute to elevating the IOP. In almost every instance, the blood or hyphema is absorbed in 24 hours unless there has been significant filling of the anterior chamber.

Corneal endothelial burns occur if there is not enough space between the anterior surface of the iris and endothelial surface of the cornea (1 mm Nd:YAG; 0.5 mm for argon). These burns can occur with one burst of the YAG and often can occur with the argon when fired repeatedly and fast. If an endothelial burn occurs before the iridectomy is completed, it obscures the iris view and prevents further laser energy from getting to the iris. Thus a new spot on the iris will have to be chosen for treatment. These burns leave permanent scars, but do not lead to corneal decompensation.

Epithelial burns of the cornea usually are found when the cornea is still edematous or not crystal clear. In those instances, the cornea absorbs the laser energy as it passes through, and if enough heat is generated, will coagulate the corneal tissue (Fig. 8-3). These epithelial burns should be debrided and

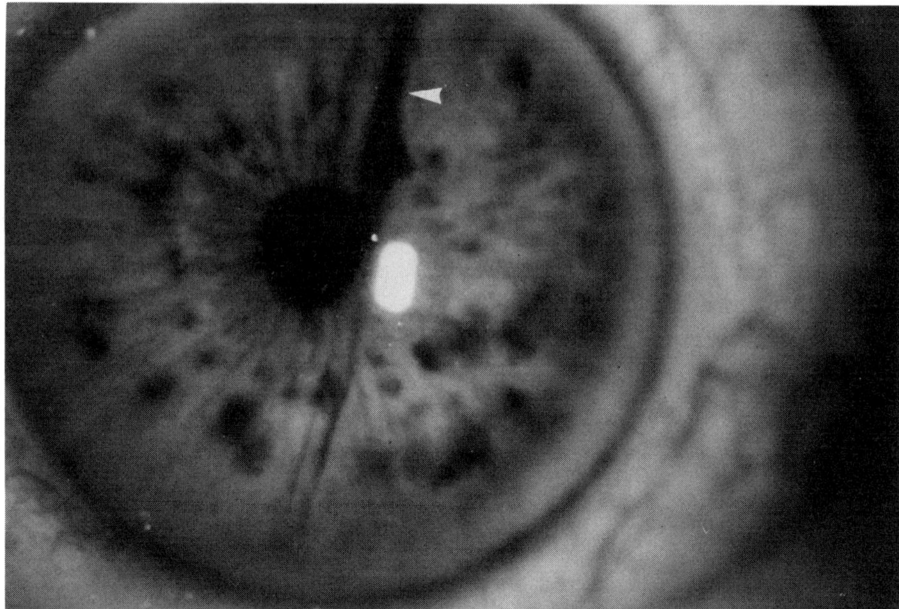

Figure 8-2. Blood streaming from YAG iridectomy (arrow).

treated as any corneal burn. When an epithelial burn develops, it obscures the iris and a new treatment site needs to be started. If corneal clouding is the cause, however, the treatment should be stopped until the cornea is cleared by lowering the IOP or decreasing the inflammation. Glycerin on the cornea might help, especially for YAG laser iridectomies, but often is not sufficient for the argon laser treatment.

Iritis itself is a contraindication to perform an argon laser iridectomy, although an iridectomy can be made with the Nd:YAG when iritis is present. However, the only YAG iridectomies that have closed were in patients with uveitis. Iritis is more likely to occur with argon laser iridectomy because heat is absorbed by and is more irritating to the iris. The diagnosis is made when flare and cells persist longer than 24 hours after the iridectomy. Pain, flush, and a miotic pupil become evident. Late sequella include posterior synechiae at the pupil or synechiae at the iridectomy. The further the iridectomy is in the periphery, the less likely synechiae will develop around the iridectomy site, because the lens is convex and falls away from the iris (Fig. 8-4). To prevent posterior synechiae, the pupil should be dilated and prednisolone acetate 1% given more frequently at the first signs of iritis.

Lenticular opacities are seen frequently after argon laser iridectomy (Fig. 8-5) but do not progress to a generalized cataract. They are seen as white spots on the surface of the lens. In time, new cortical fibers are laid down over these spots and they appear deeper in the lens cortex. They are formed by repeated firing of the laser to enlarge a small iridectomy when the iris is in contact with the lens capsule. This problem is less likely to occur if the iridectomy site is far in the periphery (Fig. 8-4) so that there is a space between lens and iris. With the Nd:YAG laser, so much energy is generated in the mechanical disruption

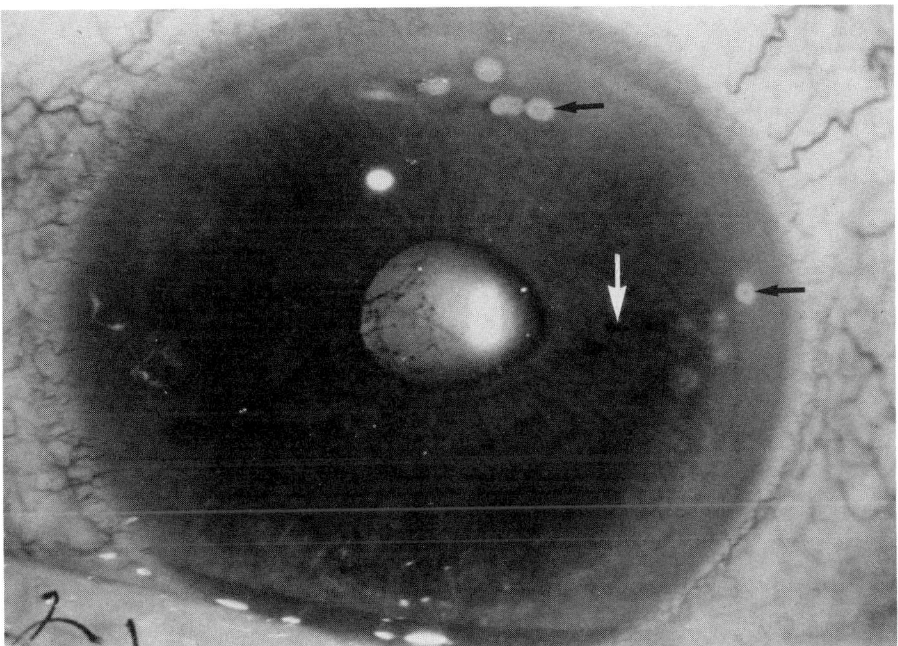

Figure 8-3. Complications of laser iridectomy: note pupil distortion toward laser site (white arrow), corneal burns (black arrow), and pigment dispersed on fibrin network. (Reprinted with permission from Schwartz L, Spaeth GL, Brown G. Laser Therapy of the Anterior Segment: A Practical Approach. Thorofare, N.J.: Slack, 1984.)

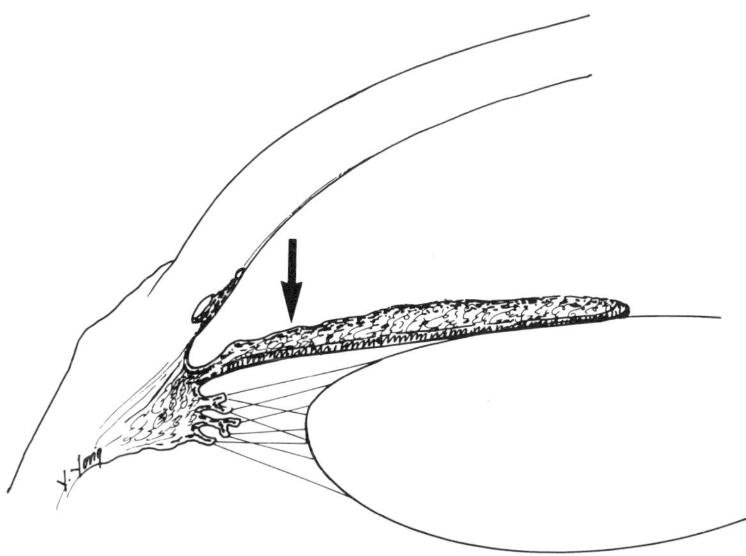

Figure 8-4. The laser should be aimed near the arrow to avoid the lens. (Reprinted with permission from Schwartz L, Spaeth GL, Brown G. Laser Therapy of the Anterior Segment: A Practical Approach. Thorofare, N.J.: Slack, 1984.)

of the iris, that the iridectomy only should be made in the far periphery. Experiments with rabbits have illustrated that if enough energy is utilized by the Nd:YAG to perform an iridectomy where the iris is in contact with the lens capsule, the anterior capsule can be torn and a synechia develop between the less and iris (Fig. 8-6). In rabbits, a generalized cataract never developed, however, even though the anterior capsule was disrupted.

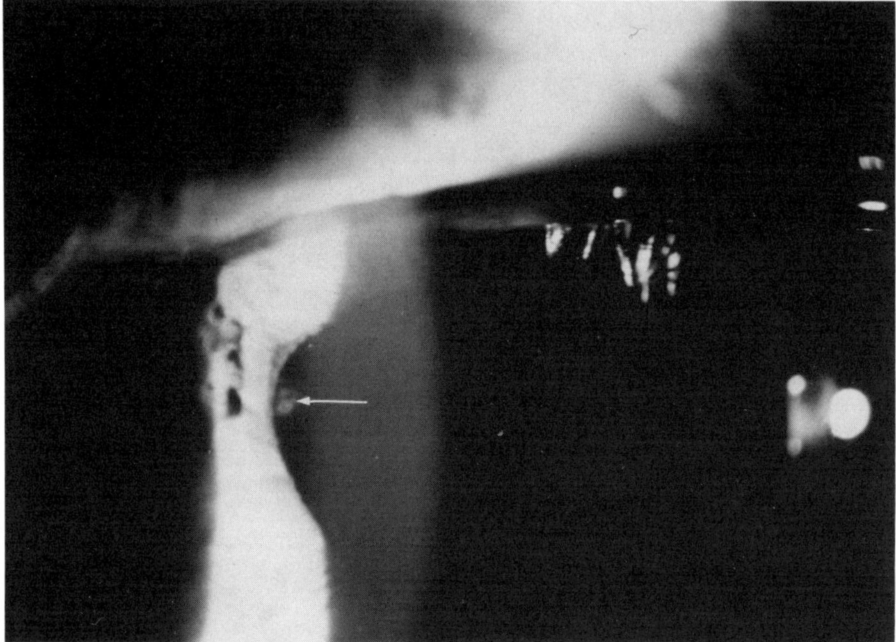

Figure 8-5. Lens opacity after argon laser iridectomy (arrow) with pupil dilated. (Reprinted with permission from Schwartz L, Spaeth GL, Brown G. Laser Therapy of the Anterior Segment: A Practical Approach. Thorofare, N.J.: Slack, 1984.)

Once an iridectomy is made, approximately 20% of the argon iridectomies will fill in with pigment and close. This is more likely to occur in light colored irides. They are easily reopened, but it is necessary to watch for this complication, as an angle closure attack can occur if the iridectomy closes. The only Nd:YAG iridectomies that have closed once a good opening is made in the iris have been in cases of uveitis or neovascular glaucoma.

Retinal burns (Fig. 8-7) have been seen after argon laser iridectomy. This problem has not been seen with the Nd:YAG. To avoid a macular burn, aim the laser toward the periphery and preferably in the superior nasal quadrant of the iris. If a retinal burn is made in the peripheral retina, no clinically significant symptoms have become apparent. One case of macular burn has been reported and obviously the visual outcome was poor.

Monocular diplopia can be significant if a large iridectomy is made below the level of the upper eyelid. To avoid this complaint, keep the iridectomy underneath the upper eyelid.

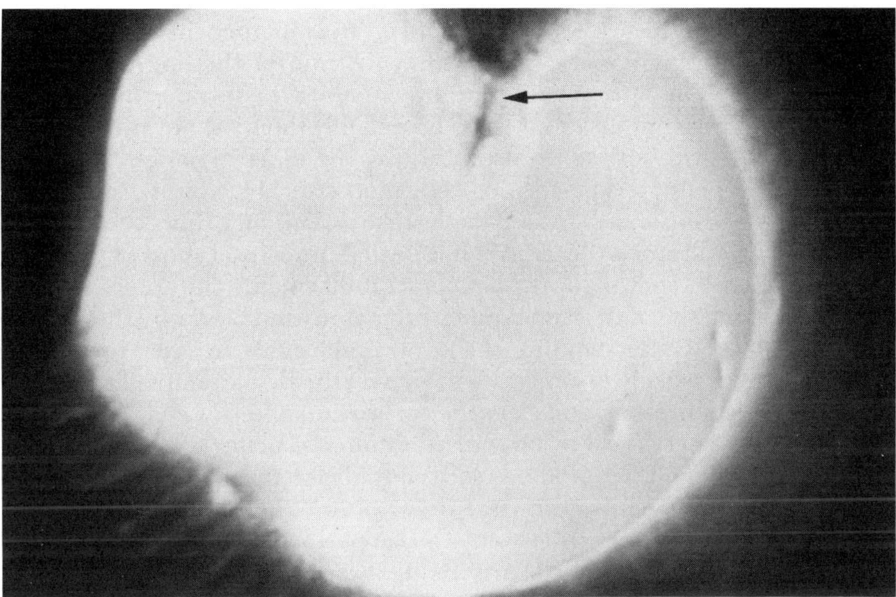

Figure 8-6. Iris synechia to ruptured lens in a rabbit after experimental high energy Nd: YAG iridectomy.

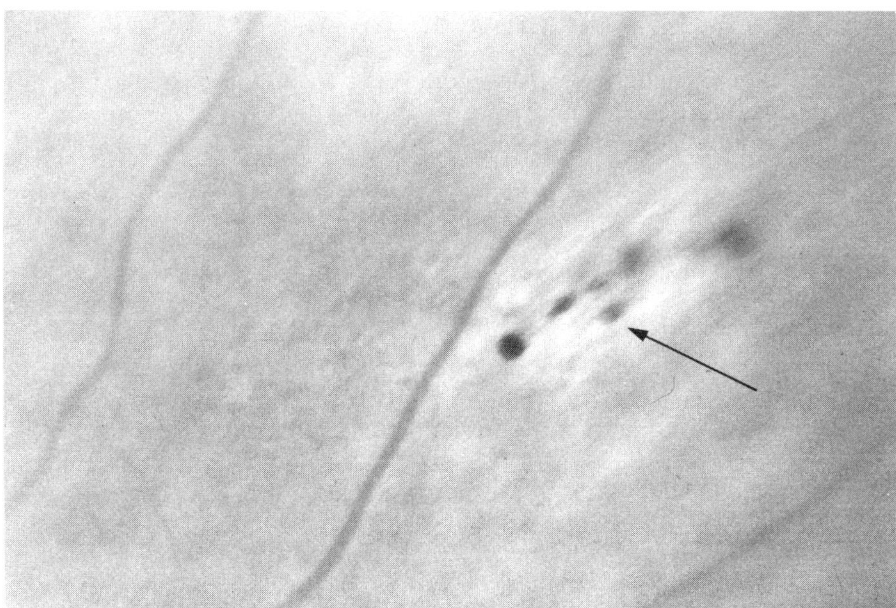

Figure 8-7. Peripheral retinal burn (arrow) after argon laser iridectomy.

One case of lens dislocation has been reported after Nd:YAG laser iridectomy. However, this was in an eye with previous trauma and one which had more than the usual number of shots to open an iridectomy.

Trabecular meshwork damage has been documented in owl monkeys when an iridectomy is performed within 0.8 mm of the limbus with the Nd:YAG laser. This appears to be localized to the area of iridectomy.

The last of the complications listed is probably the most obvious—failure of patency. As with any surgical procedure, the more experience one has the easier and better it is performed. The most critical factor in using a laser successfully is being able to focus it on the tissue. Without proper focus, insufficient energy will reach the iris. With repeated unfocused shots of the laser, the iris is irritated spewing forth pigment and fibrin into the anterior chamber. The treated site of the iris becomes edematous and blocks further efforts to penetrate it. Understanding the contraindications to laser iridectomy also make it more likely to penetrate the iris on the first attempt. Thus, quiet the eye if iritis is present, and clear the cornea and anterior chamber so that all of the laser energy will reach the iris. Often it is better to break an acute attack medically and treat the eye with steroids for three days until the eye is quiet and then perform the laser iridectomy. While waiting for the eye to quiet, however, a laser iridectomy can be performed on the fellow eye if the angle is felt capable of closure. Being aware of the complications and contraindications make penetration of the iris more likely. However, the most important thing to remember when performing a laser iridectomy is proper focus!

Acknowledgment

Much of this material is based on Chapter 3: Laser Iridectomy. In Schwartz, L.W., Spaeth, G.L., Brown, G. Laser Therapy of the Anterior Segment. Thorofare, N.J.: Slack, 1984.

Bibliography

Aron-Rosa D: Pulsed YAG Laser Surgery. Thorofare, N.J: Slack, 1983.

Berger BB: Foveal photocoagulation from laser iridotomy. Ophthalmol 91:1029-1033, 1984.

Fankhauser F, Lortscher H, Van der Zyper E: Clinical studies on high and low power laser radiation upon some structures of the anterior and posterior segments of the eye. Int Ophthalmol 5:15-32, 1982

Gaasterland DE, Rodrigues MM, Thomas G: Threshold for lens damage during Q-switched Nd:YAG laser iridectomy. A study of rhesus monkey eyes. Ophthalmol 92:1616-1623, 1985.

Gailitis R, Peyman GA, Pulido J, Mitchell MD, Weinreb RM: Prostaglandin release following Nd:YAG iridotomy in rabbits. Ophthalmic Surg 17:467-469, 1986.

Gieser DK, Wilensky JT: Laser iridectomy in the management of chronic angle closure glaucoma. Am J Ophthalmol 98:446-450, 1984.

Hirst LW, Robin AL, Sherman S, Green WR, D'Anna S, Dunkelberger G: Corneal endothelial changes after argon laser iridotomy and panretinal photocoagulation. Ann Ophthalmol 93:473-481, 1982.

Hodes BL, Bentivegna JF, Weyer NJ: Hyphema complicating laser iridotomy. Arch Ophthalmol 100:924-925, 1982.

Karmon G, Savin H: Retinal damage after Argon laser iridotomy. Am J Ophthalmol 101:554-560, 1986.

Klapper RM: Q-switched Neodymium: YAG laser iridotomy. Ophthalmology 91:1017-1021, 1984.

Krupin T, Stone RA, Cohen BH, Volker AE, Kass MA: Acute intraocular pressure response to argon laser iridotomy. Ophthalmology 92:922-926, 1985.

Martin NF, Gaasterland DE, Rodrigues MM, Thomas G, Cumming CE: Endothelial damage from retrocorneal modelocked Neodymium:YAG laser pulses in monkeys. Ophthalmol 92:1376-1381, 1985.

Martin NF, Gaasterland DE, Rodrigues MM, Thomas G, Cumming CE: Endothelial damage thresholds for retrocorneal Q-switched Neodymium:YAG laser pulses in monkeys. Ophthalmol 92:1382-1386, 1985.

McCallister JA, Schwartz LW, Moster M, Spaeth GL: Laser peripheral iridectomy comparing Q-switched Neodymium:YAG with argon. Trans Ophthalmol Soc UK 104:67-69, 1984.

Melamed S, Burraquer E, Epstein DL: Neodymium:YAG laser iridotomy as a possible contribution to lens dislocation. Ann Ophthalmol 18:281-282, 1986.

Moster MR, Schwartz LW, Salz A, Caprioli J, Spaeth GL: The effect of Nd:YAG laser iridectomy on the rabbit lens. ARVO Abstracts Supplement to Invest Ophthalmol Vis Sci. Philadelphia: J.B. Lippincott, 1984, p. 95.

Moster MR, Schwartz LW, Wilson RP, Spaeth GL, McCallister JA, Poryzees EM: Laser iridectomy. A controlled study comparing argon and neodymium:YAG. Ophthalmology 93:20-24, 1986.

Moyer KT, Pettit TH, Straatsma BR: Corneal endothelial damage with Neodymium:YAG laser. Ophthalmol 91:1022-1028, 1984.

Richardson TM, Brown SV, Thomas JV, Simmons RJ: Shock-wave effect on anterior segment structures following experimental neodymium:YAG laser iridectomy. Ophthalmol 92:1387-1395, 1985.

Rivera AH, Brown RH, Anderson DR: Laser iridotomy vs. surgical iridectomy. Have the indications changed? Arch Ophthalmol 103:1350-1354, 1985.

Robin AL: Intraocular pressure elevation following anterior segment laser surgery. Ophthalmic Laser Therapy 1:101-106, 1986.

Robin AL, Arbell S, Gilbert SM, Goosseus AA, Werner RP, Korshin, OM: Q-switched Neodymium:YAG laser iridotomy. A field trial with a portable laser system. Arch Ophthalmol 104:526-530, 1986.

Robin, AL, Pollack, IP: A comparison of argon and neodymium:YAG laser iridotomies. Ophthalmology 91:1011-1016, 1984.

Robin AL, Pollack IP: Q-switched Neodymium: YAG laser iridotomy in patients in whom the Argon laser fails. Arch Ophthalmol 104:531-535, 1986.

Robin AL, Pollack IP, de Fallen JM: Effects of Topical ALO 2145 (p-Aminoclonidine Hydrochloride) on the Acute Intraocular Pressure Rise After Argon Laser Iridotomy. Arch Ophthalmol 105:1208-1211, 1987.

Rodrigues MM, Spaeth GL, Moster M, Thomas G, Hackett J: Histopathology of Neodymium:YAG laser iridectomy in humans. Ophthalmology 92:1696-1700, 1985.

Rostron CK: Acute angle-closure glaucoma: Surgery or laser? Glaucoma 7:268-274, 1985.

Schwartz LW: Laser iridectomy. In Schwartz L, Spaeth G, Brown G: Laser Therapy of the Anterior Segment. A Practical Approach. Thorofare, N.J.: Slack, pp 46-57, 1984.

Schwartz LW, Moster MR, Spaeth GL, Wilson RP, Poryzees E: Neodymium:YAG laser iridectomies in glaucoma associated with closed or occludable angles. Am J Ophthalmol 102:41-44, 1986.

Schwartz LW, Rodrigues MM, Spaeth GL, Streeter B, Douglas C: Argon laser iridectomy in the treatment of patients with primary angle closure or pupillary block glaucoma: a clinicopathologic study. Ophthalmology 85:294-309, 1978.

Schwartz LW, Spaeth GL: Argon laser iridotomy in primary angle closure or pupillary block glaucoma. Trans Ophthalmol Soc UK 99:257-263, 1979.

Seedor JA, Greenidge RC, Dunn MW: Neodymium: YAG laser iridectomy and acute cataract formation in the rabbit. Ophthalmic Surg 17:478-482, 1986.

Smith J, Whilted P: Corneal endothelial changes after argon laser iridotomy. Am J Ophthalmol 98:153-156, 1984.

Spaeth G: Use of the YAG laser in performing peripheral iridectomies. In March WF (ed.): Ophthalmic Lasers. Current Clinical Uses. Thorofare, N.J.: Slack, pp 57-59, 1984.

Trokel SL: YAG Laser Ophthalmic Microsurgery. Norwalk: Appleton-Century-Crofts, 1983.

Welch DB, Apple DJ, Mendelsohn AD, et al: Lens injury following iridotomy with Q-switched neodymium:YAG laser. Arch Ophthalmol 104:123-125, 1986.

Wise J, Munnerlyn CR, Erickson PJ: A high efficiency laser iridotomy—sphincterotomy lens. Am J Ophthalmol. 101:546-553, 1986.

CHAPTER 9

Complications of Argon Laser Iridoplasty and Coreoplasty

Louis W. Schwartz, MD

Complications of Argon Laser Iridoplasty and Coreoplasty

Argon Laser Iridoplasty

Indications

Argon laser iridoplasty (laser iris retraction, laser gonioplasty) is a treatment of the peripheral iris that alters its configuration so that the iris retracts, widening the approach to the angle (Figs. 9-1 and 9-2). It can prevent acute angle closure or intermittent angle closure attacks as well as treat subacute or chronic angle closure (Table 9-1). When there is an acute attack of angle closure and the central cornea is bedewed, this technique can be utilized on the peripheral iris, even with some corneal edema present, to break the acute attack.

The technique is useful in plateau iris syndrome where there is an anterior iris insertion and the iris folds up in the chamber angle blocking the trabecular meshwork at the time of pupil dilatation. The iris appears flat centrally rather than bowed forward. An iridectomy is of no value with this syndrome, but flattening the peripheral iris will allow pupil dilatation without angle closure. In addition, when one needs to perform argon laser trabeculoplasty in an individual with open angle glaucoma, but narrow angles, in many instances adequate treatment of the angle structures is impossible because of the peripheral iris. Under these conditions, iridoplasty can flatten the peripheral iris and allow treatment of the trabecular meshwork. This technique can also be combined with local pupilomydriasis in one segment to break an acute pupillary block angle closure attack.

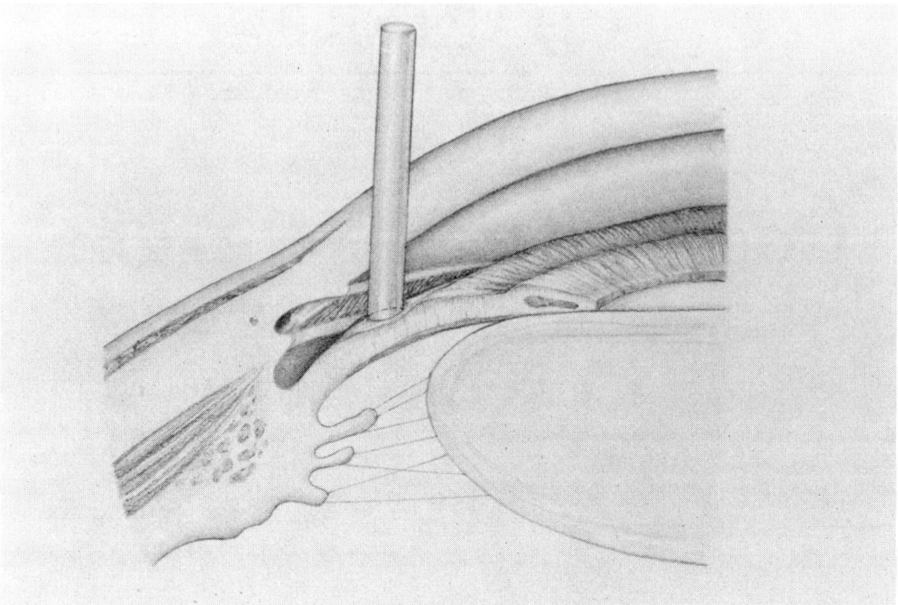

Figure 9-1. Argon laser iridoplasty. Diagram of closed angle with proper position of laser beam. (Reprinted with permission from Schwartz L, Spaeth GL, Brown G. Laser Therapy of the Anterior Segment: A Practical Approach. Thorofare, N.J.: Slack, 1984.)

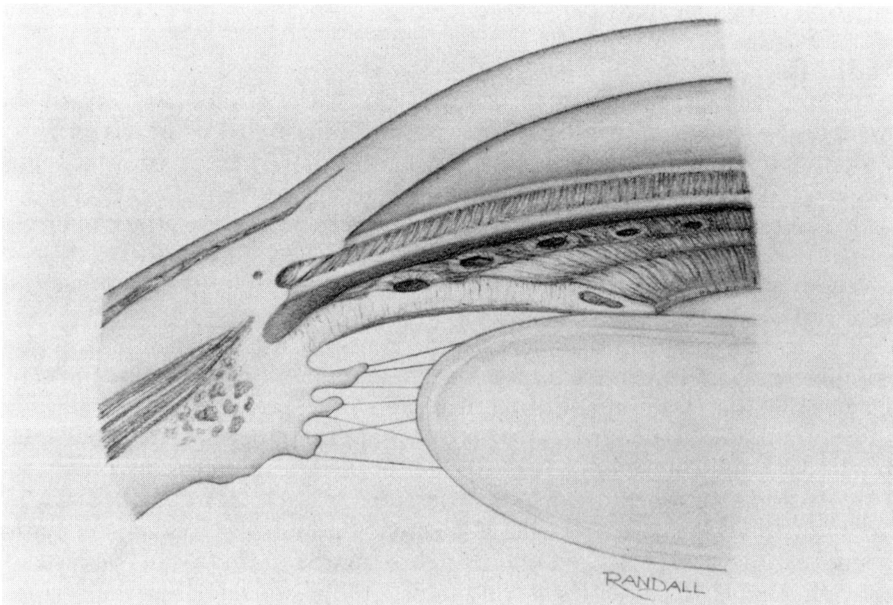

Figure 9-2. Argon laser iridoplasty. Angle open and scars on iris after argon laser iridoplasty. (Reprinted with permission from Schwartz L, Spaeth GL, Brown G. Laser Therapy of the Anterior Segment: A Practical Approach. Thorofare, N.J.: Slack, 1984.)

Table 9-1. Indications for Argon Laser Iridoplasty
Acute angle closure glaucoma
Intermittent angle closure glaucoma
Subacute or chronic angle closure glaucoma
Plateau iris syndrome
Open angle glaucoma with narrow angles before ALT to visualize the angle

Technique

The technique for argon laser iridoplasty is listed in Table 9-2. The laser can be aimed through the center lens alone at the peripheral iris just inside the arcus, or it may be directed through the angle mirror. The initial laser settings are 500 μm spot size, 0.2 seconds, and 150 to 400 mW power. The cornea may be cleared with glycerine if necessary. A test burn should be applied at the most peripheral part of the iris as possible. A sustained contraction of the iris stroma should be noted. If a dense burn with pigment liberation is seen, decrease the power or duration. If the iris reaction is inadequate, increase the power or duration. The power needed varies with the amount of corneal and anterior chamber clarity as well as iris pigmentation. When an adequate burn is made, the iris will stay in the desired position and on gonioscopy the angle will appear more open. About 10 burns per quadrant should be adequate (Figs. 9-1 and 9-2).

Table 9-2. Technique for Argon Laser Iridoplasty
Topical anesthetic
Anti reflective Goldmann 3-mirror lens
Spot size—200-500 μm
Duration—0.2-0.5 sec
Power—150-400 mW
Check angle to see that open
10 burns per quadrant

Argon Laser Coreoplasty

Indications

Argon laser coreoplasty (photomydriasis or pupilomydriasis) might be useful in several conditions (Table 9-3). We have all had patients who complain bitterly of decreased vision because of miotic therapy. "Everything looks darker," night driving is a problem, or the vision becomes blurred because cataracts are present and the constricted pupil will not allow vision around a central opacity. If visual fields are abnormal, a miotic pupil can make them seem worse.

Doubling the diameter of the pupil will allow four times the amount of light to enter the eye. Thus, being able to keep the pupil relatively dilated, in spite of miotic therapy, might be beneficial to the patient (Figs. 9-3 and 9-4).

Table 9-3. Indications for Argon Laser Coreoplasty

Miotic pupil
Updrawn pupil
Pupil block: (a) Aphakic with vitreous
(b) Aphakic with IOL
(c) Alone

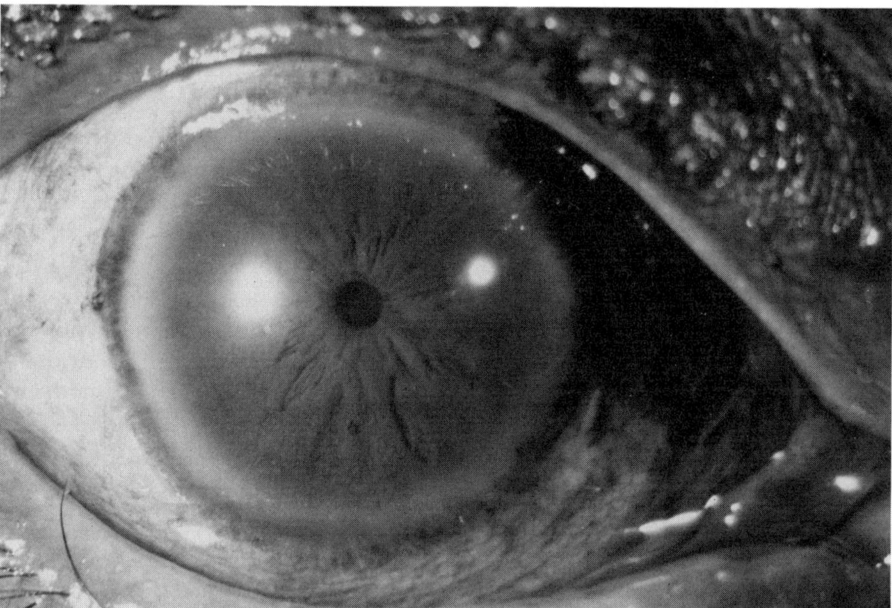

Figure 9-3. One millimeter pupil secondary to strong miotic eyedrops. (Reprinted with permission from Schwartz L, Spaeth GL, Brown G. Laser Therapy of the Anterior Segment: A Practical Approach. Thorofare, N.J.: Slack, 1984.)

The vision might be greatly compromised in an individual having an updrawn pupil with or without miotics. If the iris opening is not in the visual axis or if some opacities in the lens or vitreous face preclude good vision, it might be possible to improve the sight by retracting, dilating, or pulling the updrawn iris into the visual axis (Figs. 9-5 and 9-6). Before the laser is utilized to permanently dilate an updrawn or miotic pupil, it is important to verify that the procedure will help the individual by first dilating the pupil with mydriatics. Once the patient states "I can see better now" after mydriasis, then one can feel confident the procedure will be beneficial.

In some instances of pupil block, when a laser iridectomy might be impossible because of corneal edema or iritis, the block might be broken by just dilating the pupil with the laser. Once the inflammation and cornea have cleared, the definitive treatment of iridectomy can be performed. The laser has been utilized successfully for this purpose in pupillary block glaucoma alone, aphakic pupillary block secondary to vitreous occluding the pupil, and in pseudophakic pupil block where the intraocular lens is blocking the pupil.

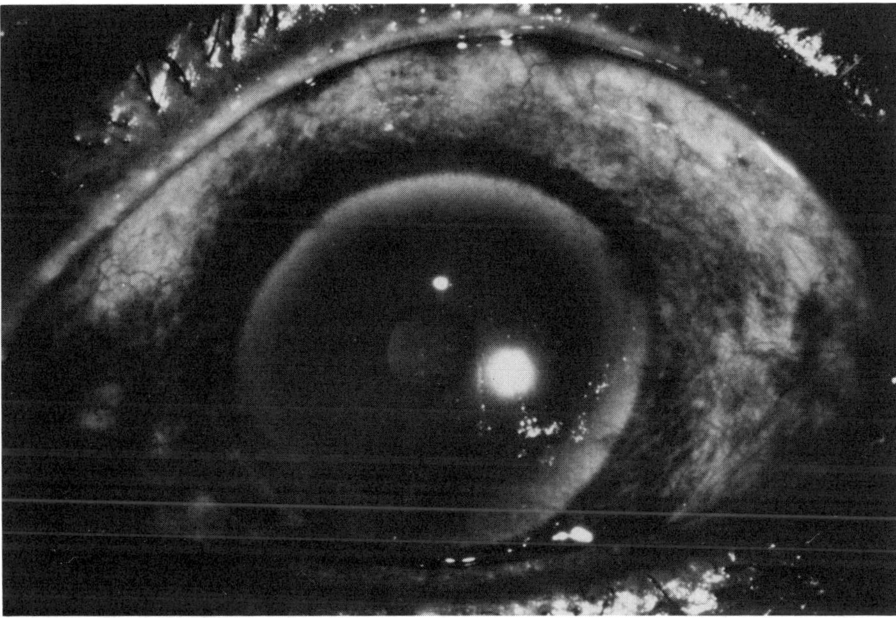

Figure 9-4. Same patient as Figure 9-3 after argon laser coreoplasty. The pupil is now two millimeters. (Reprinted with permission from Schwartz L, Spaeth GL, Brown G. Laser Therapy of the Anterior Segment: A Practical Approach. Thorofare, N.J.: Slack, 1984.)

Technique

Several drops of a local anesthetic are instilled. No retrobulbar anesthesia is required unless the patient is extremely uncooperative or has nystagmus. When dilating a miotic pupil, two rows of laser burns are made at the pupil margin (Fig. 9-7). The first row is made approximately 1 mm from the pupil margin. Each burn is made with a 200 μm diameter spot, at 0.5 W for 0.2 second. These burns are contiguous and made for 360°. As each burn is made, the iris shrinks away from the pupil margin toward the limbus, therefore, it is important to be far enough from the pupil margin so that no laser light enters the pupil. Each iris reacts differently so test burns should be made even further from the pupil margin to see how much the iris shrinks and judge the position of the first row accordingly so that the pupil will not shrink under the burn and thus allow the laser light to pass through the pupil. After the first row is complete, a second row concentric but peripheral to the first row is made using settings of 500 μm spot, 0.2 second, at 0.5 W. Further stretching of the iris peripherally should take place with each burn. Because each iris responds differently, the power may be increased in either row if necessary to get the desired stretching effect. The object of the treatment is to destroy the sphincter muscle, but leave the dilator muscle fibers intact. If this is accomplished, the pupil will stay dilated in spite of miotic therapy.

The technique for dilating an updrawn pupil is similar (Fig. 9-7). However, it is often more difficult to accomplish and thus a larger spot size is required for the first row. Settings for both rows are 500 μm spot, 0.2 second,

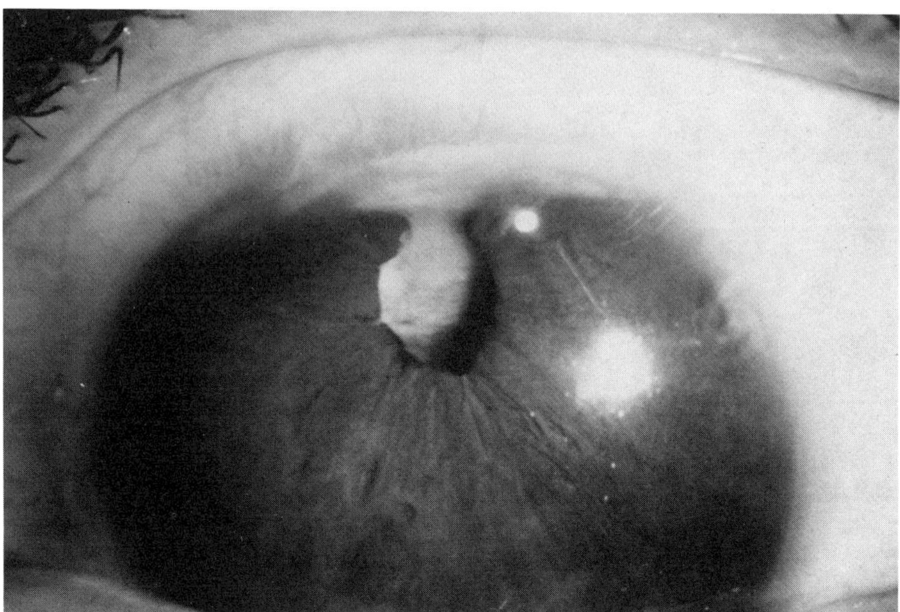

Figure 9-5. Updrawn pupil in a patient requiring strong miotics for IOP control. A secondary membrane is present. Vision on miotics was 20/400. (Reprinted with permission from Schwartz L, Spaeth GL, Brown G. Laser Therapy of the Anterior Segment: A Practical Approach. Thorofare, N.J.: Slack, 1984.)

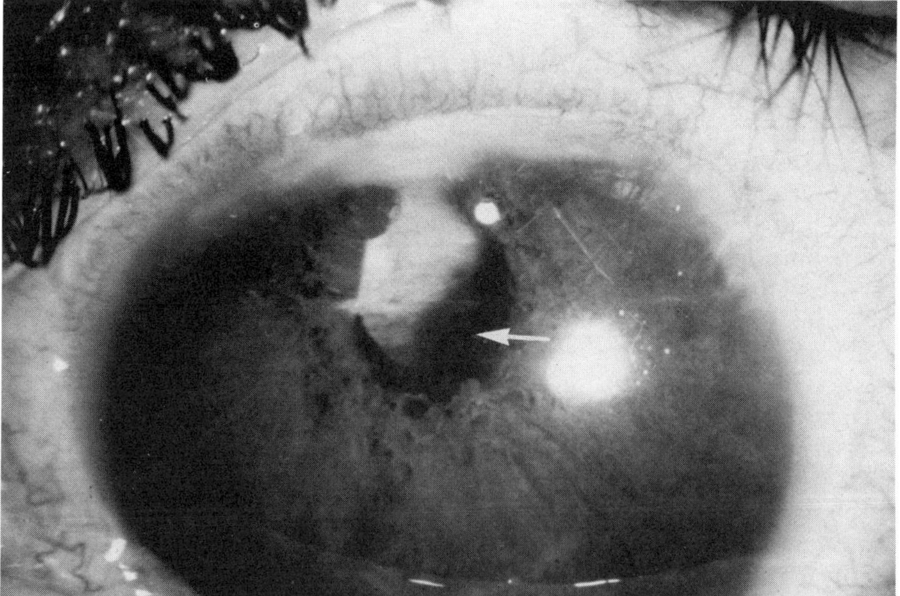

Figure 9-6. Same patient as Figure 9-5 after argon laser coreoplasty, still on the same miotic therapy. Notice iris pulled down enough so patient can see through break in secondary membrane (arrow). Vision now 20/40. (Reprinted with permission from Schwartz L, Spaeth GL, Brown G. Laser Therapy of the Anterior Segment: A Practical Approach. Thorofare, N.J.: Slack, 1984.)

and 0.5 W. The power might need to be increased up to 0.7 watt. With experience, the settings are varied according to the response of the iris. To get the updrawn pupil into the visual axis, it might be necessary to apply a few extra rows of burns at the apex while doing fewer burns to either side. After the procedure is completed the patient continues on his prior therapy, but a steroid eye drop is given four times a day for one week.

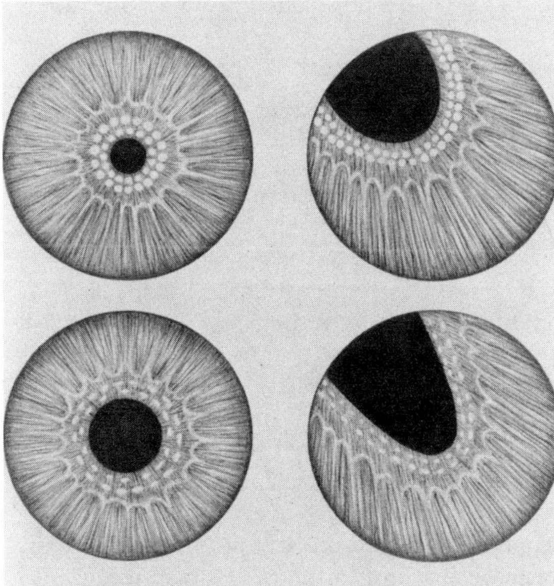

Figure 9-7. Technique of argon laser coreoplasty. Upper left: Miotic pupil. White spots indicate area of laser burns. Lower left: Pupil larger after treatment. Faded white spots indicate scarring of iris. Upper right: Updrawn pupil. White spots indicate area of laser burns. Lower right: Pupil pulled more into visual axis after treatment. Faded white spots scarring of iris. (Reprinted with permission from Schwartz L, Spaeth GL, Brown G. Laser Therapy of the Anterior Segment: A Practical Approach. Thorofare, N.J.: Slack, 1984.)

Complications of iridoplasty and coreoplasty

The major complications of argon laser iridoplasty and coreoplasty are similar and are listed in Table 9-4. As in any technique, the surgeon should be aware of the dangers and be careful to minimize the potential for ocular damage.

Table 9-4. Complications of Argon Laser Iridoplasty and Coreoplasty
Irritation (pain)
Blurred vision
Pigment dispersion
Elevation of IOP
Corneal epithelial burns
Corneal endothelial burns
Iritis
Recurrence of iris to natural position
Macular burn

Irritation or pain can occur as the iris is stretched by the burn. If iritis develops, a longer lasting pain might develop but the etiology is obvious.

Frequently, superficial punctate keratitis develops from the Goldmann contact lens and causes a foreign body sensation although a corneal abrasion could cause a more pronounced pain as could a significant rise in IOP.

All patients have markedly blurred vision for the first 10 minutes due to the goniosol and dazzling effect of the bright light. By the next day, however, the vision returns to prelaser levels unless iritis occurs or corneal edema develops from high IOP or a corneal abrasion. If the IOP rises enough to damage the optic nerve, permanent visual loss might ensue, and can be documented in the visual field.

Pigment dispersion is noted in all cases and can be seen by particles in the anterior chamber immediately following the laser treatment. Within a few hours the pigment precipitates into the inferior angle. This has not been known to cause any long-term problem with pressure or outflow facility, except in the immediate postlaser period, and may contribute to the etiology of the transient rise in pressure that occurs within the first 24 hours in many patients.

Significant elevation of the IOP occurs frequently after iridoplasty or coreoplasty and should be watched for carefully if the optic nerve is at risk from prolonged increase in the IOP. The reason for the increased IOP is unclear, but as in laser iridectomies might be related to particulate matter released from the iris surface, clogging the trabecular meshwork or possibly inflammation in the trabecular meshwork caused by the shock wave of the laser bursts. Pretreating the patient with oral acetazolamide or oral or IV osmotic agents, as well as giving pilocarpine 2% eye drops for several doses postlaser treatment might be beneficial. In addition, steroid drops posttreatment might help because iritis can be a complication of the treatment, and this might decrease the inflammatory cells and fibrin that can contribute to a decreased outflow facility.

Corneal endothelial burns occur if the iris is too close to the corneal endothelium in laser iridoplasty. Consequently, the laser burns should be placed so that at least 0.5 mm of aqueous is between the two surfaces. Corneal epithelial burns are found if the cornea is edematous or not crystal clear. In those instances, the corneal epithelium absorbs the laser energy as it passes through, and if enough heat is generated, will coagulate the epithelial tissue. Glycerine on the cornea might help, but if the IOP is too high it might have to be lowered medically to clear the cornea before laser treatment.

Iritis can occur because of the irritating effect of heat absorption by the iris. The diagnosis is made when flare and cells persist longer than 24 hours after treatment. Pain and flush become evident. Late sequella include posterior synechiae at the pupil or peripheral anterior synechiae. Since iritis is a common occurrence, prednisolone acetate 1% should be given frequently posttreatment to prevent it. At the first sign of iritis, the pupil should be dilated and a cycloplegic given if the angle on gonioscopy is adequately open and not capable of closure.

The major problem in both iridoplasty and coreoplasty seems to be the return of the iris to its original configuration. If this occurs in a case of intermittent angle closure or chronic angle closure glaucoma, the patient might be at great risk. For this reason, if at all possible, a laser iridectomy should be performed in these cases at a later date. In plateau iris syndrome, because laser iridoplasty is the treatment of choice, it might be necessary to repeat the procedure if the iris returns to its plateau configuration. In coreoplasty, if the iris returns to its original position the procedure can be repeated or else a laser or surgical sphincterotomy might be performed.

Macular burns can occur if the laser energy is focused through the pupil. This is more likely with the coreoplasty—and as mentioned previously—great care must be taken to aim the laser at least 1 mm from the pupil margin at the initial burn, because the iris will shrink toward the periphery under the burns. If the focus is too close to the pupil margin, the laser beam will enter the pupil and could be focused by the patient's own lens on the macula.

Acknowledgment

Much of this material is based on Chapter 5: Other Uses of Argon Laser in the Anterior Segment. In Schwartz L.W., Spaeth, G.L., Brown, G.: Laser Therapy of the Anterior Segment. Thorofare, N.J.: Slack, 1984.

Bibliography

Blumenthal A, Floman N, Treister G. Laser iris retraction for narrow-angle glaucoma. Glaucoma 4:47-49, 1982.

L'Esperance FA, James WA. Argon Laser photocoagulation of iris abnormalities. Trans Am Acad Ophthalmol Otolaryngol 79:321-339, 1975.

Obstbaum SA, Barasch KR, Galin MA, Baras I. Laser photomydriasis in pseudophakic pupillary block. J Am Intraocular Soc 7:28-30, 1981.

Ritch R. Argon laser treatment for medically unresponsive attacks of angle closure glaucoma. Am Ophthalmol 94:197-204, 1982.

Robin AL. Intraocular pressure elevation following anterior segment laser surgery. Ophthalmic Laser Ther 1:101-106, 1986.

Schwartz LW, Spaeth GL. Laser treatment of the anterior segment. Trans PA Acad Ophthalmol Otolaryngol 33:33-39, 1980.

Shin D: Argon laser iris photocoagulation to relieve acute angle-closure glaucoma. Am Ophthalmol 93:348-350, 1982.

Sobel LI, Ritch R, Prince A. Argon laser sphincterotomy. Ophthalmic Laser Ther 1:87-92, 1986.

Thomas JV. Pupilloplasty and photomydriasis, in *Photocoagulation in Glaucoma and Anterior Segment Disease.* C.D. Belcher III, J.V. Thomas, R.V. Simmons (eds). Baltimore: Williams & Wilkins, 1984, Chapter 11.

Wise JB. Iris sphincterotomy, iridotomy, and synechiotomy by linear incision with the argon laser. Ophthalmol 92:641-645, 1985.

CHAPTER 10

Nd:YAG Laser Transscleral Cyclophotocoagulation

Marlene R. Moster, MD

Introduction

Nd:YAG transscleral cyclophotocoagulation (CPC) has proved to be an effective method of lowering IOP in advanced glaucomatous eyes. The purpose of this procedure is to discreetly destroy areas of the ciliary body (Fig. 10-1), thereby decreasing aqueous production and lowering IOP. The ciliary body destruction might be related to alteration in blood supply as well as direct destruction of non-pigmented epithelial cells.

History

The concept of lowering IOP by destroying isolated areas of ciliary body was introduced by Vogt in 1936 with the electrodiathermy procedure.[1] This was associated with a high percentage of failures and a 7% incidence of atrophy or phthisis. In 1950, Bietti[2] introduced cyclocryotherapy as a means of lowering IOP in advanced glaucomatous eyes. Success was variable, however, because of inconsistent freezing techniques and the complication rate was high. With the advent of the xenon arc, transscleral photocoagulation became possible, but lesions that lowered IOP were associated with severe complications, such as phthisis and hemorrhage.[3] As an alternative to the xenon arc, the ruby laser was successful in lowering intraocular pressure with fewer complications.[4,5] Because of the lack of suitable ruby lasers, however, ophthalmologists did not widely adopt this technique. The commercial availability of Nd:YAG laser, combined with the properties needed to deliver energy transsclerally, made the neodymium energy suitable for cyclocoagulation in advanced glaucomatous eyes.[6,7]

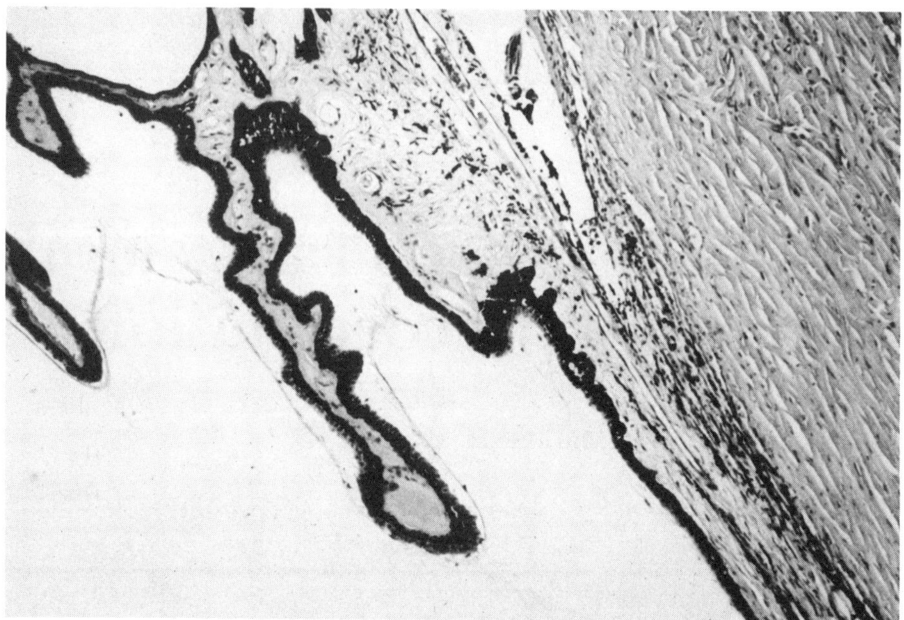

Figure 10-1. A. Normal ciliary body of pigmented (Dutch-belted) rabbit.

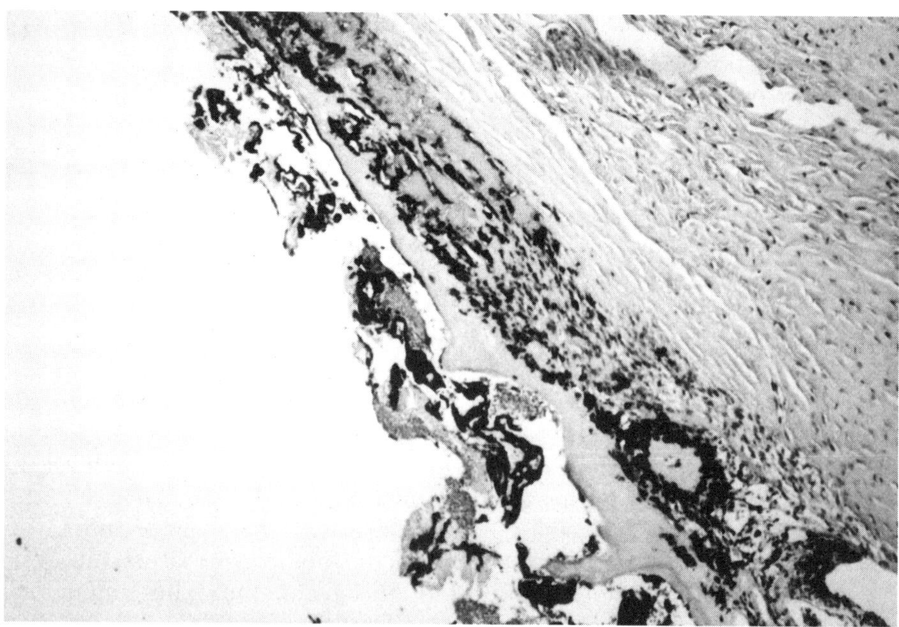

Figure 10-1. B. One week status post-Nd:YAG CPC in pigmented rabbit eye. Hemorrhagic necrosis evident with marked pigment disruption.

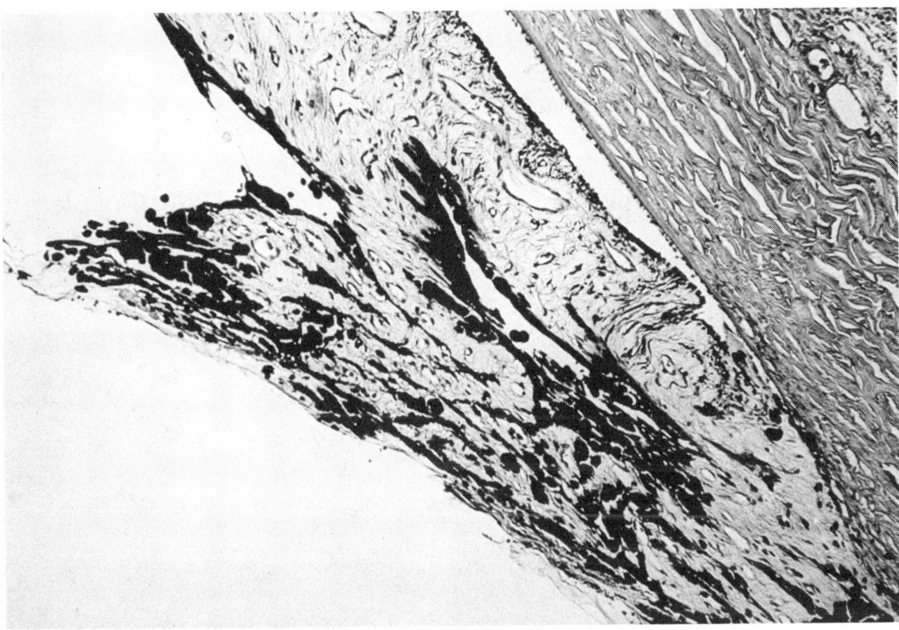

Figure 10-1. C. One month status post-Nd:YAG CPC in pigmented rabbit eye. Necrosed fibrotic ciliary body region with pigment hyperplasia and minimal residual inflammation. (Courtesy of Louis Cantor, M.D.)

Technique

A Nd:YAG laser with a thermal mode capability is required to perform Nd:YAG cyclophotocoagulation. The procedure is performed in an outpatient setting and requires a retrobulbar anesthetic block of bupivacaine or Carbocaine with hyaluronidase. No facial block is necessary. Topical anesthetics alone are not recommended because of unacceptable discomfort to the patient. The Lasag Microruptor II Nd:YAG laser is pulsed (20 milliseconds) in the thermal free running mode. The thermal mode emits infrared light that allows better absorption and penetration into tissues. Although the helium-neon beam is focused on the conjunctiva, the energy is delivered more deeply into the bulk of the ciliary body by retrofocusing the Nd:YAG beam by 3.6 mm. This amount of defocusing is necessary to compensate for the tangential rather than perpendicular angle of the beam to the sclera. Unlike argon laser photocoagulation, the energy level is chosen beforehand and not titrated to a tissue response. The optimal energy setting for the best results with fewest complications is still under investigation. Energy settings in the range of 1.2 to 8.0 joules have been associated with pressure lowering effects, but we now recommend using between 4.0 and 6.5 joules. Higher power settings tend to be associated with increased inflammation and postoperative pain.

Thirty-two to 40 discreet lesions are placed transsclerally 2 to 3 mm from the limbus for 360° over the pars plicata. The globe is transilluminated to delineate the pars plicata and the helium-neon beam is focused directly over it. Transillumination allows for exact placement of the beam over the pars plicata, compensating for the difference between large myopic eyes and smaller hyperopic eyes where the pars plicata might be closer to the limbus. The major vessels at the 3 o'clock and 9 o'clock positions are avoided in order to decrease the possibility of anterior ischemia. A contact lens is not necessary for the CPC, but a lid speculum might facilitate the procedure. If the cornea dries during the CPC, a wetting solution of balanced salt can be sprayed on the eye. After treatment, a rosary of conjunctival burns are visible for approximately 24 hours (Fig. 10-2).

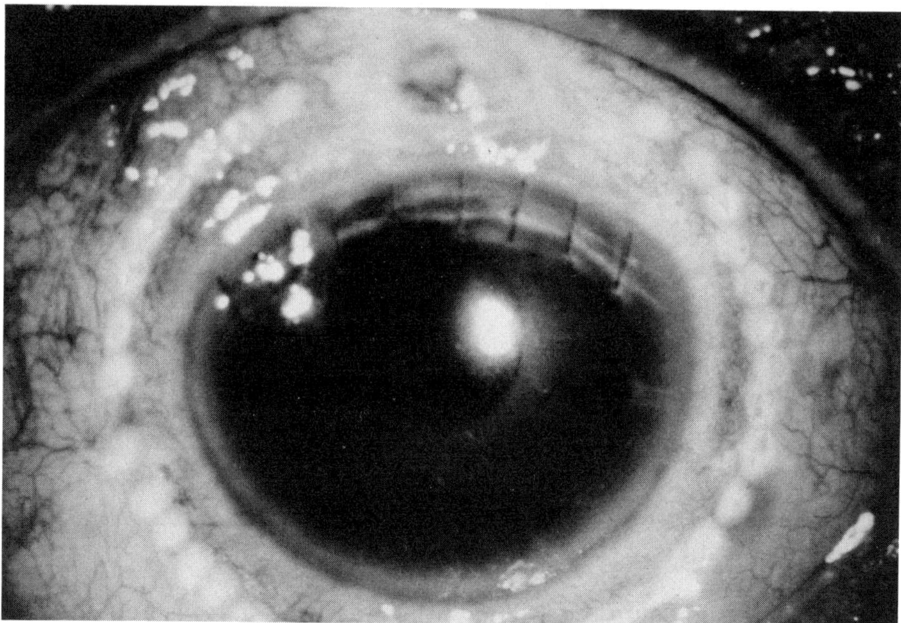

Figure 10-2. Rosary of discrete conjunctival lesions directly over the pars plicata.

Immediately after the procedure patients are given a drop of a topical betablocker, a steroid drop and a single oral dose of a carbonic anhydrase inhibitor, unless contraindicated. The IOP is measured for 1-2 hours post procedure. If the IOP rises 5-10mm above baseline, patients are given an oral osmotic agent and monitored for an additional 2 to 3 hours. Postoperatively patients are placed on topical steroids, mydriatics, and their preoperative glaucoma medication, except for miotics. Miotics may be reintroduced after the initial inflammation has subsided.

Results

The results of studies by various authors with Nd:YAG cyclophotocoagulation are summarized in Table 10-1. One can readily see that CPC results in a clinically important IOP decrease for many patients.

Factors that might affect the results include iris pigmentation, diagnosis, energy level used, and area of ciliary body treated. In rabbit models, Wilensky[8] has shown that as little as 1.5 joules of energy produces histologic evidence of acute hemorrhagic necrosis in the ciliary body as well as sustained lowering of IOP. Iris pigmentation, however, appears to play a role in the amount of destruction noted within the ciliary body. Cantor and coworkers[9] found that albino rabbits demonstrated less necrosis within the ciliary body than pigmented rabbits. In contrast, iris pigmentation has not affected the IOP response in humans. Schwartz,[10] Flack,[11] and Klapper[12] noted no difference in success or complications when comparing blue- and brown-eyed patients.

Diagnosis might play a role in the ultimate outcome. Patients with neovascular glaucoma appear to have more complications and visual loss than other types of glaucoma, but larger sample sizes are necessary to confirm this.[11]

Total energy used during the procedure may affect the ultimate IOP response. Initially, with a mean of 2.1 joules of energy, 41% required a second CPC and 8% required a third CPC for persistently elevated IOP.[13] Between 4.0 and 6.5 joules of thermal energy which leads to fewer repeat procedures without further increase in complications is suggested. When increasing the energy to 7.0 to 8.0 joules, patients note more pain, the eyes are more inflamed and hypopyon is more common. When comparing the treatment of 180° vs. 360° around the limbus, the 360° treatment produced a significant decrease in the percentage of patients requiring additional laser intervention.

When a poor pressure lowering response to the initial cyclophotocoagulation occurs, a repeat CPC is performed. The CPC can be repeated as early as one week later—and as often as five times within a two-year period—without adverse effect. It is advisable, however, to wait one month before repeating the Nd:YAG CPC to allow the initial inflammation to subside.

Complications

The major benefit of Nd:YAG cyclophotocoagulation over cyclocryotherapy is its much lower complication rate. For instance, the serious complications of cyclocryotherapy — such as early IOP rise phthisis and visual loss — are rare with CPC. The common complications of CPC are transient and include: persistent cell and flare, chemosis, microhyphema, fibrin clot, and air bubbles in the anterior chamber. The complication rates are summarized in Table 10-2 and a comparison with complications of cyclocryotherapy is provided in Table 10-3.

Phthisis, the most serious complication of cyclocryotherapy, has been reported in between 9.4 to 34% of cases following the procedure.[14-17] In contrast, phthisis is a rare complication of Nd:YAG CPC utilizing energy levels below 6.5 joules. Beckman[7] in initial work with the Ruby laser, found chronic hypotony and phthisis a frequent complication (24%) with energy levels of 7.5 joules. The Nd:YAG laser, initially using 8.5 joules of energy, was equally effective, while minimizing complications of hypotony and phthisis.[7] In our series, one patient out of 37 (3%) developed phthisis at 6 months.[10]

A decrease in visual acuity is common after cyclocryotherapy. For instance Caprioli and coworkers,[14] reported worsening vision in 41% of aphakic

Table 10-1.

Author	Laser	Laser Energy	Success Rate	Distance From Limbus	Comments
		(Joules)			
Beckman, et al[7]	Ruby	4-8	53%	3-6mm	
Klapper, et al[12]	Nd:YAG	3.8 (mean)	86%	2 or 3mm	3mm Required, fewer retreatment
Schwartz & Moster[10]	Nd:YAG	2.0 (mean)	69%	2-3mm with transillumination over pars plicata	48% Required, repeat CPC
Devenyi, et al[20]	Nd:YAG	1.8-3.0	62.5%	2-3mm	46% Required, retreatment IOP ≤ 25 mm Hg
Flack, et al[11]	Nd:YAG	4.9 (mean)	33% in 180° group 40% in 360° group	2-3mm with transillumination over pars plicata	After 1 CPC only Success equals: – 10P 5-21mm Hg. – no change in vision – 10P decrease 30% from base-line – no additional surgical procedures

Table 10-2. Complications of Nd: YAG CPC

	Frequency[6,10-13,20]
Flare	66 - 100%
Iritis	52 - 100%
Corneal Edema	3 - 100%
Air Bubble in Anterior Chamber	38%
Pain	33%
Hyphema	3 - 29%
Vitreous Hemorrhage	3 - 13%
Hypopyon	0 - 21%
Phthisis	0 - 14%
IOP Spike greater than 5mm following CPC	9%
Hypotony	5%
Retinal Detachment	2 - 7%
Vitritis	2 - 7%
Progressive Cataract	3 - 4%
Dellen	3%
Choroidal Detachment	3%

Table 10-3.
Comparison of Complications With Nd:YAG CPC and Cyclocryotherapy

0 = None 1 = Minimal 2 = Moderate 3 = Severe

	CPC[6,7,10-13,20]	CCT[14-17]
Phthisis	0-1	2-3
Increased IOP following procedure	0-1	2-3
Visual Loss	0-1	0-3
Chemosis	0-2	2-3
Pain	0-2	1-3
Hyphema	0-2	0-3
Cataract	0-1	0-3
Hypotony	0-2	0-3
Iris Atrophy	0	0-1
Anterior Ischemia	0	0-1
Retinal Detachment	0-1	0-1
Loss of Light Perception	0-1	0-3

patients with open angle or angle closure glaucoma and 70% with neovascular glaucoma. Fifteen percent of patients progressed to no light perception vision. In contrast, the visual acuity decrease following Nd:YAG CPC is usually transient and returns to baseline when the inflammation subsides. Klapper[12] found no significant loss of vision in 30 eyes.

An early IOP rise often occurs with cyclocryotherapy. Caprioli and colleagues[18] noted an IOP spike to 60 to 80 mm Hg during the procedure while Moster and coworkers[19] noted that 32% of patients had an IOP rise with a mean of 25 mm (range 12 to 14 mm Hg), fifteen minutes after cyclocryotherapy. A similar early IOP rise following Nd:YAG CPC does not occur. Flack and colleagues noted an IOP rise of 5 mm in 7% and of 10mm in only 2% of patients one hour after CPC.[11] When an early pressure rise is noted, the patient may be treated with oral isosorbide, a drop of a betablocker, atropine, dipivefrin, intensive topical steroids, and I.V. acetazolamide.

Prolonged and severe pain has been described after cyclocryotherapy, which might require retrobulbar alcohol injection for its control. Postoperative pain occurs in 33% with CPC. It varies dramatically from patient to patient but is usually mild and transient. In most cases, 600 to 1,000 milligrams of acetaminophen every four hours with ice compresses controls discomfort. In eyes with high IOP, pain, and poor vision without potential for improvement, 1.0 cc absolute alcohol can be injected following the retrobulbar block. Often, preoperative pain from high IOP is alleviated following cyclophotocoagulation without retrobulbar alcohol when the IOP returns to the normal range.

Most complications of CPC with the Nd:YAG laser are transient. In the series of Klapper and coworkers these included iritis, hyphema, dellen, and sterile hypopyon.[12] The notable complications experienced with this technique at Wills Eye Hospital include flare, present in 66% of patients, and iritis in 52% at one month. By three months, although flare was still common, profound iritis was limited to the patients with sustained uveitic glaucoma. A fibrin clot in the anterior chamber overlying the lens was often encountered in phakic patients after CPC, but most often resolved within 1 week (Figure 10-3). Air bubbles appeared in the anterior chamber during the procedure, but resolved within 24 hours. Microhyphema was common in eyes with

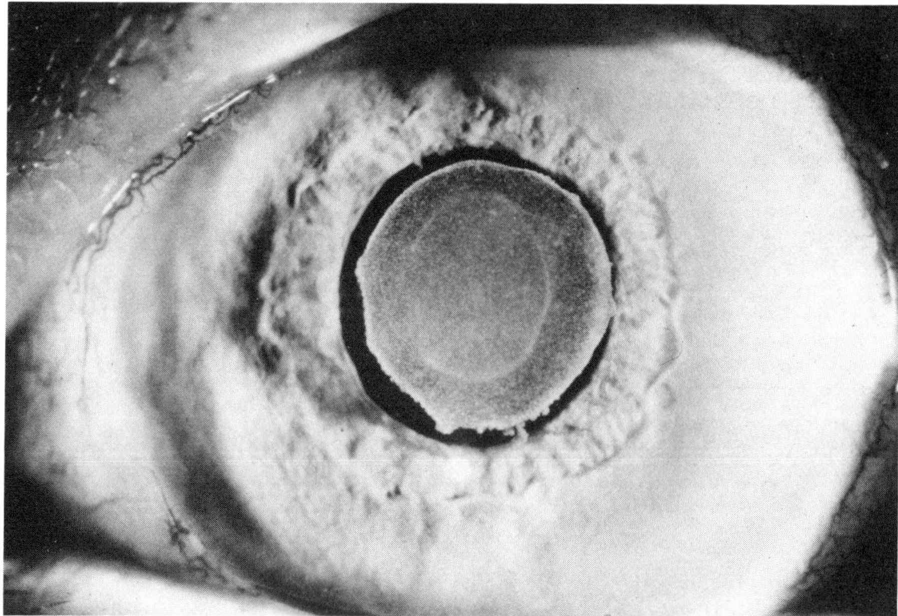

Figure 10-3. Fibrin clot over lens in an eye with neovascular glaucoma twenty-four hours after Nd:YAG CPC.

neovascular glaucoma and usually resolved within 1 month. Vitreous hemorrhage rarely occurred. Chemosis developed in most eyes but was less severe than following cyclocryotherapy. Other complications encountered were one patient each with retinal detachment, severe vitritis, and prolonged hypotony without phthisis at 6 months. Anterior chamber ischemia was not noted, which may be related to sparing of the long ciliary arteries at the 3 o'clock and 9 o'clock positions.[13]

In early experiences using 7.0 to 8.0 joules per application, the eyes displayed greater inflammation, postoperative pain, hypopyon, hyphema and debris from the ciliary body visible in the vitreous cavity. Beckman and coworkers routinely used Nd:YAG energy levels above 7.0 joules, but did not note any increase in the complication rate. Recently, Devenyi[20] suggested that variable laser energy output might be responsible for the differences noted.

In conclusion, Nd:YAG cyclophotocoagulation is a viable alternative to cyclocryotherapy in the treatment of refractory glaucoma. It is associated with a reasonable rate of success, is simple to perform in an outpatient setting, and has a lower complication rate than cyclocryotherapy.

References

1. Vogt A. Versuche zue intraokularen druckherabset zung mittelst diathermine schedt gung des corpus ciliare. Klin Monatsbl Augenhelkd 97:67, 1936.
2. Bietti G. Surgical intervention on the ciliary body. JAMA 142:889, 1950.
3. Weekers R, Lavergne G, Watillon M, et al. Effects of photocoagulation of ciliary body upon ocular tension. Am J Ophthalmol 52:156-163, 1961.
4. Beckman H, Kinoshita A, Rota A. Transscleral ruby laser irradiation of the ciliary body in the treatment of intractable glaucoma. Trans Am Acad Ophthalmol Otolaryngol 76:423-436, 1972.
5. Beckman H, Weltermann J. Transscleral ruby laser cyclocoagulation. Am J Ophthalmol 98:788-795, 1984.
6. Beckman H, Sugar S. Neodymium laser cyclocoagulation. Arch Ophthalmol 90:27-28, 1973.
7. Beckman H. Transscleral laser cyclocoagulation. Trans of New Orleans Aca Ophthalmol 148-153; 1985.
8. Wilensky J, Welch D, Mirolovich M. Transscleral cyclocoagulation using a neodymium:YAG laser. Ophthalmol Surg 16:95-98, 1985.
9. Cantor L, Katz, LJ, Nichols, et al. Nd:YAG cyclodiathermy; the role of pigmentation. Invest Ophthalmol Vis Sci (Suppl): (28)32:273, 1987.
10. Schwartz L, Moster M. Neodymium:YAG transscleral cyclodiathermy. Ophtalmol Laser Ther 1:135-141, 1986.
11. Flack NJ, Moster MR, Schwartz LW, et al. Comparison of Neodymium:YAG transscleral cyclophotocoagulation in the treatment of advanced glaucoma—180 degrees vs. 360 degrees. Invest Ophthalmol Vis Sci (Suppl) 29:234, 1988.
12. Klapper R, Wandel T, Donnenfeld E, et al. Transscleral Nd:YAG thermal cyclophotocoagulation in refractory glaucoma. Presented at Academy of Ophthalmology, November, 1986.

13. Moster MR, Schwartz LN, Cantor L, et al. Treatment of advanced glaucoma with Nd:YAG laser cyclodiathermy. ARVO Abstracts. Invest Ophthalmol and Vis Sci (Suppl) 27:P253, 1986.
14. Caprioli J, Strang S, Spaeth G, et al. Cyclocryotherapy in the treatment of advanced glaucoma. Ophthalmology 923:947-954, 1985.
15. Kaiden J, Serniuk R, Bader B. Choroidal detachment with flat anterior chamber after cyclocryotherapy. Ann Ophthalmology 1111-1113, 1979.
16. Bellows AR. Cyclocryotherapy for glaucoma. Int Ophthalmol Clin 21:99-111, 1981.
17. Krupin T, Mitchell KB, Becker B. Cyclocryotherapy in neovascular glaucoma. Am J Ophthalmol 896:24-26, 1978.
18. Caprioli J, Sears M. Regulation of intraocular pressure during cyclocryotherapy for advanced glaucoma. Am J Ophthalmol 101:542-545, 1986.
19. Moster M, Simmons S, Feldman R, et al. Cyclocryotherapy: acute intraocular pressure rise and long term results. Invent Ophthalmol Vis Sci (Suppl) (28)32:273, 1987.
20. Devenyi R, Trope G, Hunter, et al. Neodymium:YAG transscleral cyclocoagulation in human eyes. Ophthalmology 94:1519-1522, 1987.

SECTION III

Complications of Operative Surgical Procedures — Their Prevention and Management

CHAPTER 11

Complications of Ophthalmic Anesthesia

Richard P. Wilson, MD

Adequate anesthesia is a requirement of all surgical procedures. The quality of the anesthesia is crucial to the general outcome of the surgery and continued well being of the patient. In ophthalmology, this is especially true because of the older age of the majority of patients and the requirements for fine manipulation of tissues inherent in ophthalmic surgery. Both local and general anesthesia have kept pace with the advancements in ocular surgery, and provide generally excellent circumstances for the surgeon while surprising patients with the comfort and ease of their surgery. In spite of the improvements in anesthesia science, complications occasionally occur. This chapter will discuss the circumstances where anesthetic complications take place, the reasons for their occurrence, and how they can be avoided. It is not meant to be a text on ophthalmic anesthesia and those interested in a more complete look at the subject should consult other works, such as the chapter on anesthesia in *Ophthalmic Surgery* edited by George L. Spaeth.

Local Anesthesia

Topical Anesthesia

The topical anesthetics (Table 11-1) in wide use in this country are proparacaine, benoxinate, tetracaine, and cocaine. The first two have a rapid onset of action and cause only a brief stinging sensation. These attributes make them an excellent choice for applanation tonometry. Tetracaine penetrates more deeply into tissue, but has a longer (up to 30 seconds) stinging sensation after instillation. The deeper anesthesia it effects makes tetracaine useful in the operating room and in minor surgery. Cocaine, the first local anesthetic to be used clinically[1] provides excellent surface anesthesia with a 1 to 4% solution. In addition, it causes conjunctival as well as scleral vasoconstriction.

Table 11-1. Topical Anesthetic Agents*

Agent	Trade Name	Concentration
Proparacaine HCl	Ak-taine	0.5%
	Alcaine	0.5%
	Ophthaine	0.5%
	Ophthetic	0.5%
Benoxinate HCl	Fluress	0.4%
	(combined with fluorescein sodium 0.25%)	
Tetracaine HCl	Anacel	0.5%
	Pontocaine	0.5%
Cocaine HCl		1-4%
Onset within 1 minute Duration of action 10 to 20 minutes		

*Only presently-marketed topical anesthetics in United States. From Physicians' Desk Reference for Ophthalmology. Oradell, N.J., Medical Economics Company, 1987.

Side effects from these topical agents are dose related,[2] and except for cocaine, consist mainly of the delay in healing of epithelial defects caused by inhibition of cell division and migration. This topical toxicity limits the use of these agents to surgery or diagnostic tests.[3,4] Repeated use, as during surgery, results in cumulative toxicity. Corneal drying and trauma should be minimized in order to prevent epithelial slough. When used in conjunction with a facial nerve block, the eye is patched postoperatively to prevent corneal damage. Patients with keratitis sicca are most susceptible to postoperative superficial corneal problems. Corneal erosion or massive superficial punctate keratitis often follow exposure to the operating room microscope or contact with gonioscopic solutions for extended periods, as during panretinal photocoagulation or laser trabeculoplasty. The frequent use of ocular lubricants for weeks, and in rare cases, months, can be required to return the cornea to its normal state.

Localized hypersensitivity can develop either to the agent itself or to preservatives in the vehicle. Systemic complications, however, are limited to the use of cocaine. Since it acts to block the reuptake of norepinephrine at the neuron level, cocaine can produce hypertensive crises in patients also on reserpine, guanethidine, methyldopa, or monoamine oxidase inhibitors.[5] More localized side effects include mydriasis without cycloplegia,[6] potentially more of a problem with occludable angles than when cycloplegia deepens the anterior chamber, and a marked loosening of the corneal epithelium, which might lead to large erosions.

Regional Anesthesia

Local anesthetics (Table 11-2) generally belong to one of two groups, differentiated by structural differences. Procaine and chloroprocaine contain an ester linkage between the benzene ring and the intermediate chain and therefore are called aminoesters. They are characterized by low toxicity and rapid onset of action. Their short duration of action, however, limits their usefulness in ophthalmic surgery.[7] The aminoamides include bupivacaine, etidocaine, lidocaine, mepivacaine, and prilocaine and have an amide link between the benzene ring and the intermediate chain. These agents have a longer duration of action, but greater toxicity.[8] Structural differences also dictate the rate and route by which the agents are metabolized. The aminoester anesthetics are hydrolyzed in plasma by the enzyme pseudocholinesterase. The amide-linked anesthetics undergo enzymatic degradation in liver microsomes.

Table 11-2. Regional Anesthetic Agents*

Agent (Trade name)	Chemical Class	Concentration	Maximum Dose	Relative Potency	Onset of Action	Duration of Action
Procaine (Novocaine)	Ester	1%, 4%	500 mg	1	7-8 min	30-40 min
Chloroprocaine (Nesacaine)	Ester	1%, 3%	800 mg	1	6-12 min	60 min
Mepivacaine (Carbocaine)	Amide	1%, 2%	500 mg	2	3-5 min	120 min
Lidocaine (Xylocaine) (Dalcaine)	Amide	1%, 2%	500 mg	2	4-6 min	40-60 min
Bupivacaine (Marcaine) (Sensorcaine)	Amide	0.25%, 0.75%	175 mg	8	5-11 min	4-12 hours
Etidocaine (Duranest)	Amide	1%, 1.5%	400 mg	8	3-5 min	5-10 hours

*Modified from Raj PP: Handbook of Regional Anesthesia. New York, Churchill Livingstone Inc., 1985; Physicians' Desk Reference for Ophthalmology. Oradel, N.J., Medical Economics Company, 1987; Crandall DC: Pharmacology of Ocular Anesthetics. In Duane TD, Jaegar EA (eds.) Biomedical Foundation of Ophthalmology, Philadelphia, Harper and Row, 1986.

Selective practical aspects of local anesthetic pharmacology include the fact that they produce a nonpolarized block which effects the smaller fibers that are autonomic in nature first followed by the sensory fibers and last the largest fibers that are motor and proprioceptive. Therefore, low concentrations of anesthetic (e.g., bupivacaine 0.25% versus 0.75%) might give a sensory block without paralysis.[9,10] Regional anesthetics also cause peripheral vasodilation by relaxing vascular smooth muscle. This effect is directly related to the strength of the anesthetic and encourages vascular absorption of the agent leaving less drug available in the tissue. Epinephrine in dilute concentrations (1:200,000)[11,12] added to the anesthetic solution will counteract the vasodilation of the local anesthetic and produce a longer-acting block with reduced peak blood levels. The addition of epinephrine allows a greater amount of anesthetic to be used without systemic toxicity. Epinephrine's effect on duration of action depends upon the agent used with lidocaine's duration of action being greatly extended, prilocaine and mepivacaine moderately prolonged, but no change in the duration of action of bupivacaine and etidocaine.[13,14] Additional benefits of epinephrine are the inhibition of local bleeding and the counteraction of the depressive effects of local anesthetics on the cardiovascular system. On the other hand, however, it introduces risks of its own, especially increased cardiac excitability and hypertension. Patients with hypertension, diabetes, cardiovascular disease, or a thyrotoxicosis are more susceptible to the side effects and patients undergoing halothane anesthesia have a greater risk of cardiac fibrillation with its use.[6] A significant decrease in ophthalmic artery pulse pressure also has been reported when epinephrine was added to the anesthetic for retrobulbar anesthesia. This should at least make epinephrine a theoretic contraindication for retrobulbar anesthesia in patients with glaucoma.

Hyaluronidase is an enzyme often added to the local anesthetic mixture to promote rapid diffusion of the agent and a greater area of block with the same amount of anesthesia. Conversely, hyaluronidase also increases the absorption of the drug into the blood stream and can cause systemic toxicity with a dose that would usually be tolerated if not absorbed so quickly.

Toxicity

Excitation of the central nervous system and depression of the cardiovascular system are the major side effects of local anesthetics. (Table 11-3). These effects are dose related. Since the concentration required to produce neuronal blockade is nearly 600 times that required to cause serious systemic side effects, toxicity is linearly related to systemic absorption. This, in turn, is related to the quantity of drug used, the rate of injection, the vascularity of the area receiving the injection, the vasoactive properties of the drug, the toxicity of the drug, and its rate of deactivation and excretion. Neurologic side effects are secondary to penetration of the anesthetic through the blood-brain barrier with blockage of inhibitory pathways resulting in central nervous system excitation. Cardiac effects result from the stabilizing effect of local anesthetics on the cell membranes of the myocardium. This leads to a drop in conduction rate, contraction force, and excitability.

Systemic toxicity as a consequence of overdose, unintentional intravascular injection of the usual dose, or unusually quick absorption from a highly vascular tissue produces a typical pattern. The prodrome consists of garrulousness, perioral numbness and tingling, diplopia, and tinnitus. Tremors and muscle twitching often progress to a generalized myoclonic seizure with depression of the nervous system if blood levels are high. The depressant effect of the local anesthetic on the myocardium and peripheral dilation can result in loss of consciousness and respiratory depression with circulatory collapse. Hypoxia and acidosis accompany these changes.[15]

Table 11-3. Signals of Local Anesthetic Toxicity

Central Nervous System	
Mild	**Severe**
Tingling	Muscle twitching
Drowsiness	Generalized myoclonic seizure
Tinnitus	Respiratory depression
Disorientation	Unconsciousness
Cardiovascular System	
Mild	**Severe**
Sinus bradycardia	Hypotension
Decreased cardiac output	Cardiac failure
Falling blood pressure	Asystole

Grand mal seizures and respiratory arrests have been reported following retrobulbar injection of marcaine and marcaine combined with lidocaine or mepivacaine.[16,17] The suggested mechanism for this complication is the direct injection of anesthetic into the subdural space surrounding the optic nerve allowing a small amount of drug direct access into the subdural space surrounding the pons and midbrain.[18,19] Because of the direct access to the brain stem, respiratory arrest without prior cardiovascular symptoms can result.[20] Supporting the mechanism suggested is a report of three cases of reversible contralateral amaurosis after retrobulbar anesthesia. The most likely explanation for this phenomenon is the dissection of anesthetic solution along the subdural space of the optic nerve back to the chiasm and to the contralateral nerve.[21,22]

An alternative explanation is the rupture of an arterial wall in the presence of a large volume of retrobulbar anesthetic under sufficient pressure to force the drug to enter the arterial system and flow in a retrograde manner to the cerebral circulation.[23] Several studies support this possibility.[24,25] Injection of an anesthetic into the venous system should not cause serious adverse effects, as the total dose given with retrobulbar anesthesia is less than the toxic intravenous dose.

Postoperative diplopia is occasionally seen after retrobulbar anesthesia. This can be secondary to gross intraorbital hemorrhage or isolated intramuscular hemorrhage, both mechanical etiologies and also to direct toxicity of the local anesthetic on the extraocular muscles. Lidocaine and bupivacaine have been shown to cause a toxic degeneration of muscle fibers with later regeneration. A transient diplopia in the postoperative period can result.[26] The incidence of serious side effects with the use of local anesthetics in ophthalmology is thankfully low. One study found 9 of 1,000 patients for cataract surgery developed a complication of local anesthesia. Eight had hypotension requiring intervention with pressure agents or other intravenous drugs. One case of respiratory arrest occurred five minutes after a retrobulbar block employing 0.75% bupivacaine and 2% lidocaine. Another study reported 3 cases of respiratory arrest out of 1,500 consecutive cases.

The seriousness of the side effects when they occur, however, emphasizes the necessity for prevention and detection. Because the most frequent cause of toxicity is overdosage, the smallest volume of the lowest effective concentration should be employed, never exceeding the recommended dose-to-weight ratio. Aspiration before injection, and where feasible, movement of the needle during injection will minimize intravascular injection. Lidocaine and mepivacaine, nonester anesthetics that are degraded in the liver at a slower rate than the ester anesthetics are hydrolyzed, must be used with caution whenever large doses are required.[27,28]

Optimally, all patients prior to the administration of local anesthesia have an intravenous infusion with monitoring of their electrocardiogram, blood pressure, and pulse. The addition of oxygen via nasal cannula is also helpful. When symptoms of toxicity appear, drug administration must be stopped. Oxygen should be given at a high flow rate to raise the patient's oxygen reserve should convulsions follow. If tremors or muscle twitching appears, and clearly if a convulsion should occur, intravenous diazepam (5 to 10 mg.) or rapid-onset barbiturates (thiopental sodium, 50 to 100 mg.) should be administered. If the seizure cannot be controlled, succinylcholine, intubation, and oxygen are necessitated. Intravenous fluids and vasopressors are used as needed for hypotension. If cardiac arrest occurs, it is treated in the usual manner.[29]

Regional Blocks

Infiltrative blocks with local anesthetic for intraocular surgery include the supraorbital block, Van Lint block, Atkinson block, O'Brien block, Nadbath block, Spaeth block, and retrobulbar block (Fig. 11-1through 11-8). Any of these blocks can result in hemorrhage or nerve trauma with secondary tenderness for several weeks at the site of injection. Facial blocks into the area of the temporomandibular joint usually violate the parotid gland as well. Continued tenderness in this area and pain on jaw movement often can be present postoperatively.

The Nadbath block (See Fig. 11-5), which utilizes an injection into the concavity between the mastoid process and the posterior border of the mandibular ramus, occasionally has the side effect of a bitter taste in the mouth as the parotid gland secretes the anesthetic.[30] Dysphonia, swallowing difficulty, and respiratory distress have been reported in 3 out of 300 blocks by several authors. In these reported cases, 5 cc of anesthetic were used rather than the 3 cc recommended by Nadbath and a 16 mm needle was used rather than a 12 mm needle as recommended. This complication is predominantly seen in very thin patients and seems to spread from the spread of anesthetic to the jugular foramen 1 cm deeper than the stylomastoid foramen. The length of the needle and the depth of the injection are therefore critical. The Nadbath block should never be done bilaterally or in patients with preexisting unilateral oropharyngeal or vocal cord dysfunction to avoid bilateral vocal cord paralysis. If dysphonia or difficulty with swallowing or respiration occurs, positioning the patient on the side of paralysis will allow the paralyzed vocal cord to swing free, opening a clear airway.[31,32,33]

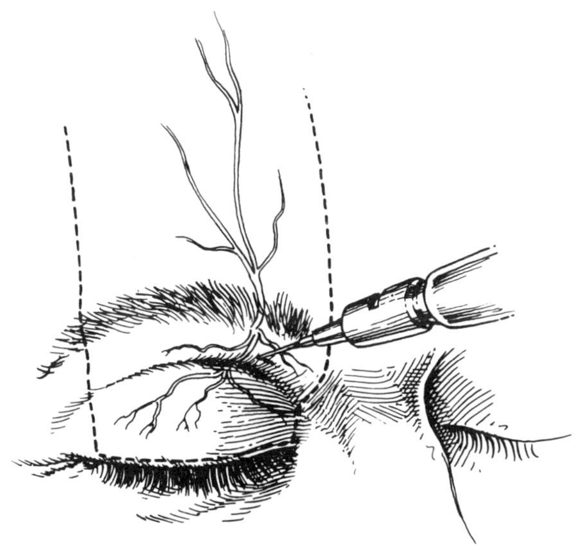

Figure 11-1. A block of the supraorbital branch of the frontal nerve is obtained by injection of anesthetic just lateral to the supraorbital notch to a depth of 1¼ inches along the roof of the orbit. Anesthesia of the outlined area will result. (Figures 11-1 to 11-7, and Figure 11-9, reprinted with permission from: Wilson RP: Anesthesia in ophthalmic surgery. In Spaeth GL (ed.): Ophthalmic Surgery: Principles and Practice. Philadelphia, W.B. Saunders, 1982.)

A safer block is one described by Spaeth (See Fig. 11-6), where the injection is into the posterior ramus of the mandible at the level of the tragus of the ear.[34] The O'Brien block chiefly anesthetizes the superior most branches of the facial nerve, which are the upper, lower, and zygomatic. These three branches themselves can swing inferior to the point at which the O'Brien block is effective and peripheral branches of the facial nerve intercommunicate distal to this area. Rami communicates spread up from the buccal and even the mandibular branches to the zygomatic branches that innervate the orbicularis oculi. If the inferior branches of the facial nerve are not blocked, akinesia of the orbicularis might be incomplete. The Spaeth block, however, provides a complete unilateral facial palsy usually within 30 seconds.[34]

Because the retrobulbar block is a blind thrust behind the eye, hemorrhage is an infrequent but unfortunate complication. The globe becomes progressively proptotic and subconjunctival blood might become evident as the hemorrhage extends anteriorly. It might not become visible, however,

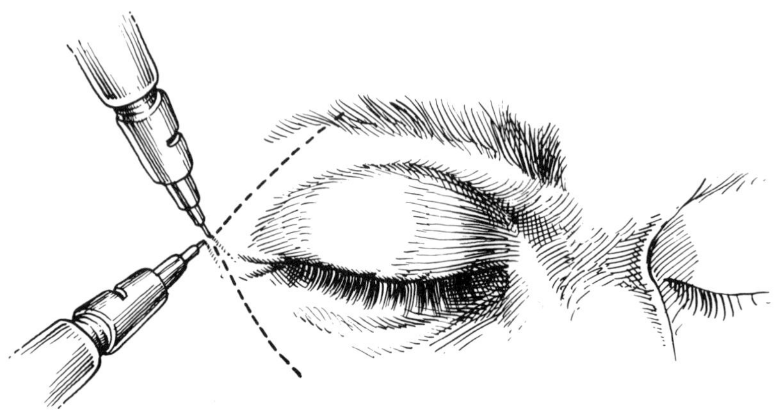

Figure 11-2. The Van Lint block can anesthetize the facial nerve branches to the orbicularis muscle as they run over the periosteum just lateral to the orbit.

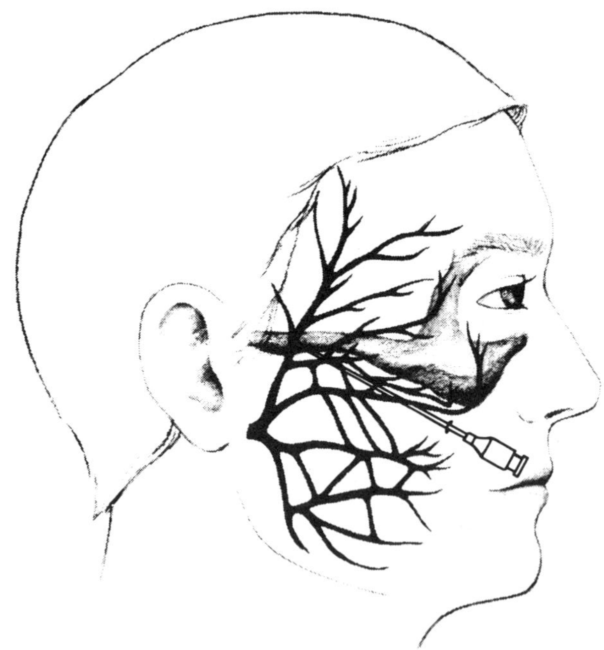

Figure 11-3. An alternative method of providing paralysis of the orbicularis muscle proposed by Atkinson intercepts the facial nerve fibers as they cross the zygomatic arch.

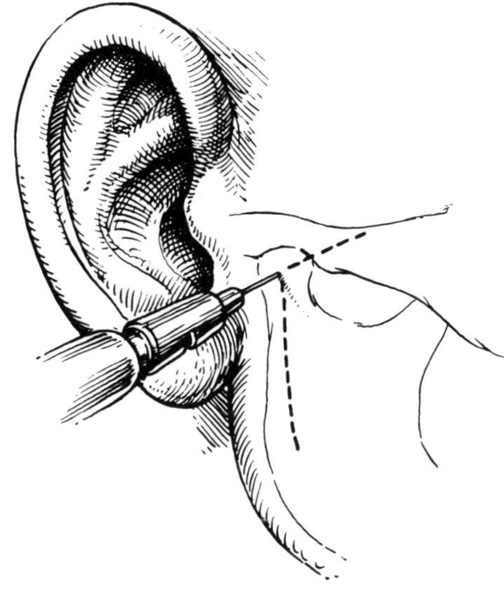

Figure 11-4. The O'Brien block of the facial nerve with its anterior and interior extensions will provide paralysis of the orbicularis muscle. It can be combined with the Van Lint block to ensure complete paralysis.

until the first postoperative day. Bleeding in a closed space increases orbital pressure and limits further hemorrhage, but IOP is elevated and surgery generally must be postponed. Even if the IOP can be reduced to normal with digital ocular massage, a significant retrobulbar clot will impede venous return resulting in engorgement of the ciliary body and much increased bleeding and an increased chance of vitreous loss if the surgeon chooses to proceed. In most instances, surgery can be performed two to three days later, preferably under general anesthesia. In cases where the presence of blood in the episcleral tissues will interfere with surgery, as with glaucoma filtering operations, the procedure usually should be deferred for at least one week.

Although retrobulbar injection, with or without retrobulbar hemorrhage, is usually associated with few sequelae it has rarely led to total permanent loss of vision and optic atrophy. Direct needle injury to the optic nerve, damage to its blood supply, or injection into the optic canal with compressive ischemia of the optic nerve have all been reported as the etiology for this complication. Disc and retinal edema, intraretinal, preretinal, and vitreous hemorrhage are usually evident on examination. Combined central retinal artery and vein occlusions have been described secondary to hemorrhage into the optic nerve sheath. Occasionally, this hemorrhage can evolve slowly over several days. Diagnosis with computerized tonography or B-scan ultrasonography allows optic nerve sheath decompression that can improve the prognosis.[35,36,37,38] When the mechanical mechanisms of optic nerve injury are added to the previously mentioned toxic manifestations of presumed intraoptic nerve sheath injection, it is clear that there are significant problems with retrobulbar injections. There have been numerous modifications in technique proposed to

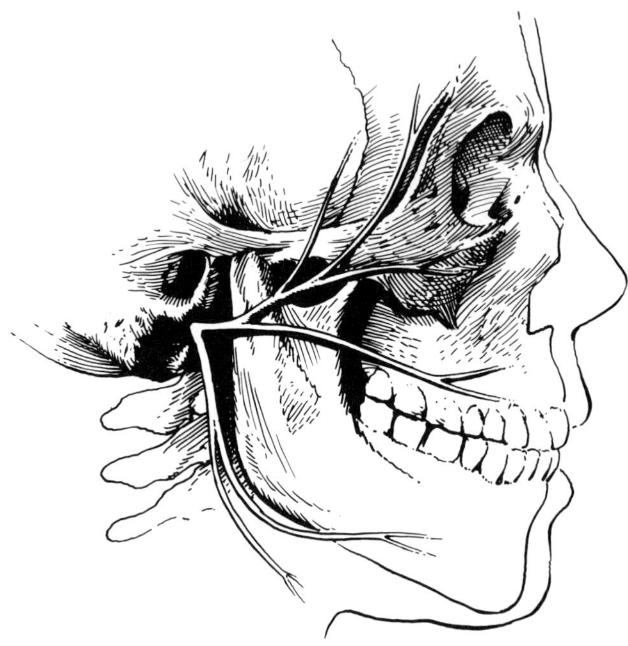

Figure 11-5. The facial nerve in relation to the mastoid process and inferior auditory canal. Complete facial block is obtained by blocking the facial nerve as it emerges from the stylomastoid foramen before the nerve divides.

avoid complications. Several authors have advocated a change in the traditional Atkinson ocular position, with the patient looking upward and inward at the time of the retrobulbar block. Atkinson recommended positioning the globe in this manner "to move the inferior oblique muscle and the facia between the lateral and inferior rectus muscles forward and upward, out of the way."[39] One study used computerized scanning of a cadaver orbit as a retrobulbar needle was introduced to show that the Atkinson position moves the optic nerve, the ophthalmic artery, the superior orbital vein, and the posterior pole of the globe adjacent to the needle tip and places the optic nerve on stretch so that it can be more easily stabbed. The authors of this study[40] recommend that the patient's gaze be directed straight ahead or slightly downward and outward and that the needle be directed toward the inferior part of the superior orbital fissure rather than toward the orbital apex as recommended by Atkinson.

Several authors have suggested directing the needle through the inferior orbit in the sagittal plane of the lateral limbus and remaining in that plane at all times. If maintained in the plane of the lateral limbus, the needle lies just nasal to the lateral rectus within the muscle cone and inferior to the globe. This places it well away from the optic nerve.[20]

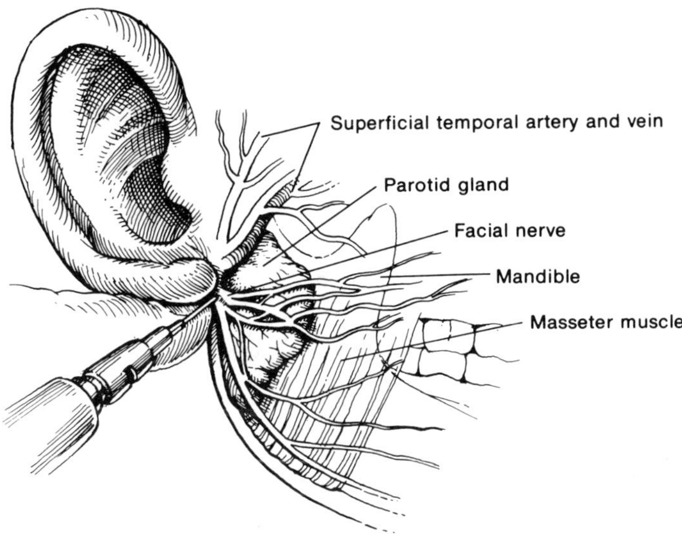

Figure 11-6. In the Spaeth modification of the O'Brien technique, the facial nerve is blocked where it crosses the posterior edge of the mandible, thus catching the nerve before it divides. This provides more complete paralysis of the inferior orbicularis muscle.

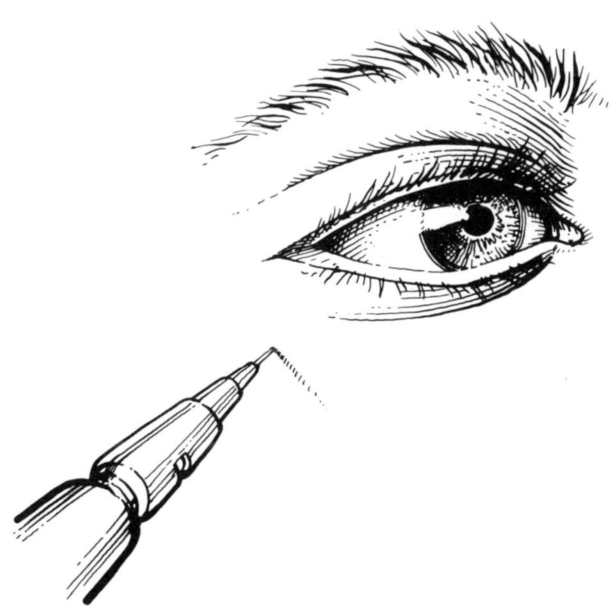

Figure 11-7. Modification of traditional Atkinson ocular position.

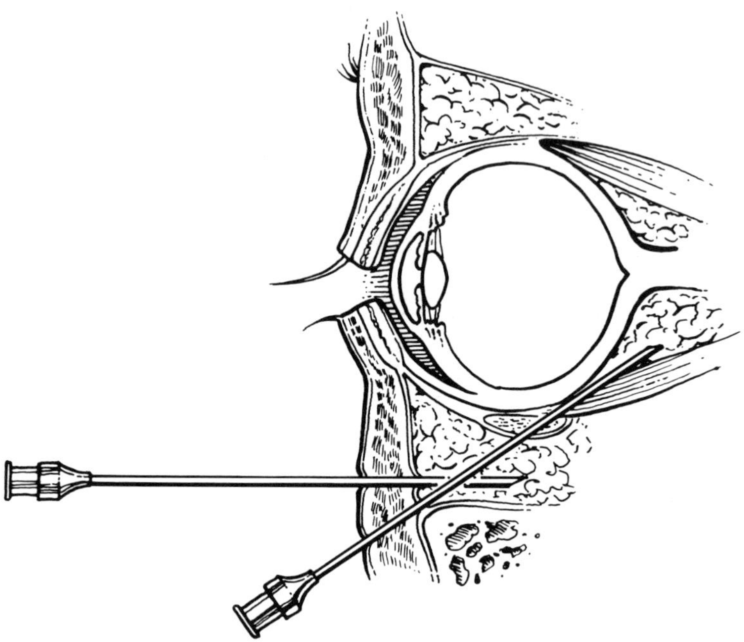

Figure 11-8. Placement of retrobulbar (A) and peribulbar (B) injection. (Figures 11-8 through 11-10 reprinted with permission from: Davis DB, Mandel MR: Posterior peribulbar anesthesia. J Cataract Refractive Surg 1986: 12, 183.)

Some authors feel that the traditional approach is acceptable as long as needle insertion is stopped and injection accomplished as soon as the surgeon feels the pop of the needle tip as it penetrates the muscle cone. The use of a 1.3 cm needle assures that the needle tip will not penetrate far enough to endanger the optic nerve.[41] When the eye is looking down and out and the muscle cone is relaxed in the inferotemporal quadrant, the surgeon can have a more difficult time ascertaining when the needle tip is within the cone and might therefore have to push further into the orbit to ensure that the needle tip is within the cone. The deeper intrusion of the needle predisposes to retrobulbar hemorrhage and undermines the reason for positioning the eye in this fashion.

Another alternative that has proven safer than the retrobulbar block and provides adequate orbicularis akinesia without the addition of a facial block is the posterior peribulbar block. This technique, introduced by Kelman and modified by others (Table 11-4) (Fig. 11-9 and 11-10), employs two stepped injections, one above the inferior orbital rim 1 cm medial to the lateral canthus and one just below the supraorbital notch. Anesthetic is deposited at the level of the skin, the orbicularis muscle just beneath the muscle and in the posterior orbit (See Table 11-4). The proponents of this block argue that is it safer, causes less pain on injection and postoperatively, does not result in loss of vision in one-eyed patients in the early postoperative period, and is easy to teach to aspiring ophthalmologists and anesthesiologists. A major disadvantage is the time between administration of the block and when it is effective. This has been described as 12 to 25 minutes and usually is in conjunction with the "super pinkie" or other ocular compression methods.[42]

Table 11-4. Procedure for Posterior Peribulbar Block

With IV going or heparin lock in, and after desired sedation and eyelid prep:

1. Make small skin wheal in lower eyelid one cm medial to lateral canthus over inferior orbital rim.
2. Make small skin wheal in upper eyelid in the skinfold directly inferior to the supraorbital foramen.
3. Through inferior skin wheal with 27 g[2] needle, inject 1/2 cc lidocaine 1% in orbicularis and inject 1 cc deep to the muscle.
4. Through upper lid skin wheal, repeat as in step 3.
5. Through lower lid skin wheal, inject 1 cc lidocaine 1%/bupivacaine 3/4%/hyaluronidase solution in the orbicularis muscle and 1 cc immediately deep to it. Advance along the floor of the orbit to the equator of the eye; aspirate and inject 1 cc; aiming slightly supermedially, advance the needle to its full depth and inject 2 to 1.5 cc.
6. Pushing globe inferiorly with free index finger, enter through upper lid skin wheal and inject 1 cc 1/2 inch deep to the orbicularis muscle and slightly nearer the canthus than in the original skin wheal; direct needle along orbital roof (without engaging periostium) to the equator, where 1 cc is injected, then to the superior orbital fissure and inject a final 1 cc of solution.
7. Pressure on the globe/orbit and time are essential to a good block; after 8 minutes, if incomplete akinesia remains, 3 to 4 cc of additional anesthetic solution is injected by the lower approach if lateral or inferior movement is seen, or by the superior approach if superior or medial movement is seen. (Always perform lower lid injections before upper lid injections.)

Adapted from Nugent CC: Peribulbar anesthesia, a safe, simple, effective and relatively painless technique. Obtained from the author at Medical Surgical Center, Hayward, CA 94541.

Preoperative Preparation

The preoperative preparation of patients undergoing surgery with local anesthesia includes not only a thorough assessment of the patient's physical preparedness for the possible rigors of the anesthesia and surgery, but also the allowance of time for the person who will be monitoring the patient to develop rapport with the patient and offer reassurance. A thorough explanation of what will happen to the patient, as well as reassurance that the support person will be with him and adjust medications as necessary will go far to ensure a relaxed and cooperative patient. The type of preoperative medication to be used must be individualized according to the type of surgery and the nature of the patient. Too much sedation can produce loud snoring with marked head movement and occasional jerks as the patient awakes. In the elderly, too much sedation can paradoxically cause excitation and diminish the surgeon's and anesthetist's ability to reason with the patient.

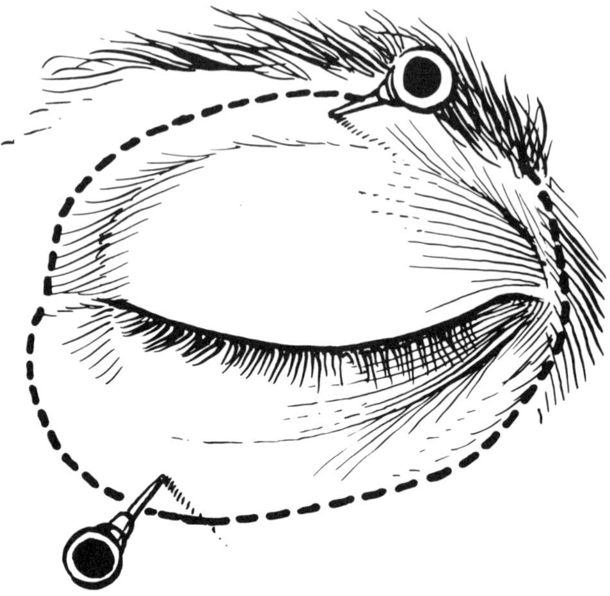

Figure 11-9. Injection sites for posterior peribulbar block.

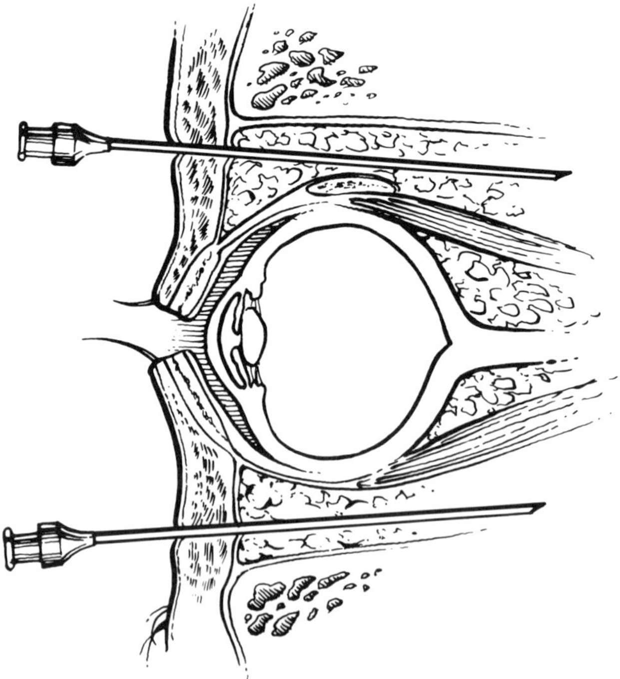

Figure 11-10. Lateral view of posterior peribulbar injeciton sites, including injections inferior and superior to the globe.

Where pain might not be completely blocked as in a reoperation to repair a retinal detachment that cannot be done under general anesthesia because of the patient's poor health, a narcotic will add helpful analgesic. If the patient is quite anxious, an agent such as diazepam or midazolam will add a calming effect. Barbiturates provide sedation and minimize toxic reactions to local anesthetics. For those patients who cannot face the pain of local anesthetic injections or if multiple procedures will be required and the surgeon does not want any memory of the injections, one of three agents can be used. An intravenous injection of thiopental sodium (50 to 100 mg.), ketamine (10 to 25 mg.), or the use of 70% nitrous oxide inhalation will abolish the pain and memory of the injections. For most patients, however, the amnesic effect of intravenous diazepam or midazolam usually is satisfactory.

General Anesthesia

Improvements in anesthetic agents and techniques have resulted in a marked reduction in operative and postoperative complications with general anesthesia. Present anesthetic practice allows a smooth, rapid induction of anesthesia, an uneventful course, and quiet emergence with few adverse drug reactions. Operating conditions for the surgeon are excellent because the anesthetist has complete control of the patient. Nervous or confused patients and those with whom communication will not be possible, (e.g., deaf, foreign) are much more easily handled under general than local anesthesia. The surgeon and operating room personnel are usually more relaxed with freer flow of communication. The risks of mechanical injury with the injection and toxic reactions to the local anesthetic are avoided. Additionally, many patients prefer general to local anesthesia. Attractive as these advantages are, they must be weighed against the greater risks inherent in using a potentially lethal drug to produce unconsciousness. The ease of administration, short turn around time between patients, and the relatively slight physiologic alteration produced by local anesthesia with sedation argue for local anesthesia. The postoperative period is also more pleasant with local anesthesia with less nausea and residual malaise. Depending upon the local anesthetic agent chosen, there can be a prolonged period of pain relief as well.

Medical Conditions Affecting the Use of General Anesthesia

The majority of ophthalmic patients are either under 10 years of age or older than 55. This places them at increased risk for any kind of anesthesia. A study at the Manhattan Eye, Ear, Nose and Throat Hospital[43] showed that the majority of patients had some form of cardiovascular disease: hypertension ischemic heart disease with a history of mild cardiac infarction, atrial fibrillation, or past cerebral vascular accidents. Diabetes mellitus, chronic bronchitis, and psychiatric disorders are also common. Clearly, the preoperative evaluation and optimization of the patient's health by his personal physician is crucial to uneventful anesthesia without surprises. The cooperation of an internist on staff is usually required for less stable patients.[44] Several general guidelines seem appropriate. Diabetics who are insulin controlled can be handled in a variety of ways. One standard regimen is to omit the routine insulin dose on the day of surgery. The blood sugar is drawn on arrival and an intravenous drip of 5% dextrose in normal saline solution started. Regular insulin is administered subcutaneously to cover the amount of glucose given (10 to 15 U/1000 D5NS). Dextrostix during and after surgery are used to determine if additional amounts are needed. When the patient's oral diet is resumed, so is his usual insulin regimen.

Hypertensive patients need to be as well controlled as possible[45,46] and should continue their medications on the day of surgery, taking them with a sip of water as necessary. Hypertension on intubation can usually be prevented with an adequate induction dose of anesthetic agent along with laryngotracheal lidocaine (2 mg./kg of a 4% solution).[47,48,49]

Most patients with severe pulmonary disease are often safer having local anesthesia. Patients with chronic bronchitis, however, are prone to coughing at inopportune times and this can result in serious consequences. Therefore, these patients are often best treated under general anesthesia where the anesthetist can eliminate coughing entirely. It is essential to have the patient enter the operating room in the best condition possible for him. Intermittent positive pressure breathing with bronchodilator drugs and, if needed, postural drainage with physiotherapy and including specific antibiotic treatment should all be employed prior to the time of surgery as necessary. An anesthetic technique that provides a high oxygen availability and minimal postanesthetic respiratory depression will minimize complications.

Drug Interactions

Drug interactions are a common cause of anesthetic complications.

Atropine. For years, atropine was not given as a premedication to patients with occludable angles for fear of causing an acute angle closure attack. These fears have proven groundless.[50] It has been found that 0.4 mg. of atropine distributed evenly in a 70 kg patient results in only about 0.0001 mg. of the drug reaching the eye. This is far less than the 0.6 mg. found there after the instillation of one drop of 1% solution. If the patient's angles are extremely narrow and it is feared that a combination of excitement and atropine will cause pupillary dilation, then pilocarpine 1% instilled once or twice in the eye one hour prior to the administration of atropine is adequate to prevent pupillary dilatation.

Psychiatric Drugs. Monoamine oxidase inhibitors, tricyclic antidepressants, and lithium are the only commonly used psychiatric drugs that complicate anesthesia. MAO inhibitors increase the effects of meperidine and might give rise to dangerous hypertensive attacks if sympathomimetics are used during anesthesia. They should be stopped two weeks prior to surgery.

Tricyclic antidepressant drugs block the reuptake of neurotransmitters and can cause fatal dysrhythmias in combination with halothane and pancuronium.[51,52] Lithium carbonate decreases the release of neurotransmitters centrally and peripherally and can prolong neuromuscular blockade.

Because lithium carbonate blocks the release of norepinephrine, epinephrine, and dopamine in the brain stem, it might decrease anesthetic requirements.[53,54,55]

Cholinesterase Inhibitors. Eye drops containing long acting anticholinesterase agents, such as echothiophate and demecarium, are absorbed systemically to the extent that there is a marked decrease in pseudocholinesterase, up to 95% after 4 to 6 weeks of use. This effect can last up to 8 weeks after the discontinuation of the drug. Even small doses of succinylcholine used to facilitate anesthesia will not be rapidly inactivated in patients with low pseudocholinesterase. The transient apnea produced by succinylcholine can last up to 5 hours in such patients. If the surgery requires general anesthesia and is elective, the anticholinesterase agent should be stopped at least a month prior to surgery and the anesthetist informed. If this is not feasible, then another muscle relaxant should be chosen. Intravenous atropine should be given preoperatively to block muscarinic effects and prevent vagal responses.[47]

Steroids. After a prolonged course of oral steroids, steroid production in the adrenals is suppressed for 6 months or more. As surgery constitutes a stressful period, supplemental steroids should be given pre- and postoperatively.

Propranolol. Sudden discontinuation of propranolol can precipitate unstable angina and even myocardial infarction. Modest doses of up to 180 mg. of propranolol over a 24-hour period can be administered up to the time of surgery. Higher doses should be tapered to the minimum therapeutic level and the morning dosage omitted the day of surgery.[56]

Control of Intraocular Pressure

Present knowledge suggests that two-thirds or more of the aqueous humor exiting the eye leaves via the trabecular meshwork to the canal of Schlemm and out through the aqueous veins to the collecting venous system and eventually back to the right side of the heart. Any blockage of venous return, (e.g., retrobulbar hemorrhage) or any cause of elevated central venous pressure, (e.g., coughing) will result in elevation of episcleral venous pressure. Any increase in episcleral venous pressure results not only in a 1:1 rise in IOP, but also an expansion of the venous volume in the choroid. Thus straining, coughing, and vomiting can produce sudden increases in IOP and choroidal volume, predisposing to positive pressure and expulsive hemorrhage. Hypoventilation with secondary increase in PCO_2 also raises the IOP. Hyperventilation and hypocapnia reduce it.[47]

Most general anesthetics cause a decrease in IOP unless there is $C0_2$ retention or hypoxemia to counteract the fall. Almost all narcotics, tranquilizers, neuroleptics, hypnotics, and barbiturates also decrease IOP 10 to 15% if there are no counterbalancing influences.[47] Nitrous oxide also lowers intraocular pressure. When it is used alone, however, patients can become overly sensitive to airway manipulation. At such times, intratracheal intubation can cause a transient rise of IOP that can be as great as 40 mm mercury.

Ketamine (Ketalar) is one general anesthetic agent that tends to elevate IOP. This rise is of the same magnitude as the decrease caused by other anesthetics and is thought to be secondary to an increase in extraocular muscle tone. When mixed with another general anesthetic, the pressure elevating effect of ketamine is balanced to a large degree by the depressing effect of the other drug. This might provide a more accurate assessment of awake IOPs in patients undergoing evaluation under anesthesia.[57] Succinylcholine, and to a lesser extent, decamethonium usually causes a transient increase in IOP. This rise is dose related and averages about 10 mm mercury. It lasts l to 10 minutes after injection with a peak at 2 to 4 minutes.[58,59] Special muscle fibers, known as Felderstruktur, are found only in extraocular muscles. These fibers react to depolarizing muscle relaxants with a slow clonic contraction that is thought tc be the cause of the pressure rise. The deeper the general anesthesia at the time of administration, the less marked the rise in IOP. Studies aimed at abolishing succinylcholine-induced fasciculations in the extraocular muscles with drugs have produced controversial results.[60,61,62,63,64] Prior treatment with acetazolamide and propranolol, however, can prevent IOP rises caused by succinylcholine.[65] The other class of muscle relaxant, nondepolarizing agents, either lower IOP by blocking extraocular muscle tone, or have no effect on it.[66,67,68,69,70] Endotracheal intubation in a lightly anesthetized, but paralyzed patient, however, can still lead to a sudden rise in IOP. This reflex can be minimized with topical tracheal anesthesia, a well-anesthetized patient (relaxed with obtunded reflexes), and if necessary, intravenous lidocaine.[47,71]

Anesthesia and Ocular Emergencies

The patient with a penetrating eye injury requires general anesthesia and meticulous control of IOP to prevent expulsion of the ocular contents. If the patient has recently eaten the problem is compounded. Optimally, there should be an eight-hour interval from the time food was ingested until the start of general anesthesia. If from the ocular point of view, however, surgery cannot be safely postponed, the following technique can be employed to prevent a sudden rise in IOP or pulmonary aspiration of stomach contents. Mannitol can be given intravenously 45 minutes prior to surgery. At the time of induction, 3 to 6 mg. of D-tubocurare or 10 to 20 mg. of gallamine are given intravenously. After preoxygenating the patient for 3 to 4 minutes, sodium pentothal, 4 to 6 mg./kg. is given, followed immediately by succinylcholine 80 to 120 mg. As soon as consciousness is lost, cricoid pressure is applied to prevent esophageal reflux and is continued until placement of the endotracheal tube.[72] This technique allows rapid intubation and prevents aspiration while minimizing the intraocular pressure elevating effects of succinylcholine through the combined use of preoperative mannitol, a defasciculating dose of curare or gallamine, and induction with sodium pentothal.[73]

Malignant Hyperthermia

Malignant hyperthermia is a rare, but feared, complication of general anesthesia. It is a reaction in which a familial defect in muscle metabolism generates more heat than the body can dissipate. If the reaction is not controlled, temperatures can rise to 110° F (43° C) with a fatal outcome. It has most commonly been triggered by succinylcholine, or even halothane and is said to be most prevalent in children, especially those who have strabismus and/or myotonia. However, at Wills Eye Hospital in the last 40,000 cases, there have been three cases of malignant hyperthermia. These involved a 17-year-old male having retinal detachment surgery and two adults undergoing penetrating keratoplasty.

It is crucial that the surgeon and anesthetist be aware of the clinical findings so that the reaction can be recognized early and treatment started. These findings include increased temperature, sweating, unstable blood pressure, a lack of response to succinylcholine, muscle rigidity, tachypnea and tachycardia, cardiac arrhythmias, mottling of the skin, cyanosis, respiratory and metabolic acidosis, and remarkable oxygen consumption. Treatment (Table 11-5) must begin before body temperature has reached 105° F (40° C) or success is unlikely. Anesthesia and surgery are immediately stopped and the patient is hyperventilated with 100% oxygen. Dantrolene should be given intravenously, 2 mg./kg. as an initial dose and repeated every 5 minutes until 10 mg./kg. total dose has been reached or symptoms disappear. In order to maintain arterial pH, sodium bicarbonate is administered, 100 mEq immediately and up to 600 mEq as necessary. In order to achieve maximum cooling, iced intravenous saline (not Ringer's lactate) solution is administered and stomach and colon irrigation with ice water accompanied by packing in ice or immersion in an ice water tank should be instituted. Ten units of regular insulin and 10 ml of 50% dextrose in water can be given slowly as a bolus to reduce potassium. Slowly must be emphasized, as hypokalemia frequently follows this period of hyperkalemia. Mannitol and furosemide are used to maintain urine output and procainamide used to control arrhythmias. If the onset of treatment is not delayed, the survival rate with this regimen is excellent.[74,75,76,77,78] The introduction of dantrolene has revolutionized the treatment of malignant hyperthermia and its administration should not be delayed while attention is diverted to control of other systemic factors.

Preoperative screening for susceptibility if positive, can alert operating room personnel and ensure early recognition of malignant hyperthermia. A family history of anesthetic exposure going back two generations can be helpful. Screening with blood CPK has been used in the past, but a recent study has shown that there are too many false positive and false negative results for this to be a useful test.[79] The most valuable test is in vitro contracture testing of muscle biopsy tissue. This is more than 90% reliable, but is only done in 10 centers in the United States and four in Canada. It therefore may be impractical to obtain. Patients with suspicious history can be treated as if they have the disease. Intravenous dantrolene (2 mg./kg.) may be given just prior to the induction of anesthesia, avoiding the uncertainty in blood levels associated

Table 11-5. Malignant Hyperthermia

Symptoms
Increasing temperature, sweating
Unstable blood pressure
Muscle rigidity
Tachypnea and tachycardia
Cardiac arrhythmias
Respiratory and metabolic acidosis
Treatment
Stop anesthesia and surgery
Hyperventilate with 100% oxygen
Administer Dantrolene: 2 mg/kg initially and repeat as needed according to symptoms every 5 minutes until 10 mg/kg total dosage is reached
Administer sodium bicarbonate: 100 mEq stat and up to 600 mEq as needed to maintain arterial pH
Institute packing in ice, cold intravenous saline, and stomach and colon irrigation with ice water
Administer 10 units regular insulin
Maintain urine output with mannitol and furosemide
Administer procainamide for arrythmia control

with the oral route.[80] Anesthesia should consist of nitrous oxide, barbiturates, narcotics, opiates, tranquilizers, and nondepolarizing muscle agents to minimize triggering the reaction. Potent volatile agents and depolarizing muscle relaxants are avoided even after pretreatment with dantrolene.[77,81,82]

Pediatric Anesthesia

To avoid complications in the pediatric age group a thorough understanding of the physiologic and pharmacologic differences between adults, neonates, and children is required. A surface-to-volume ratio, which is 70 times greater for a neonate than an adult, allows for quick cooling and hypothermia. This requires rigorous monitoring of the infant's temperature and often warming devices. The therapeutic drug range is much more narrow in this age group. Meticulous attention to dosages is required.[83]
Infants are easily dehydrated and are best scheduled early in the day. An appropriate regimen allows solid food and milk until 8 hours preoperatively and clear liquids until 6 hours before surgery.[44]

When surgery is required for infants of less than 44 weeks gestation, oxygen concentrations greater than those in room air are relatively contraindicated unless required for life. Retinopathy of prematurity has been reported as a possible sequelae.[84] An enzymatic defect seen in children, as well as adults, is congenital atypical pseudocholinesterase. Since pseudocholinesterase is responsible for hydrolyzing succinylcholine, these patients are subject to prolonged apnea if administered the drug and exhibit varying responses to muscle relaxants and anesthetic agents.

A common but difficult decision is seen in the child with a low grade fever. This can signal an oncoming illness, mild dehydration, or emotional stress and crying. If an obvious upper respiratory infection is present, then surgery should be postponed until the child is free of symptoms for two weeks, allowing laryngeal edema to subside.

The Oculocardiac Reflex

The oculocardiac reflex is more exaggerated in children and results in a slowing of the pulse in response to traction on the extraocular muscles or pressure on the eye. It can be associated with arrhythmias and even periods of asystole. Without anesthesia, these maneuvers have much less effect except in the presence of paroxysmal atrial tachycardia. Anesthesia, however, affects vagal sympathetic balance and 85% of patients will show a reflex bradycardia in response to pressure on the globe. Serious arrhythmias are much less frequent. Traction on the medial rectus is the most common stimulus, but even retrobulbar injections can cause enough ocular compression to elicit the reflex in almost 50% of patients.[85,86,87,88] Bradycardia persists for 10 to 15 seconds after the stimulus is stopped and is less likely to occur again if the stimulus is restarted.[89] Children under 12 years of age and individuals with brown irides are more susceptible. All anesthetics produce the reflex with approximately the same frequency and hypercarbia may exacerbate this incidence.[90] The pathway for the oculocardiac reflex has an afferent limb through the trigeminal nerve and an efferent limb through the vagus nerve.[91] Prevention and treatment can address both ends of this loop. A retrobulbar block reduces the incidence by one-half,[92,93 94,95] but the risk of complications inherent in the retrobulbar block probably exceeds the slight risk from the arrhythmias caused by the oculocardiac reflex. Gallamine can be used to increase the heart rate and thereby decrease the oculocardiac reflex, but is not consistently effective.[96] Atropine has long been used to prevent and treat the oculocardiac reflex, but its use is still controversial.[97,98] Intravenous atropine given in 0.007 mg./kg. increments and glycopyrrolate are effective in preventing bradycardia, although glycopyrrolate has a much slower onset time.

Current recommendations are to provide anticholinergic protection, keep the patient well ventilated to avoid hypercarbia and provide constant electrocardiographic monitoring. Gentle manipulation by the surgeon and an adequate depth of anesthesia are both helpful in preventing the oculocardiac reflex. If an arrythmia develops and persists, surgical manipulation should be halted until the heartbeat is regular again. If severe bradycardia persists, atropine is titrated. Smaller doses of atropine might have no effect, or paradoxically, worsen the arrhythmia. If the reflex cannot be abolished with atropine and more surgical stimulation is necessary, infiltration of the recti with local anesthetic may block the stimulus.[47]

Emotional and psychological support and careful preparation of the patient by the anesthetist is always important at any age, but is crucial in dealing with a child. Strong arm tactics will allow induction with the uncooperative child, but leave a deep-seated fear of medical personnel and surgery, a complication more serious than many ocular ones. This is often avoided if time is set aside for the anesthetist to establish rapport before surgery and instruct the child on what is to come. Allowing the parent to stay with the child in the preoperative room as long as possible can supply additional reassurance.

Conclusion

The quality of a patient's anesthesia plays a major role in not only the success of the procedure, but also in the stress levels of the surgeon and patient. The patient's memory of an easy comfortable surgical procedure ensures both the surgeon's reputation and the patient's willingness to return for other procedures. Combining optimum operating conditions for the surgeon and the greatest safety for the patient requires close cooperation between the surgeon and the anesthetist. This is most easily achieved if each has an understanding of the other's task and problems.

References

1. Koller K. Uber die verwendung des cocain zur anasthesierungam auge. Wine Med Bl 7:1352, 1884.
2. Maurice DM, Singh T. The absence of corneal toxicity with low-level topical anesthesia. Am J Ophthalmol 99:691, 1985.
3. Man WG, Wood R, Senterfit L, et al. Effect of topical anesthetics on regeneration of the corneal epithelium. Am J Ophthalmol 43:606, 1957.
4. Duffin RM, Olson RJ. Tetracaine toxicity. Ann Ophthalmol Sept 1984, p. 836.
5. Smith RB, Everett WG. Physiology and pharmacology of local anesthetic agents (anesthesia in ophthalmology). Int Ophthalmol Clin 13:56, 1973.
6. Havener WH. Ocular Pharmacology. St. Louis, CV Mosby, 1978, Chapter 5.
7. Ritchie JM, Cohen PJ. Cocaine procaine and other synthetic local anesthetics. In Goodman LS, Gilman A (eds). The Pharmacological Basis of Therapeutics. New York, Macmillan, 1975, Chapter 2.
8. Frayer, WC. Local anesthesia: Indications and techniques. In Duane TT, (ed). Clinical Ophthalmology, Vol. 5. Philadelphia, Harper and Row, 1978, Chapter 2.
9. Crandall DC. Pharmacology of ocular anesthetics. In Duane TD, Jaeger EA (eds). Biomedical Foundations of Ophthalmology, Vol. 3. Philadelphia, Harper and Row, 1983, Chapter 35.
10. Carolan JA, Cerasoli JR, Houle TV: Bupivacaine in retrobulbar anesthesia. Ann Ophthalmol 6:843-847, 1974.
11. Adriani, J. Newer anesthetics, sedatives, Therapeutics: Transactions of the New Orleans Academy of Ophthalmology. St. Louis: C.V. Mosby, 1970, Chapter 20.
12. Bryant JA. Local and topical anesthetics in ophthlamology. Surv Ophthlamol 13:263, 1969.

13. Lufstrom B. Aspects of pharmacology of local ansethetic agents. Anaesth 42:194, 1970.
14. Lufstrom B., Green K, Jansson O, et al. An evaluation of bupivacaine (Marcaine) without adrenaline. Acta Anaesth Scand 37 (suppl):282, 1970.
15. Alper MH. Toxicity of local anesthetics. N Engl J Med 295:1432, 1976.
16. Meyers EF, Ramirez RC, Boniuk I. Grand mal seizures after retrobulbar block. Arch Ophthlamol 98:847, 1978.
17. Smith JL. Retrobulbar bupivacaine can cause respiratory arrest. Ann Ophthlamol 12:1005, 1982.
18. Drysdale DB. Experimental subdural retrobulbar injection of anesthetic. Ann Ophthalmol 16(8):716, 1984.
19. Lombardi G. Radiology in Neurophthalmology. Baltimore, Williams and Wilkins, 1967, page 6.
20. Hamilton RC. Brain stem anesthesia following retrobulbar blockade. Anesthesiology 63:688, 1985.
21. Friedberg HL, Kline DR. Contralateral amaurosis after retrobulbar injection. Am J Ophthalmol 101:688, 1986.
22. Follette JW, LoCasiscio JA. Bilateral amaurosis following unilateral retrobulbar block. Anesthesiology 63:238, 1985.
23. Chang J, GonxalexAbola E, Larson CE, et al. Brainstem anesthesia following retrobulbar block. Anesthesiology 61:789, 1984.
24. Beltranea H, Vega MJ, Garcia JJ, et al. Complications of retrobulbar marcaine injection. J Clin Neuroophthalmol 2:159, 1982.
25. Wittpen JR, Rapoza P, Sternberg Jr P, et al. Respiratory arrest following retrobulbar anesthesia. Ophthalmology 93:867, 1986.
26. Chostain, GM. Acute blood levels of lidocaine following paracervical block. J Med Assoc Ga 158:426, 1969.
27. Keating V. Anesthetic Accidents, 2nd ed., Chicago, Year Book Publishers, 1961, p. 176.
28. Arimes, DA, Cotes, Jr, W. Deaths from paracervical anesthesia used for first trimester abortion. 1972, 1975, N Eng J Med 295:25, December 1966.
29. Kaplan LJ, Jaffe NS, Clayman HM. Ptosis and cataract surgery, a multivariant computer analysis of a prospective study. Ophthlamology 92:237,1985.
30. Wilson CA, Ruiz RS. Respiratory obstruction following the Nadbath facial nerve block. Arch Ophthalmol 103:1454, 1985.
31. Shoch D. Complications of the Nadbath facial nerve block. Arch Ophthalmol 104:1114, 1986.
32. Rabinowitz L, Livingston M, Schneider H, Hall A. Respiratory obstruction following the Nadbath facial nerve block. Arch Ophthalmol 104:1115, 1986.
33. Spaeth GL. A new method to achieve complete akinesia of the facial nerve muscles of the eyelids. Ophthalmic Surg 7:105, 1976.
34. Sullivan KL, Brown GC, Forman AR, Sergott RC, Flanagan, JC. Retrobulbar anesthesia and retinal vascular obstruction. Ophthalmology 90:373, 1986.

35. Pautler SE, Grizzaard WS, Thompson LN, Wing GL. Blindness from retrobulbar injection into the optic nerve. Ophthalmic Surgery 17:334, 1986.
36. Klein ML, Jampol LM, Concon PI, Rice TA, Serjeant GR. Central retinal arter occlusion without retrobulbar hemorrhage after retrobulbar anesthesia. Am J Ophthalmol 93:573, 1982.
37. Bolder PM, Norton ML. Retinal hemorrhage following anesthesia. Anesthesiology 61:595, 1984.
38. Atkinson WS. The development of ophthalmic anesthesia. Am J Ophthalmol 51:114, 1961.
39. Unsld R, Stanley JA, DeGroot, J. The CT topography of retrobulbar anesthesia. Graefes Arch Clin Exp Ophthalmol 217:125, 1981.
40. Laval J. Retrobulbar block. Arch Ophthalmol 104:22, 1986.
41. Davis II DB, Mandel MR. Posterior peribulbar anesthesia: An alternative to retrobulbar anesthesia. J Catarct Refract Surg 12:182, 1986.
42. Wolf GL, Lynch S, Berlin I. Intraocular surgery with general anesthesia. Arch Ophthalmol 93:323, 1975.
43. PrysRoberts C, Meloche R, Foex P. Studies of anesthesia in relation to hypertension. 1. Cardiovascular responses of treated and untreated patients. Br J Anaesth 43:122, 1971.
44. Goldman L, Caldera DL. Risks of General anesthesia and elective operastion in the hypertensive patient. Anesthesiology 50:285, 1979.
45. Donlon Jr JV. Anesthesia for eye, ear, nose and throat. In Miller RD (ed). Anesthesia, Vol. 3, New York, Churchill Livingstone, 1986, Chapter 52.
46. Adams A, Fordham RMM. General anesthesia in adults. Int Ophthalmol Clin 13:83, Summer 1973.
47. Stoelting RK. Endotracheal intubation. In Miller RD (ed). Anesthesia, Vol. 1, New York Churchill Livingstone, 1986, Chapter 16.
48. Rosen DA. Anesthesia in ophthalmology. Canad Anesth J 9:545, 1962.
49. Edwards RE, Miller RD, Roizen MF, et al. Cardiac effects of imipramine and pancuronium during halothane and enflurane anesthesia. Anesthesiology 50:421, 1979.
50. Kosanin R. Anesthetic considerations in patients on chronictricyclic antidepressant therapy. Anesthesiol. Rev. 8:38, 1981.
51. Hill GE, Wong KC. Lithium carbonate and neuromuscular blocking agents. Anesthesiology 46:122, 1977.
52. Martin BA, Kramer PM. Clinical significance of the interaction between lithium and a neuromuscular blocker. Am J Psychiatry 139:1326, 1982.
53. Martin BA, Kramer PM. Clinical significance of the interaction between lithium and a neuromuscular blocker. Am J Psychiatry 139:1326, 1982.
54. Haidinzak JG, Didier EP. Case history number 95: Anesthetics and propranolol, anesthesia and analgesia. Curr Res 56(6):283, 1977.
55. Corssen G, John JE. A new parenteral anesthetic CL581: Its effect on intraocular pressure. J Ped Ophthalmol 4:20, 1962.
56. Pandey K, Badola RP, Kumar S. Time course of intraocular hypertension produced by suxamethonium. Br J Anaesth 44:191, 1972.

57. Magora F, Collins VJ. The influence of general anesthetic agents on intraocular pressure in man. Arch Ophthalmol 66:806, 1962.
58. Eakins KE, Katz RL. The action of succinylcholine on the tension of extraocular muscle. Br J Pharmacol 26:205, 1966.
59. Miller RD, Way WL, Hickey RF. Inhibition muscle relaxants. Anesthesiology 29:123, 1968.
60. Bowen DJ, McGrand JC, Palmer RJ. Intraocular pressure after pretreatment with pancuronium. Br J Anaesth 48:1201, 1975.
61. Meyers EF, Krupin T, Johnson M, et al. Failure of nondepolarizing neuromuscular blockers to inhibit succinylcholine induced increased intraocular pressure. Anesthesiology 48:149, 1978.
62. Giala MM, Balamoutsos NG, et al. Failure of gallamineto inhibit succinylcholine induced increase in IOP.
63. Carballo AS. Succinylcholine and acetazolamide in anesthesia for ocular surgery. Can Anaesth Soc J 12:486, 19865.
64. Goldsmith E. An evaluation of succinylcholine and gallamineas muscle relaxants in relation to intraocular tension. Anaesthanalg 46:557, 1967.
65. Litwiller RW, DiFazio C, Rushia EL. Pancuronium and intraocular pressure. Anesthesiology 42:750, 1975.
66. Balamoutos NG, Tsakona H, et al. Alcuronium and intraocular pressure. Anesth Analg 62:521, 1983.
67. Cunningham AJ, Kelly PC, et al. Effect of metocurine pancuronium combination on IOP. Can Anaesth Soc J 29:617, 1982.
68. Agarwal LP, Mathur SP. Curare in ocular surgery. Br J Ophthalmol 36:603, 1952.
69. Van Aken H. Prevention of hypertension at intubation with intravenous lidocaine. Anaesthesia 37:82, 1982.
70. Sellick BA. Cricoid pressure to control regurgitation of stomach contents during induction of anesthesia, preliminary communication. Lancet 2:404, 1961.
71. Libonati MM, Leahy JJ, Ellison N. The use of succinylcholine in open eye surgery. Anesthesiology 62:637, 1985.
72. Sedwick LA, Romano PE. Malignant hyperthermia considerations for the Ophthalmologist. Surv Ophthalmol 25:378, 1981.
73. Gromert GA. Malignant hyperthermia. In Miller RD (ed.) Anesthesia, New York, Churchill Livingstone, 1986, Vol. 3, Chapter 56.
74. Herschel EO (ed.). Malignant hyperthermia, current concepts. New York, Appleton Century Crofts, 1977.
75. Gromert GA. Malignant hyperthermia. In Miller RD (ed.) Anesthesia, New York, Churchill Livingstone, 1986, Vol. 3, Chapter 56.
76. Gronert GA. Malignant hyperthermia. Seminars in anesthesia 2:197, 1983.
77. Paasuke RT, Brownell KB. Serum creatine kinase level as a screening test for susceptibility to malignant hyperthermia. JAMA 255:769, 1986.
78. Flewellen EH, Nelson TE, Jones WP, et al. Dantrolenedose response in awake man: implications for management of malignant hyperthermia. Anesthesiology 59:275, 1983.

79. Ruhland G, Hinkle AF. Malignant hyperthermia following preoperative oral administration of dantrolene. Anesthesiology, 60:159, 1984.
80. Fitzgibbons DC. Malignant hyperthermia following preopoerative oral administration of dantrolene. Anesthesiology, 54:73, 1981.
81. Gregory GA. Pediatric anesthesia. In Miller RD (ed.) Anesthesia, New York, Churchill Livingstone, 1986, Vol. 3, Chapter 49.
82. Belts E. Dumes JJ, Shaeffer D, Johns R. Retrolental firboplasia and oxygen administration during general anestheisa. Anesthesiology, 47:518, 1977.
83. Potinen PJ. The importance of the oculocardiac reflex during intraocular surgery. Acta Ophthalmol 86:1, 1966.
84. Newell FW. Current trends in ophthalmic anesthesia. Ophthalmic Surg 6(2):125, Summer 1975.
86. Alexander JP. Reflex disturbance of cardiac rhythm during ophthalmic surgery. Br J Ophthalmol 59:518, 1975.
87. Mirakhur RK, Jones CJ, Dundee JW, et al. Atropine orglycopyrrolate for the prevention of OCR children undergoing squint surgery. Br J Anaesth 54:1059, 1982.
88. Blanc VF, Hardy JF, Milot J, et al. The OCR: A graphic and statistcal analysis in infants and children. Can Anaesth. Soc J 30:360, 1983.
89. Forestner JE, Imbrech P. Controlled respiration does not inhibit OCR during strabismus surgery. Anesthesiology 59:A457, 1983.
90. Atkinson WS. Anesthesia in Ophthalmology. Springfield, IL, Charles C. Thomas, 1955, p. 42.
91. Monnie GT, Rees DI, Elton D. The oculocardia reflex during strabismus surgery. Canad Anesth Soc J, 11:621, 1964.
92. Berler D. The oculocardiac reflex. Am J Ophthalmol, 56:954, 1963.
93. Mendelblatt F, Kirsch RE, Lemberg L. A study comparing methods of preventing the oculocardiac reflex. Am J Ophthalmol 53:506, 1962.
94. Alexander JP. Reflex disturbance of cardiac rhythm during ophthalmic surgery. Br J Ophthalmol 59:518, 1975.
95. Linn JG Jr, Smith RB. Intraoperative complications and their management. Int Ophthalmol Clin 13:149, Summer 1973.
96. Blanc VF. The effect of anticholinergic premedication for infants and children on the OCR. Can Anaesth Soc J 30:683, 1983.
97. Steward D. The effect of anticholinergic premedication in infants and children on the OCR. Can Anaesth Soc J 30:684, 1983.

CHAPTER 12

Filtering Procedures: The Patients

Mark B. Sherwood, MD

Studies have shown that for patients with phakic primary open angle glaucoma, standard filtration surgery—either full thickness or guarded—has a successful rate of approximately 60 to 85%.[1-4] Success has been variously defined by the different series but is perhaps best described as attainment of a suitable IOP, such that there is no further progression of field loss or optic nerve damage. The specific level of IOP required to achieve this varies among patients. Patients with far advanced optic nerve damage generally require a lower final pressure to prevent further nerve damage. Abrupt lowering of pressure in these patients, however, particularly in those with splitting of fixation or a small central island of visual field, can also present problems; "snuff out" of the central field with marked decrease in visual acuity has been recorded following surgery.[5]

Techniques

Every experienced surgeon has a filter technique that he or she prefers and that gives good results. We routinely perform a guarded trabeculectomy, originally described by Cairns,[6] in cases with a hypertensive glaucoma. This procedure offers a suitable lowering of IOP in most cases and is associated with less postoperative complications than full-thickness filters.

The amount of drainage obtained from the guarded trabeculectomy can be greatly varied in response to the needs of the patient. For those in whom a low IOP is required, less sutures are placed in the scleral flap and they can be tied less tightly. Further, the deep trabeculectomy block can be excised so that its side borders are only minimally overlapped by the overlying scleral flap. This will increase flow through the nasal and temporal margins of the flap. Patients with a shallow anterior chamber, especially if they have preexisting peripheral anterior synechiae, might need a more conservative filter procedure to reduce the chance of postoperative flat chamber and possible aqueous misdirection.

An oblique, self-sealing paracentesis tract through clear cornea is recommended at an early stage in the operation (Fig. 12-1). Besides allowing the anterior chamber to be left well inflated at the end of the surgery, this also permits the amount of fluid flow through the filter site to be directly accessed. After two corner sutures have been placed in the rectangular, partial-thickness scleral flap the anterior chamber is reformed with balance salt solution, via the paracentesis tract (Fig. 12-2). The aqueous egress, if insufficient, can be increased by careful diathermy to the nasal or temporal borders of the scleral flap or by loosening the flap sutures. Alternatively, if excessive, it can be decreased by the placement of extra sutures. The result of each maneuver is reviewed by refilling the anterior chamber with further balanced saline until the flow through the filter site appears correct. The amount of drainage is adjusted for each individual.

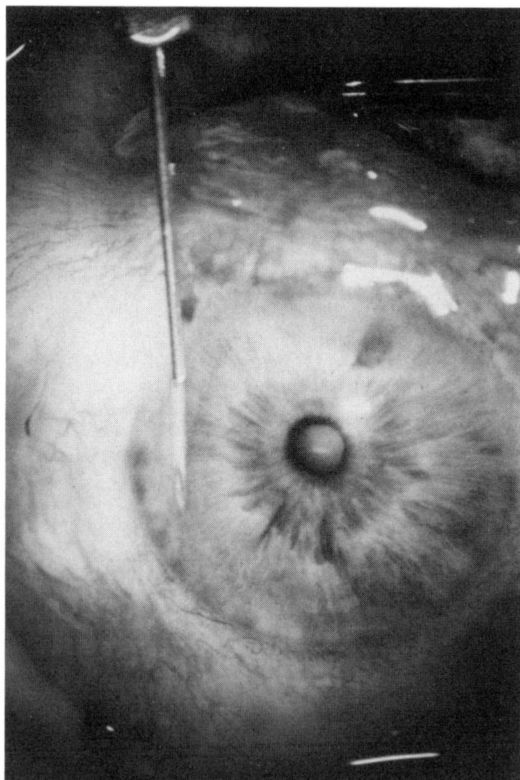

Figure 12-1. Self-sealing peripheral paracentesis tract made with round 25- or 27-gauge needle.

Modification for the Individual

In patients with advanced field loss, where the surgeon desires to obtain low pressures, a greater leakage through the filter site can be allowed. The need for increased leakage, however, must be weighed against the added risk

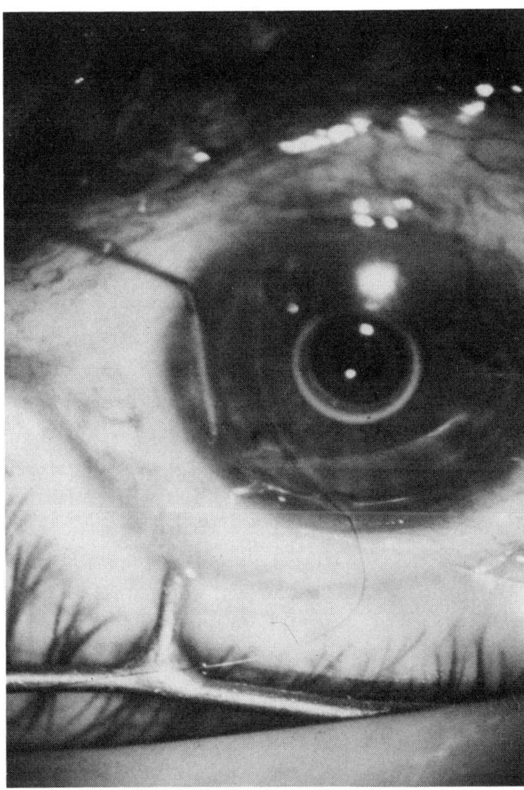

Figure 12-2. 30-gauge blunt tipped canula introduced into the anterior chamber via the 27-gauge needle tract. The chamber can be repeatedly reformed using this and the amount of flow through the filter site tested.

of postoperative flat anterior chamber and serous choroidal detachment. If a particularly low final IOP is required, the guarded trabeculectomy can be further modified either by the placement of releasable sutures at surgery (See Chapter 13), or postsurgically by early cutting of the scleral flap sutures using a Hoskins-style lens and the argon laser. In the latter case, should the Tenon's capsule be thick, a tenonectomy might be required to allow adequate visualization of the scleral flap sutures. These techniques have the advantage of decreased risk of early hypotony and flat anterior chamber, from an initially tightly sutured scleral flap, together with later high aqueous flow from an unsutured or only partially sutured flap.

In patients with progressive "low-tension" glaucoma, where low-normal or even subnormal pressures are needed, a thermal sclerostomy, trephine, or unsutured scleral flap is recommended by many.[7] The postoperative IOP is, in general, lower with these than with other techniques. Full-thickness techniques have also been recommended for black patients.[8] These methods can be combined with the immediate postoperative use of a Simmon's compressions shell[9] to reduce the risk of complications from excessive drainage (See Chapter 13). Although it has been demonstrated that greater optic nerve damage is seen in the eye with the higher IOP, in patients with asymmetric low-tension glaucoma,[10] there is still no clear evidence that reducing IOP in patients with low-tension glaucoma to subnormal levels will prevent further progression of field loss.[11] Surgery to one eye and continued medical therapy to the other are recommended in these cases until the results of the initial surgery are established.

Several authorities have suggested that early surgery for glaucoma might be beneficial.[12,13] Recent evidence indicates that there is an increase in the number of inflammatory cells in conjunctival and tenon's capsule tissue in patients who have received long-term medical therapy.[14] Preliminary data has further shown that patients undergoing primary trabeculectomy surgery for POAG might have a higher success rate than those who have received several years of medical antiglaucoma treatment before surgery,[15] although it is difficult to strictly compare the two patient groups.

For each individual the surgeon must evaluate the likelihood of a successful outcome using a standard filtration technique. Some patients might be unwilling to consider further, repeat surgery. The importance of a good result at the first procedure cannot be overstressed, both from the patient's psychological standpoint and with regard to the final ocular prognosis. The success rate at reoperation is much reduced,[16,17] mainly because each surgical manipulation of the eye causes inflammation and increases fibrous tissue formation. Both will increase the likelihood of external scarring of the bleb. Additionally, first-time success is important, since the best site for filtration surgery is usually utilized at the first procedure, leaving only more difficult areas available for reoperation. Also, the conjunctiva and tenon's capsule will be more adherent to underlying tissues at reoperation, thus increasing the risks of complications, such as button-hole formation. Although serious, sight-threatening complications are rare, every additional procedure adds to these risks.

There are certain individual patient factors that have a significant influence on the outcome of standard filtration surgery. These are presented in Table 12-1.

Table 12-1. Patient Factors Influencing Success of Surgery
Age of Patient
Race
Type of glaucoma
Aphakia or pseudophakia
Previous ocular surgery
Extent of optic nerve damage
Duration of medical antiglaucoma therapy
Other ocular disease — uveitis, cataract (combined procedure)

Young patients,[18] blacks,[19] those with a secondary or a developmental glaucoma,[18,20,21] aphakes,[22,23] and patients who have undergone previous surgery involving the conjunctiva[16,17] have a higher risk of subsequent bleb failure. In most cases this is because of external fibrosis of the filtration fistula.[24-26] A number of intra- and postoperative modifications to the standard technique have been proposed for patients with a poor prognosis. These include drainage devices to shunt aqueous, via a biologically inert tube, to an area where fibrosis is less likely to occur, and the use of chemical antifibrotic agents.

Preliminary data suggest that subconjunctival 5-fluorouracil given postoperatively can improve the success rate of trabeculectomy in patients with aphakia, those with a previously failed filter, those with an inflammatory glaucoma, and in those with neovascular glaucoma.[27-30] A larger, multicenter, prospective study is in progress to verify these findings. The use of 5-fluorouracil is not without risks. Vision-impairing corneal stroma ulcers have been reported.[31] Lower dose 5-fluorouracil regimens have been proposed to reduce the incidence of side effects[29,30] but these do not eliminate the problems of corneal toxicity or wound leakage nor the need for careful patient monitoring. At this time the use of 5-fluorouracil is recommended only in certain selected patients with a poor prognosis, and at centers where an adequate, daily review of the patient can be undertaken during the initial postoperative period. Other adjunctive chemical agents, such as beta-aminopropionitrile and D-penicillamine, are being investigated but use of these drugs is still experimental.[32,33]

Drainage devices have been described by a number of authors.[34-37] Each employs a narrow silicone or silastic tube to shunt aqueous to a protected area. Results obtained using these tubes have been especially impressive in patients with neovascular glaucoma. They are recommended by some as a first line of surgical treatment in these eyes, providing the eye has a reasonable visual potential. They might also be considered for the management of other poorly responsive glaucomas, particularly in those cases with a history of multiple previous failed surgeries.

These modifications might enhance the chance of success in cases with refractory glaucoma, but they carry risks of possibly increased postoperative morbidity. These are discussed in Chapters 13 and 15. The surgeon's familiarity with the particular modified technique is a further factor to consider. For these reasons, standard filtration surgery is still preferred, at present, for phakic patients with a primary glaucoma undergoing their first surgery.

Patients with certain conditions bear special consideration because they often respond poorly to filtration surgery.

Nanophthalmos

The term "nanophthalmos" has been coined to describe a pure form of microphthalmos in which there are no other related structural or developmental abnormalities of the eye or body.[38] The eye is short and has a small overall volume, but is otherwise normal. The anterior chamber is shallow, but the crystalline lens is of normal size. There might be scleral thickening. Arrested development after the stage of embryonic fissure closure is responsible for the condition. There is an associated high hyperopia and a predisposition to angle closure glaucoma. Miotics can worsen angle obstruction by producing a relative pupillary block and by relaxing the lens zonules.

Filtration or cataract surgery in these patients is often followed by choroidal detachment and secondary, nonrhegmatogenous retinal detachment (uveal effusion).[39] Choroidal detachment can also develop spontaneously before any surgery.[40] Systemic steroids[39] or surgical vortex vein decompression[41] have been suggested for the management of these posterior segment complications. There is a high risk also of malignant (ciliary block) glaucoma following trabeculectomy, because of the shallow anterior chamber.[42]

The management of these nanophthalmic patients is initially medical. Topical beta blockers and systemic carbonic anhydrase inhibitors are the most effective drugs for IOP control. Surgical intervention is avoided whenever possible.

At the earliest stage, when there is no glaucoma, the angles are regularly examined for evidenced of progressive narrowing. If the risk of angle closure is large, laser therapy is recommended. This includes argon laser gonioplasty (iridoplasty) to contract the peripheral iris and thereby widen the angle, together with argon or Nd:YAG laser iridectomy to prevent pupillary block. The details of these procedures are discussed in Chapters 8 and 9. The effect of gonioplasty gradually can be lost with time, but the procedure can be repeated at intervals if the angle narrows. Laser iridectomy can be very difficult in nanophthalmic patients, because the iris seems thicker than usual and might be hard to penetrate. Noninvasive methods are preferred because of the high risks associated with any intraocular surgery. Surgical iridectomy is reserved for those in whom a patent iridotomy cannot be obtained with the laser. To be effective, iridectomy should be performed before significant peripheral anterior synechial closure of the angle occurs.

Filtration surgery is contraindicated in all except those patients with extensive synechial closure who have uncontrolled IOPs despite maximum medical therapy. Modification of the filtration surgery to avoid postoperative hypotony and performing prophylactic posterior sclerectomies in the lower quadrants has been recommended.[40]

Sturge Weber Syndrome

Sturge Weber Syndrome is a congenital hamartomatous malformation producing hemangiomas of the skin, meninges, and eye. Glaucoma occurs in about 30% of cases, usually (in 60%) before the age of two.[43,44] It is frequently difficult to control the IOP in these patients medically, and goniotomy has had a poor success rate.[45-47] Trabeculectomy has been advocated as a treatment of choice for patients unresponsive to medical therapy, but there is a high risk of expulsive hemorrhage,[48,49] intraoperative massive choroidal effusion,[50-53] and serous retinal detachment.[50,51] The lens, ciliary body, and iris are pushed forward with flattening of the anterior chamber. Ciliary process, which rotate anteriorly, can prolapse into the fistula site[50,54] or the peripheral iridectomy;[51] and rupture of lens zonules has been recorded with presentation of vitreous into the trabeculectomy wound.[54] The iris can prolapse and be difficult to reposit.[50]

The cause of these problems is the rapid development of uveal effusion that can occur in eyes with an elevated episcleral venous pressure when the anterior chamber is opened and the pressure in the anterior segment suddenly reduced to atmospheric level. The mechanism has been postulated to be similar to the common postoperative choroidal detachment, but the degree and speed with which it develops makes surgery difficult and potentially hazardous.[52] Angiomatous involvement of the choroid as well as of the episclera has been demonstated,[55] and a greater than normal pressure differential will exist across the capillary membranes of the ciliary body and choroid. This will encourage rapid transudation of fluid from the intravascular to the extravascular space when the IOP is lowered to zero at surgery.[50]

To reduce the risk of intraoperative complications, as well as of prolonged postoperative choroidal detachment and flat anterior chamber, it is recommended that a posterior sclerotomy be performed before the anterior chamber is opened.[50] This allows any effusion fluid formed to drain and relieves the forward pressure on the lens, ciliary body, and iris.[47]

References

1. Yashimata H, Eguchi S, Yamamoto T, et al. Trabeculectomy: a prospective study of complications and results of long-term follow-up. Jpn J Ophthalmol 29:250-262, 1985.
2. Shirato S, Kitazawa Y, Mishima S. A critical analysis of the trabeculectomy results by a prospective follow-up design. Jpn J Ophthalmol 26:468-480, 1982.
3. Lewis RA, Phelps CD. Trabeculectomy v Thermosclerostomy—a five-year follow-up. Arch Ophthalmol 102:533-536, 1984.
4. Shuster JN, Krupin T, Kolker AE, et al. Limbus— v fornix-based conjunctival flap in trabeculectomy. A long term randomized study. Arch Ophthalmol 102:361-364, 1984.
5. Cairns JE. Surgical methods currently in use in the glaucomas. In Cairns JE, (ed): Glaucoma, London, Grune and Stratton pp 173-190, 1986.
6. Cairns JE. A preliminary report of a new method. Amer J Ophthalmol 66:673-679, 1968.
7. Abedin S, Simmons RJ, Grant WM. Progressive low-tension glaucoma. Treatment to stop glaucomatous cupping and field loss when these progress despite normal intraocular pressure. Ophthalmol 89:1-6, 1982.
8. Shingleton, BJ, Distler JA, Baker BH. Filtration surgery in black patients: early results in a West Indian population. Ophthalmic Surg 18:195-199, 1987.
9. Simmons RI, Singh OS. Shell tamponade technique in glaucoma surgery. In Symposium on Glaucoma, Transactions of the New Orleans Academy of Ophthalmology. St Louis: CV Mosby, 1981.
10. Cartwright MJ, Anderson DR. Correlation of asymmetric damage with assymetric intraocular pressure in normal-tension glaucoma (low-tension glaucoma). Arch Ophthalmol 106:898-900, 1988.
11. Sheilds MB. Textbook of Glaucoma, ed 2. Baltimore: Williams & Wilkins, 1987, p 157.

12. Watson PG, Grierson I. The place of trabeculectomy in the treatment of glaucoma. Ophthalmol 88:175-196, 1981.
13. Jay JL. Earlier trabeculectomy. Trans Ophthalmol Soc UK 103:35-38, 1983.
14. Sherwood MB, Grierson I, Hitchings RA. Long-term morphological effects of antiglaucoma drugs on the conjunctiva and tenons in glaucomatous patients. Invest Ophthalmol Vis Sci (suppl) 28:135, 1987.
15. Lavin MJ, Migdal CS, Hitchings RA. The influence of prior medical therapy on success of trabeculectomy. Submitted.
16. Schwartz AL, Anderson DR. Trabecular surgery. Arch Ophthalmol 92:134-138, 1974.
17. Cohen JS, Shaffer RB, Heatherington J, et al. Revision of filtration surgery. Arch Ophthalmol 95:1612-1615, 1977.
18. Gressel MG, Heuer DK, Parrish RK. Trabeculectomy in young patients. Ophthalmol 91:1242-1246, 1984.
19. Miller RD, Barber JC. Trabeculectomy in black patients. Ophthalmic Surg 12:46-50, 1981.
20. Portney GL. Trabeculectomy and postoperative hypertension in secondary angle closure glaucoma. Am J Ophthalmol 84:145-149, 1977.
21. Allen RC, Bellows R, Hutchinson T, et al. Filtration surgery in the treatment of neovascular glaucoma. Ophthalmol 89:1181-1187, 1982.
22. Heuer DK, Gressel MG, Parrish RK et al. Trabeculectomy in aphakic eyes. Ophthalmol 91:1045-1051, 1984.
23. Bellows AR, Johnstone MA. Surgical management of chronic glaucoma in aphakia. Ophthalmol 90:807-813, 1983.
24. Maumenee AE. External filtering operations for glaucoma: the mechanism of function and failure. Trans Am Ophthalmol Soc 58:319-328, 1960.
25. Hitchings RA, Grierson I. Clinicopathological correlation in eyes with failed fistulizing surgery. Trans Ophthalmol Soc UK 103:84-88, 1983.
26. Addicks EM, Quigley HA, Green WR, et al: Histologic characteristics of filtering blebs in glaucomatous eyes. Arch Ophthalmol 101:795-798, 1983.
27. Heuer DK, Parrish RK, Gressel MG, et al: 5-Fluorouracil and glaucoma filtering surgery. II. A pilot study. Ophthalmol 91:384-393, 1984.
28. Rockwood EI, Parrish RK II, Heuer DK, et al. Glaucoma filtering surgery with 5-fluorouracil Ophthalmol 94:1071-1078, 1987.
29. Ruderman SM, Welch DB, Smith MF, et al. A randomized study of 5-fluorouracil and filtration surgery. Am J Ophthalmol 104:218-224, 1987.
30. Weinreb RN. Adjusting the dose of 5-fluorouracil after filtration surgery to minimize side effects. Ophthalmol 94:564-570, 1987.
31. Knapp A, Heuer DK, Stern GA, et al. Serious corneal complications of glaucoma filtering surgery with postoperative 5-fluorouracil. Am J Ophthalmol 103:183-187, 1987.
32. Moorehead LC, Smith J, Stewart R, et al. Effects of beta-aminopropionitrile after glaucoma filtering surgery; pilot human study. Ann Ophthalmol 19:223-225, 1987.

33. McGuigan LJB, Mason RP, Sanchez R, et al. D-penicillamine and beta-aminopropionitrile effects on experimental filtering surgery. Invest Ophthalmol Vis Sci 28:1625-1629, 1987.
34. Molteno ACB, Straughan JL, Ancker E. Long tube implants in the management of glaucoma. S Afr Med J 50:1062-1066, 1976.
35. Krupin T, Kaufman P, Mandell AI, et al. Long-term results of valve implants in filtering surgery for eyes with neovascular glaucoma. Am J Ophthalmol 95:775-782, 1983.
36. Schocket SS, Nirankari VS, Lakhanpal V, et al. Anterior chamber tube shunt to an encircling band in the treatment of neovascular and other refractory glaucomas. Ophthalmol 92:553-562, 1985.
37. Joseph NH, Sherwood MB, Trantas G, et al. A one-piece drainage system for glaucoma surgery. Trans Ophthalmol Soc UK 105:657-664, 1986.
38. Duke-Elder S. System of Ophthalmology. St Louis: CV Mosby, 1963 Vol. 3:488-495.
39. Brockhurst RI. Nanophthalmos with uveal effusion. A new clinical entity. Arch Ophthalmol 93:1289-1299, 1975.
40. Simmons RJ. Nanophthalmos, diagnosis and treatment. In Chandler and Grant's Glaucoma 3rd ed. Philadelphia: Lea & Febiger, pp 251-256, 1986.
41. Brockhurst RJ. Vortex vein decompression for nanophthalmic uveal effusion. Arch Ophthalmol 98:1987-1990, 1980.
42. Calhoun FP. The management of glaucoma in nanophthalmos. Trans Am Ophthalmol Soc 73:97-122, 1975.
43. Font RL, Ferry AP. The phakomatoses. Int Ophthalmol Clin 12:1-50, 1972.
44. Weiss DI. Dual origin of glaucoma in encephalotrigeminal Trans Ophthalmol Soc UK 93:477-493, 1973.
45. Shaffer RN, Weiss DL. Congenital and pediatric glaucomas. Saint Louis: CV Mosby, 1970, pp 60-67.
46. Lister A. The prognosis in congenital glaucoma. Trans Ophthalmol Soc UK 86:5-18, 1966.
47. Walton ES. Hemangioma of the lid with glaucoma. In Chandler and Grant's Glaucoma 3rd ed. Philadelphia: Lea & Febiger, 1986, pp 512-514.
48. Duke-Elder S. System of Ophthalmology, St. Louis: CV Mosby, 1969, 9:637-640.
49. Christiansen GR, Records RE. Glaucoma and expulsive hemorrhage mechanism in the Sturge-Weber syndrome. Ophthalmol 86:1360-1366, 1979.
50. Bellows AR, Chylack LT, Epstein DL, et al. Choroidal effusion during glaucoma surgery in patients with prominent episcleral vessels. Arch Ophthalmol 97:493-497, 1979.
51. Board RJ, Shield MB. Combined trabeculotomy-trabeculectomy for management of glaucoma associated with Sturge-Weber syndrome. Ophthalmol Surg 12:813-817, 1981.

52. Shihab ZM, Kristan RW. Recurrent intraoperative choroidal effusion in Sturge-Weber syndrome. J Ped Ophthalmol Strabis 250-252, 1980.
53. Ruiz RS, Salmonsen PC. Expulsive choroidal effusion complication of intraocular surgery. Arch Ophthalmol 94:69-70, 1975.
54. Rosenbaum LJ: Glaucoma in Sturge-Weber syndrome. Birth Defects 18(6):645-649, 1982.
55. Witschel H, Font RL: Hemangioma of the choroid: a clinicopathologic study of 71 cases and review of the literature. Surv Ophthalmol 20:415-431, 1976.

CHAPTER 13

Filtering Procedures: The Procedures

Full-Thickness versus Guarded Procedures

Roger A. Hitchings, FRCS

Following the recognition that elevated IOP was a major cause of visual loss in glaucoma, ophthalmologists have been devising ways of controlling (lowering) it. The surgical options that have been exercised have been directed toward bypassing the resistance to aqueous outflow at the trabecular meshwork. Over the past 80 years more than 100 operations (or modifications thereof), have been described. Each of these operations was designed to establish an alternative route between the anterior chamber and the subconjunctival space. The number of operations that have been described owe more to changing fashions in surgery than to undoubted superiority of one operation over another. In recent years, two operation subtypes have predominated, the thermal, unguarded, sclerostomy and the guarded sclerostomy. The former, which uses heat to retract wound edges derives from the sclerostomy of Preziosi, modified by Scheie. The latter idea, where a deep block of tissue is removed, but bulk outflow is restricted by a superficial lamellar flap was suggested by Suger and popularized by Cairns, called by both a trabeculectomy. This introduction compares and contrasts these two types of operations. It discusses the techniques, advantages, and disadvantages of both and concludes with suggested indications.

Technique

General Points of Technique Common to Both Types of Operation

A standard approach needs to be used, involving local anesthetic or a general anesthetic according to the patients and surgeon's preference. (It should be remembered that the local anesthetic can be restricted to topically applied drops or subconjunctival injection, for the sensory nerves involved are to be found in the conjunctiva, and a few in the iris root. This maneuver is not painful if no traction is placed upon the iris root during irridectomy.

An adequate microsurgical technique for glaucoma surgery involves adequate magnification, instrumentation, haemostasis, and preoperative IOP control to allow use of 10-0 nylon sutures, microsurgery of the angle structures, avoidance of conjunctival trauma and postoperative hypotony.

Both types of operation require the reflection of a conjunctival flap. This flap can be either fornix or limbal based. (Figs. 13-1 and 13-2). Traditionally, a limbal-based flap was used and will be described first.

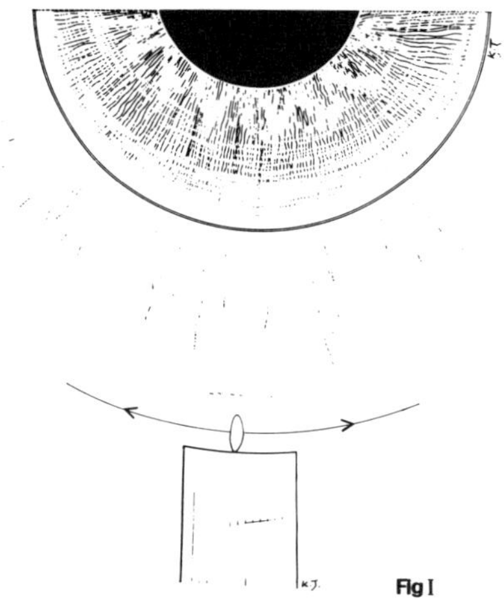

Figure 13-1. Limbus-based flap. The diagram illustrates the initial buttonhole in the conjunctiva, the arrows directed away from this show the direction of conjunctival incisions.

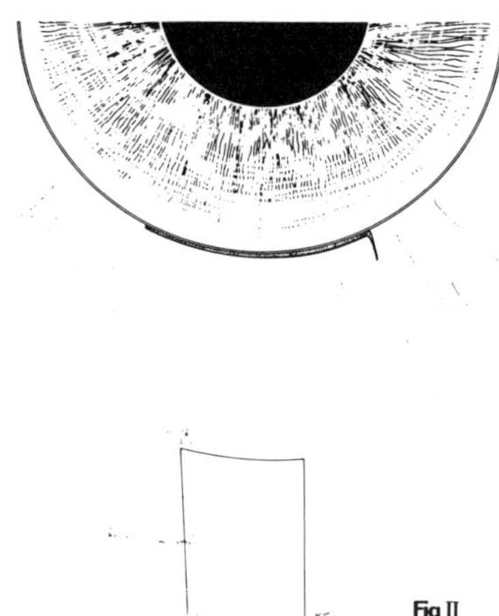

Figure 13-2. Fornix-based flap. The diagram illustrates the incision line, a peritomy centered at 12 o'clock with a radial relieving incision at one end.

Limbus Based Flap

Transfix the superior rectus with a stay suture using it to rotate the eye down from the primary position and expose the upper bulbar conjunctiva.

Grasp the bulbar conjunctiva with non-toothed or block forceps midway between the limbus and the superior rectus insertion to hold up a fold of tissue. Incise this conjunctiva and Tenons, exposing the rectus insertion. Insert curved, blunt ended spring scissors into the subtenons space, passing the closed blades circumferentially around the globe for about 2 clock hours in both directions. In each direction open the closed blades to enlarge this potential space, then withdraw the scissor blades to reinsert one blade in the space and make a full thickness cut through tenon's and conjunctiva parallel with the limbus for 2 clock hours in each direction. This semicicular conjunctival incision allows easy reflection of a conjunctival flap toward the limbus to expose the limbal tissues. This flap is most easily reflected forward with a moist cellulose swab to avoid inadvertent conjunctival damage.

Use a Tooks knife, or other blunt dissector, to clean an area 5 by 4 mm of bulbar sclera adjacent to the limbus free from episclera. Apply cautery to close any superficial scleral vessels and mark with cautery the outline of the scleral incisions. (The cautery heat should be sufficient to coagulate without charring.)

Fornix Based Flap

Transfix the superior rectus and rotate the eye as described previously.

At either the 1 or the 2 o'clock position make a 5 mm long full-thickness conjunctival and tenons incision radial to and extending to the limbus. Extend this incision as a peritomy past the 12 o'clock position for 4 clock hours. As the episclera is inserted 2 mm posterior to the conjunctiva at the limbus it will need to be incised separately. Use a blunt dissector, such as a Tooks knife, to clean episclera away from the sclera, exposing a 4 by 5 mm wide area of sclera.

Wound Closure

At the end of the procedure the conjunctival wound is closed. The fornix based flap is closed with 3 10-0 nylon sutures, on at each limbal edge of the peritomy wound, and the third to close the conjunctival edges midway along the radial incision. The sutures are inserted from the undersurface of the conjunctiva, allowing the knot to be tied beneath the conjunctival surface. In this way exposure of knots and suture ends is kept to a minimum.

The limbal based flap has a longer incision. A discrete Tenon's layer must be closed separately with two or more interrupted catgut or nylon sutures. The conjunctival wound can be closed with a continuous or interrupted suture. The continuous stitch, if nonabsorbable, will rarely free itself and has to be removed, while interrupted sutures usually fall out spontaneously.

A Comparison Between the Two Types of Conjunctival Incision

Published studies of the IOP control in operations involving these two types of wound closure do not point out differences between them. Wound leaks in the fornix based flap are uncommon and, if present, short lived. A major difference between the two types of closure is that the limbal based flaps are more congested. This appears to be a result of incising the radially oriented blood supply of the conjunctiva. The incision for a limbal based flap cuts through all the draining veins.

Conjunctival edema occurs during the postoperative period and will persist until a satisfactory alternative drainage route establishes itself. Although, under normal circumstances, this seems not to effect the long term IOP result, postoperative tissue edema can restrict aqueous absorption and influence fibroblast mobility.

Thermal Sclerostomy

The aim of a thermal sclerostomy is to create a 4 to 5 mm long full-thickness limbal incision into the anterior chamber, and by applying heat to the incision edges, retract them and so create a sclerostomy for the bulk outflow of aqueous.

Procedure: Expose and clean the limbus as described above.

Grasp the limbus at one end of the proposed incision with fine toothed forceps and with a diamond knife or fine steel blade make a partial-thickness incision through cornea anterior to the gray line dividing cornea and sclera.

Use a fine tipped cautery to retract the posterior lip of the incision by running the tip along the cut edge.Repeat the stages above, each time cutting a little deeper followed by cautery, until the anterior chamber has been entered. Care needs to be taken to ensure that the length of the incision is the same on the inside as the outside of the cornea.

A peripheral irridectomy is performed. The conjunctival wound is closed as described above.

One variant of this method is to perform a posterior lip sclerectomy. In this the corneoscleral incision is sloped anteriorly into the anterior chamber at an angle of about 45 degrees. A sclerectomy punch is used to remove the posterior lip of this incision. Care must be taken to ensure that the punch does not remove part of the adjacent ciliary body for this will create a not inconsiderable hemorrhage.

Guarded Sclerostomy

The aim is to cover a sclerostomy with a superficial flap of sclera. This lamellar flap (Fig. 13-3) acts as a valve to restrict bulk outflow of fluid from the anterior chamber in the immediate postoperative period.

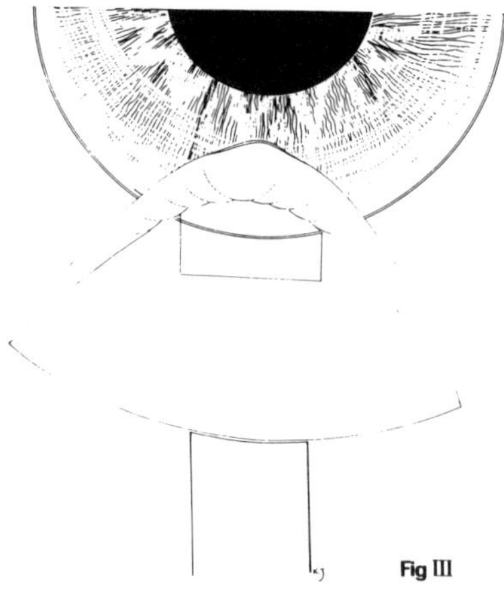

Figure 13-3. Lamellar scleral flap. Outline.

Procedure: Expose perilimbal bulbar sclera as described above. Use cautery to lightly mark out the limits of the superficial scleral flap incision. The lamellar flap is 5mm wide. It need only extend 2.5 mm posterior to the limbus, but if the "Watson modification" is being performed then it need extend 4 to 5 mm posterior to the limbus.

The superficial flap is hinged at the limbus. A thin flap is dissected free from the scleral bed (Fig. 13-4). (There is some evidence that thin flaps offer less resistance to the passage of aqueous than thick flaps). To obtain a flap of suitable thinness, grasp a posterior corner with fine toothed forceps, lifting it slightly. Using a technique of blunt dissection, (the writers preference is for the edge of a diamond blade or steel knife) lift a flap of sclera. The scleral bed should be thick enough to prevent the underlying choroid from imparting a bluish tinge to it. Continue the dissection anteriorly until the junction between translucent cornea and white sclera can be seen. (In the original descriptions of the operation one method of action was considered to be drainage of fluid circumferentially around the Canal of Schlemn, entering through the cut edges. Later studies showed that this was unlikely, and that the aqueous drained through or around the cut edges of the Scleral flap.) With that knowledge in mind then there is no need to remove trabecular meshwork at the time of operation, rather to remove a block of tissue lined by cells impervious to the passage of aqueous. This block can be anterior trabecular meshwork and the adjacent peripheral cornea. (Current ideas of failure following trabecular surgery suggested that 'excessive' conjunctival wound healing is a major cause. One factor that determines the extent of the wound healing is the extent of the postoperative inflammation. The more anterior approach avoids incising peritrabecular blood vessels, and thus exciting an inflammatory response). To ensure that deep dissection avoids intratrabecular blood vessels continue the dissection forward into clear cornea for 1.5 mm exposing a corneal strip 5 by 1.5 mm in size.

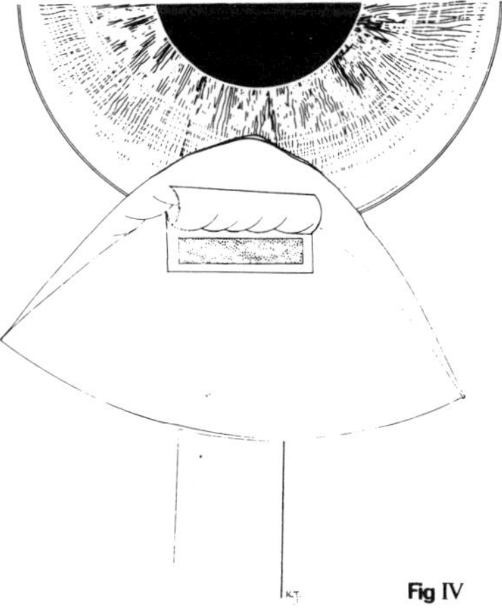

Figure 13-4. Lamellar scleral flap. Dissection.

A block of clear cornea 0.75 mm deep by 4 mm wide is removed (Fig. 13-5). To do this, grasp the left-hand edge of the lamellar scleral incision adjacent to the flap reflection with fine toothed forceps. Make a 4 mm partial-thickness incision in clear cornea parallel to the 0.75 mm anterior to the limbus leaving a 0.5 mm gap between the ends of the incision and the lamellar scleral incision. This incision leaves a shelf, 0.75 mm wide between the base of the lamellar flap and the incision. This corneal shelf is grasped with fine forceps held in the left hand and rotated toward the cornea, opening the incision. The blade can now be used to deepen the incision until the anterior chamber is entered. Once the anterior chamber has been entered the blade tip is inserted into the chamber and used to cut upward into the previously made partial-thickness incision along its complete length.

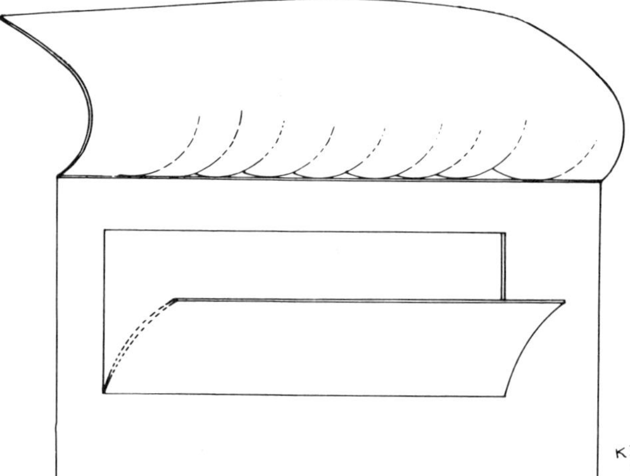

Figure 13-5. Deep corneal block: The diagram shows the lamellar scleral flap layered at the limbus and rotated forward. The deep corneal block is incised posteriorly to and hinged at the scleral spur. The block is removed by cutting it just anterior to the scleral spur.

This approach will produce a narrow rectangle parallel to the limbus, a peripheral irridectomy is performed through this. The "superficial" lamellar scleral flap is closed with two 10-0 monofilament nylon sutures, one in each corner. The tension on these sutures should suffice to appose the edges of the flap with slight flattening of the flap against the base. No gaps should be left between the cut edges and the sides of the base, for bulk outflow through these will allow postoperative hypotony and late cystic degeneration of the bleb. If scleral shrinkage occurred with cautery required for hemostatis then an extra suture to appose these gaping edges will be required.

Modifications: With an operation as popular as the trabeculectomy many modifications have been described. These can be subdivided into modifications of style and technique. Style differences are seen in the size and shape of the lamellar and deep flaps. It has been shown that within a 3 by 3 mm to 5 by 5 mm range there is little difference in the results from varying the size of the superficial flap. The shape also can vary from square to rectangular to triangular without any apparent effect on the result.

Technical differences are more subtle. One of the earliest was that introduced by Watson. His "modification" involved a longer superficial flap and excision of that part of scleral spur beneath it. In effect he added a cyclodialysis. The long-term results were comparable with the "Cairns" approach. The cyclodialysis carried the additional risk, in experienced hands, of unwanted hemorrhage.

A paracentesis performed before entering the anterior chamber has been advocated. This alternative entry route has been used to refill the anterior chamber at the end of the operation, when required, and also to gauge the resistance to the bulk outflow of fluid through the slcerostomy. For the reasons outlined above the writer has not felt that bulk outflow should play a major part in postoperative aqueous drainage. Under the operative conditions described the anterior chamber refills spontaneously by the end of the operation. Therefore, unless the trabeculectomy is part of a more complex anterior segment procedure, a paracentesis is not needed.

Advantages and Disadvantages of the Two Operations

These can be summarized under three headings:

- Early complications
- Late complications
- Long term IOP control

Early Complications

Early complications include infection, excessive aqueous drainage from the anterior chamber, and early failure to control IOP (in the first 3 postoperative months).

Pre-, peri-, and postoperative antibiotics together with an aseptic operative technique have all lowered the infection rate to very low levels. There is no evidence that either operation is more liable to postoperative infection.

Adherence to the operative technique outlined above reduces bulk outflow to a minimum. Any increase in aqueous loss above the capacity of the ciliary processes to replace it will lead to shallowing of the anterior chamber and hypotony. This was usual with the unguarded sclerostomy. This problem would persist upward of 5 days before spontaneously resolving. During this period the eye was at risk of the following: lens corneal touch, 'kissing choroidals' and suprachorodial hemorrhage. Each of these constituted an ophthalmological emergency necessitating surgical intervention. It has to be remembered that these problems do occur despite a guarded sclerostomy, the incidence is, however, considerably reduced.

Even without developing the major problems outlined here, a shallow anterior chamber can lead to the development of posterior and peripheral anterior synechiae and can also hasten the development of preexisting cataract.

The fibroblast response that induces 'early failure' (within the first three postoperative months) will develop with either type of operation. There is no evidence that either is more susceptible.

Late Complications

Late complications include cataract formation and degenerative changes in the bleb.

Cataract is a well recognized complication of glaucoma surgery. Although there is little supportive evidence it would appear likely that the eyes with pre-existing cataract and shallowing of the anterior chamber postoperation would be more likely to develop lens opacities.

Loss of conjunctival blood vessels and the deposition of 'degenerate' mucoid cells produce a pale elevated bleb. This is frequently surrounded by a row of radially arranged capillaries starkly red by contrast.

This 'cystic' bleb can 'dissect' (subconjunctivally) from the limbus toward the pupillary area. Such an enlarged avascular bleb is at risk from opportunistic bacterial infections. Once these gain entry (through a microscopic surface break) an endophthalmitis soon follows. In many instances these blebs continuously leak aqueous, a positive Seidel being detectable. These degenerate blebs develop following long-term exposure to aqueous in bulk. They are much less likely to occur with a guarded sclerostomy—unless there is a gap between the side wall of the flap and its base.

Late failure occurs with the progressive deposition of 'mucopolysaccharides' in the wall of the bleb. Comparative studies show that this occurs with equal frequency in the two types of operation.

IOP Control

From the forgoing remarks it is clear that the two types of operation have similar success rates in terms of IOP control, yet the postoperative complication rate is far higher in the unguarded sclerostomy. In the writer's practice the unguarded sclerostomy plays little part in his glaucoma management. There are, however, a number of instances when it might have a role. In the black patient with a thick layer of Tenon's capsule, the degeneration of the conjunctival tissues that follows the unguarded sclerostomy could improve the long-term success rate. In reoperations when it is desirable to remove a thick layer of episclera and Tenon's, thus allowing aqueous access to more normal surrounding tissue.

Apart from these few instances a guarded sclerostomy is the approach to be preferred.

Limbal Versus Fornix Based Conjunctival Flaps for Glaucoma Filtering Procedures

George L. Spaeth, MD

It is still not known whether, as a general rule, filtration procedures succeed better when they are preformed under a limbus-based or a fornix-based conjunctival flap.[1] There are certain situations, however, in which one technique appears to be preferable to the other; the competent "complete" glaucoma surgeon must be accomplished in performing either type of procedure (Table 13-1).

Table 13-1. Preference for limbal- or fornix-based flap

Limbal Flap Preferred		Fornix Flap Preferred
	Indications	
Routine filtration procedure by experienced surgeon		Routine filtration by by "occasional" surgeon
Filtration procedures where antifibrous treatment (5-fluorouracil, etc.) is planned		Cataract extraction with trabeculectomy or other filtration procedure
		"Tube"procedures such as Molteno implant
		Reoperation where conjunctiva is badly scarred
		Bleb revisions
	Relative Advantages	
Probably more secure		Easier to perform
Permits more vigorous compression of bleb area immediately postoperatively[4]		Less likely to cause Tenon's cyst
		Less likely to be associated with subconjunctival hemorrhage postoperatively
		Easier to release sutures in scleral flap using argon laser[3]

Some principles apply to both methods. Perhaps of most importance is the realization of the importance of proper development of conjunctival flaps in glaucoma filtering procedures, and of the direct relation between techniques and success.

One essential way to assure success is to insist upon satisfactory visualization. The conjunctival flap, whether limbal- or fornix-based, should not be performed unless the surgeon sees everything he or she is doing. Tissue should be handled only with forceps that will not penetrate, such as smooth or Pierse-Hoskins forceps. Toothed forceps should never be used. The limbus-based flap should be started as far posteriorly as possible, and the fornix-based flap should be started as far anteriorly as possible.

Limbus-Based Conjunctival Flap

The incision for the limbus-based flap should be as high in the cul-de-sac as possible. The surgeon should put the tissue on firm stretch while operating. The novice is concerned that such tension will tear the tissue; it will not, unless toothed forceps are employed. On the other hand, when the tissue is not put on firm traction, visualization is poor and technical errors will occur because of the poor visualization. Perhaps the most common mistake of the learning glaucoma surgeon is failure to insist upon seeing clearly. Probably the most common instructions I give to surgeons I am supervising is "Lift! Put the tissue on stretch! Please lift the tissue firmly!"

The limbus-based flap is a bit more difficult to perform and may be associated with a higher incidence of "Tenon's capsular cysts," those tense elevations of conjunctiva and Tenon's capsule that develop in around one third of patients having a standard trabeculectomy.[2]

The advantage of limbus-based flap is that when performed properly it provides the safest covering over the sclerostomy. This is of concern where the surgeon is trying to develop marked filtration and a very low final intraocular pressure. In such cases it is helpful to have the most secure covering over the filtering area.

Limbus-based flaps are of little value if they are not properly closed. In most instances it is appropriate to close Tenon's capsule separately, using running absorbable suture such as 8-0 chromic collagen or 8-0 polyglactin (Vicryl). Then the overlying conjunctiva is meticulously closed with multiple sutures—no further than 2 mm apart—of running absorbable suture such as 8-0 chromic or 8-0 or 9-0 polyglactin.

Fornix-Based Conjunctival Flaps

Fornix-based flaps are quicker and easier to perform; the difference in the hands of an experienced surgeon is not great, but for the "occasional" surgeon or the novice the difference is substantial. The major disadvantages of a fornix-based flap are first, that a small percent will leak persistently from the cut edge of the limbus, predisposing to hypotony, flat anterior chamber, and related complications. In addition, application of pressure in the area of the filtration site intended to encourage filtration postoperatively is more hazardous in the patient with the fornix-based flap because such pressure often disrupts the developing adhesion between the cut edge of the conjunctiva and the underlying sclera, predisposing to prolonged leak with its attendant complications.[3,4]

When performing a filtering procedure in an area where there is extensive scarring between the conjunctiva and the underlying sclera, it may be easier, technically more feasible, and perhaps more successful, to employ a fornix-based flap. There are also advantages to using a fornix-based flap when combining a filtration procedure with a cataract extraction. In this procedure visualization of the corneoscleral incision is easier with a fornix-based flap, permitting more accurate incisional closure and less subsequent astigmatism. It is also usually easier to release sutures under a fornix flap by burning them with an argon laser.[4] Additionally, there tend to be fewer hyphema in association with the fornix and as opposed to limbus-based flaps when performed in conjunction with cataract extraction.[5]

An additional indication for a fornix-based flap is the repair of a ruptured or excessively filtering conjunctival bleb. When performing a fornix-based flap, corneal epithelium should be removed where the surgeon wants the conjunctiva to adhere. There are a variety of ways of doing this; superficial cautery, alcohol, or a blade are all effective.

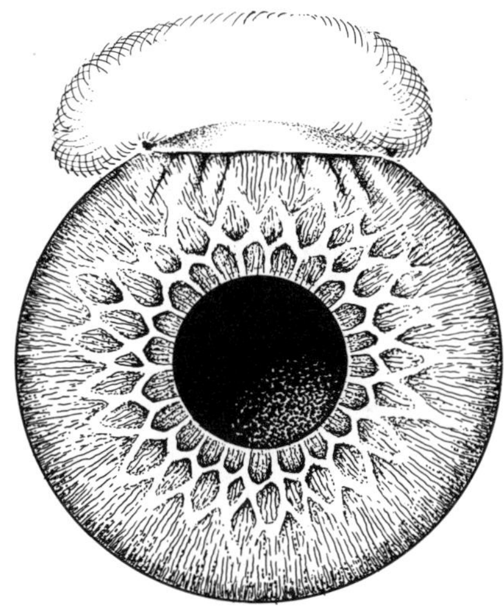

Figure 13-6. Closure fornix flap showing a very tight apposition of conjunctiva to cornea. Corneal epithelium should be denuded underneath the flap.

In most instances the fornix flap can be secured adequately by placing a suture at each end of the cut edge of the flap. The tissue is grasped with a Pierse-Hoskins forceps and put on firm stretch, so that it is pulled taut over the area where it is to adhere. It must be stressed that the tissue should be firmly anchored. The conjunctiva should be secured to the corner of the sclera, *not* to other conjunctiva. A line of indentation where the flap rests on the cornea should be present (Figure 13-6). If the length of the flap is more than 6 or 7 mm, as would be the case when using a fornix-based flap with a standard cataract extraction, it is helpful to place one or more sutures near the center, as well as each edge, in order to prevent the tissue from purse-stringing down over the cornea, covering more of the cornea than is desired (Figure 13-7).

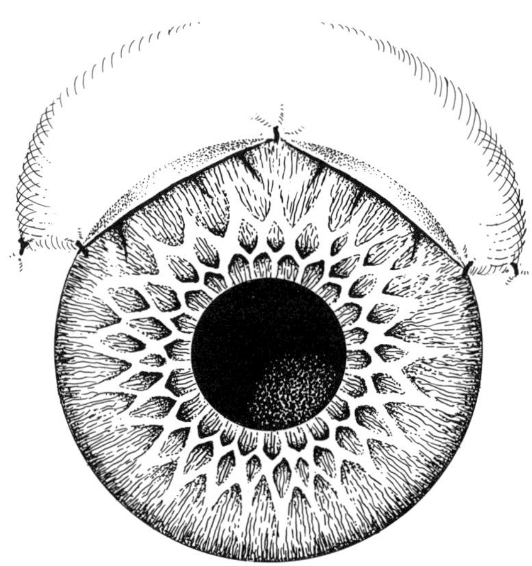

Figure 13-7. Where extensive fornix-based flap closure is necessary, it is often best to place a suture at the center portion of the flap to prevent the flap from being pulled down too far on the cornea.

In summary, the two types of flaps appear, in the routine case, to work equally well. The limbus-based flap may be slightly safer, and it is for this reason that I prefer the limbus-based approach in routine cases.

References

1. Antonios SR, Traverso CE, Tomey KF. Extracapsular cataract extraction using temporal limbal approach after filtering operations. Arch Ophthalmology 106:608, 1988.
2. Feldman RM, Gross RL, Spaeth GL, et al. Risk factors in the development of Tenon's capsule cysts following trabeculectomy. Ophthalmology 96:336-341, 1989.
3. Traverso CE, Greenbridge KC, Spaeth GL. Formation of peripheral anterior synechiae following argon laser trabeculectomy. Arch Ophthalmol 102:861, 1984.
4. Hoskins HD, Migliazzo C. Management of failing filtering blebs with the argon laser. Ophthalmic Surg 15:731-733, 1984.
5. Simmons SF, Litoff D, Nichols DA et al. Extracapsular cataract extraction and posterior chamber lens implantation combined with trabeculectomy in patients with glaucoma. Am J Ophthalmol 104:465-471, 1987.

Medical Management of Wound Healing in Filtration Surgery and Its Complications

Steven T. Simmons, MD

Medications to alter the surgical success of filtering operations have been used for decades. Corticosteroids were introduced in the early 1950s in an attempt to reduce would healing and increase the surgical success rate. Since then, a variety of topical, subconjunctival, and systemic medications have been introduced to reduce ocular inflammation, fibroblast proliferation, and collagen synthesis. With most of the agents, some success has been achieved. These new medications, however, produce new side effects and complications uncommonly seen by the ophthalmic surgeon in the past.

Corticosteroids

Cortisone was introduced in the ophthalmic literature in 1951 by Leopold[1] and was first used in filtration surgery in 1953 by Laval.[2] Since that time, local and systemic steroids have been used to reduce postoperative inflammation and cellular wound healing in filtration surgery. The anti-inflammatory effects of corticosteroids are nonspecific. Corticosteroids decrease cellular tissue infiltration and fibrinous exudation from inflamed capillaries. Corticosteroids reduce wound healing by inhibiting fibroblastic activity, reducing neovascularization, and impeding epithelial regeneration.

Over the years, controversy has remained as to which is the most efficacious method of delivering corticosteroids. Topical therapy offers many advantages. These advantages include ease of application, ability to administer high local concentrations, relatively low cost, and avoidance of systemic complications. In support of topical therapy alone, Starita[3] and Roth[4] demonstrated no clinically significant value to the addition of systemic steroids over topical prednisolone acetate in the surgical outcome of trabeculectomy in a randomized prospective trial. Over the last ten years, however, Molteno has reported excellent surgical success using oral steroids in combination with cholchicine and fluphenamic acid.[5] In addition, subconjunctival injections of triamcinolone have recently been reported to offer benefit in the surgical outcome of trabeculectomy.[6]

With each route of administration, numerous complications can occur. Systemic corticosteroids cause the greatest number of side effects. These side effects include activation of infection, mental changes, peptic ulcer disease, water retention, electrolyte imbalance, and alteration in control of diabetes and hypertension. Growth retardation and permanent facial changes can occur with long-term use in young individuals. Because of these various side effects, a detailed medical history and physical examination is necessary prior to the initiation of oral corticosteroids. In addition, a recent urinalysis, complete blood count, and electrolytes should be obtained prior to the initiation of therapy. If there is a suspicious history of tuberculosis, a tuberculine skin test and chest x-ray might be warranted as well.

The use of postoperative local steroid preparations have also been associated with some complications. As a result of the reduced wound healing and epithelial regeneration, postoperative wound leaks at the surgical incision or through inadvertent conjunctival breaks can occur more frequently. Because of these effects, steroids often need to be reduced or discontinued to allow for closure of these breaks. In the same light, when postoperative corneal abrasions occur, topical steroids should be reduced to allow for rapid epithelial regeneration. If the local steroids are continued, there is a risk of permanent stromal scarring and corneal melting related to the ability of steroids to promote collagenase production.

Because corticosteroids suppress the migration of inflammatory cells and inhibit the release of hydrolytic enzymes, corticosteroids reduce the ocular resistance to secondary bacterial, viral, and fungal infections. Reactivation of herpetic infections and secondary bacterial corneal ulcers are probably the most common complications of this type. For this reason, when steroids are used postoperatively in patients with preexisting corneal disease, the ophthalmic surgeon needs to monitor closely for secondary bacterial or fungal infections, especially when antimetabolites have been used.[7,8] Often topical antibiotic therapy is used in the initial postoperative period in an attempt to reduce this possible complication. No study, however, has been able to clearly prove the advantages of this additional therapy. If a patient has a history of previous ocular herpes, the steroid therapy should be covered with an appropriate topical antiviral agent.

Two of the complications of long-term use of steroids are cataract formation and the elevation of IOP. As a result, steroids have been implicated as the possible cause of the increased incidence of cataracts following filtration surgery and the pressure elevation that can be seen three to four weeks following trabeculectomy. These hypotheses, however, have not been confirmed in the literature and probably should not be stressed.

Antimetabolites

Fibroblast proliferation has been isolated as playing a major role in the failure of filtration surgery.[9,10] Following filtration surgery, fibroblasts migrate and proliferate in the area of filtration and produce collagen and glycosaminoglycans that provide the matrix for wound closure. For this reason, there has been extensive research in finding agents that will reduce this proliferation. Blumenkranz[11] and Kwong[12] have tested a variety of antimetabolites and have found that 5-fluorouracil, bleomycin, doxorubicin, and cytarabine were successful in inhibiting fibroblast proliferation in vitro. Subsequent animal studies have confirmed the advantages of bleomycin[13] and 5-fluorouracil[13,14]. This success has lead to the use of subconjunctival 5-fluorouracil. Prospective randomized trials are in progress studying the efficacy of subconjunctival 5-fluorouracil.

The use of 5-fluorouracil has introduced new postoperative complications. To date, the major complications have been related to corneal and conjunctival epithelial toxicity that results in corneal epithelial defects and conjunctival wound leaks. In Heuer's study,[14] 45% of the patients developed corneal ephithelial defects. Most of these defects healed within one week after the 5-fluorouracil was discontinued. Some of these defects, however, remained for four weeks. As a result of these persistent epithelial defects, three patients developed subepithelial corneal scarring. Knapp[6] has reported four cases of serious corneal complications following the administration of subconjunctival 5-fluorouracil and topical steroids in patients with preexisting corneal disease. These complications included two bacterial corneal ulcers, a sterile corneal ulcer and corneal perforation, and a keratinized corneal plaque with an underlying sterile stromal infiltrate. In each case, postoperative corneal erosions were noted and preexisting corneal disease was present.

Conjunctival wound and needle track leaks occurred in 41% of the patients in Heuer's study. The use of 9-0 monofilament or 8-0 braided vicryl sutures on a tapered vascular needle has helped eliminate some of these wound leaks by maintaining equal diameters between the needle and the suture material. In a recent update, however, conjunctival wound leaks continued to be the most significant complication with the use of 5-fluorouracil and usually occurred 3 to 5 days following surgery.[18] In addition, delayed wound leaks have been reported associated with 5-fluorouracil with subsequent bleb failure.[8] By reducing the total dose of 5-fluorouracil, Weinreb reported less epithelial toxicity without a reduction in the surgical success rate.[17]

In an attempt to minimize the toxic high peak levels of subconjunctival 5-fluorouracil and reduce the number of injections, various delivery systems have been tested for 5-fluorouracil. Collagen sponges,[13] liposomes,[19,20,21,22,23] biodegradable polymers,[24,25] and polyvinyl alcohol membranes[26] have been studied in animal models and have demonstrated initial success. To date, none of these delivery systems are available for human use. Future studies on the dosage schedule and the means of delivery will be important to help maximize the efficacy of these agents, while minimizing their toxic side effects.

Inhibitors of Collagen Cross-Linking

Because collagen plays a vital role in wound healing and scar formation, any agent that impedes the formation of mature collagen can benefit the surgical outcome by reducing the tensile strength of the scar. To date, two agents—BAPN and D-penicillamine—have been studied. Both of these agents inhibit the immature collagen fibrils from undergoing cross-linkage necessary in forming mature collagen. In preliminary studies,[27,28] these agents have shown promise in prolonging successful filtration and presently a randomized clinical trial has been initiated to investigate the efficacy of topical BAPN in filtration surgery. To date, no toxic side effects have been reported in the preliminary work.

Other Agents

In treating secondary glaucomas, Molteno has reported inadequate control of bleb inflammation and fibrosis with topical and systemic steroids alone.[29] As a result, he has advocated the use of cholchicine and fluphenamic acid in addition to topical and systemic steroids to reduce bleb fibrosis.[5] Cholchicine is an inhibitor of microtubule metabolism that prevents the release of chemotactic factors from neutrophils, and retards the proliferation of fibroblasts. Recently the efficacy of cholchicine in inhibiting fibroblast proliferation has been further supported by Lemor.[30,31,32] He has shown the successful inhibition of proliferative vitreoretinopathy with oral cholchicine in an animal model. Diarrhea, nausea, vomiting, and abdominal pain are the major adverse reactions to the use of oral cholchicine. These symptoms occur quite frequently and can limit the use of this medication in high doses. The ingestion of large doses of cholchicine can cause central nervous system depression, a burning sensation in the throat, bloody diarrhea, and leukopenia.

Fluphenamic acid and meclofenamate are members of the fenamate family of nonsteroidal anti-inflammatory agents. Molteno has recommended the use of fluphenamic acid but this agent is unavailable in the United States. The only available member of this family is meclofenamate (Meclomen). Meclofenamate, indomethacin (Indocin), and naproxen (Naprosyn) are potent nonsteroidal anti-inflammatory agents and potent inhibitors of the cyclooxygenase responsible for the biosynthesis of porstaglandins. All these agents have been shown to have a prominent inhibitory effect on leukocyte migration. Naproxen is particularly potent in this regard and has been shown to be more effective than cholchicine in vitro.[33] In addition, Blumenkranz has demonstrated that both indimethacin and meclofenamate to be potent inhibitors of fibroblast proliferation in vitro.[11]

The most common side effects of the nonsteroidal anti-inflammatory agents involve the gastrointestinal system. These gastrointestinal complications include dyspepsia, gastric discomfort, nausea, vomiting, diarrhea, and gastric bleeding. Because of the gastrointestinal complications, these agents are relatively contraindicated in those patients with a history of gastrointestinal disease. In addition, central nervous system complications that include headache, vertigo, depression, and hallucination can occur. Other complications to these medications include hepatic and renal toxicity, dermatologic abnormalities, and blood dyscrasias.

The effects of topical indomethacin on the surgical outcome of trabeculectomy was studied by Migdal and Hitchings.[34] In their prospective trial, topical indomethacin was unsuccessful in increasing the surgical success or bleb quality. In their preliminary report, they noted actually an increased inflammatory reaction immediately following surgery in the indomethacin treated group. No other complications were noted. Future studies of both systemic and topical nonsteroidal anti-inflammatory agents are necessary to further delineate their role in the modulation of wound healing following glaucoma filtration surgery.

Conclusion

Over the years, the ophthalmic surgeon has tried to increase the surgical success of glaucoma filtration surgery through the medical modulation of fibroblast proliferation and the inflammatory reaction in surgical wound healing. In the last few years, a variety of agents have been introduced. Many of these agents are new to the ophthalmic surgeon and introduce new surgical complications and systemic side effects. The ability to recognize these effects and complications is vital to the ultimate surgical outcome and the general health of the patient.

References

1. Leopold IH, Purnell JE, Cannon E, Steinmetz C, McDonald PR. Local and systemic cortisone in ocular disease. Am J Ophthalmol 34:361, 1951.
2. Laval JMD, Coles PS. Role of cortisone in glaucoma surgery. Arch Ophthalmol 49:168, 1953.
3. Starita RJ, Fellman RL, Spaeth GL, et al. Short- and long- term effects of postoperative corticosteroids on trabeculectomy. Ophthalmology 92:938, 1985.
4. Roth SM, Spaeth GL, Poryzees EM, Steinmann WC, and Starita RJ. The effects of postoperative corticosteroids on trabeculectomy; long term follow-up. Invest Ophthalmol, Vis Sci. (Suppl) ARVO Abstracts. 29:367, 1988.
5. Molteno ACB, Strachum J, Ancker E. Control of bleb fibrosis after glaucoma surgery by antiinflammatory agents. S Afr Med J 50:1062-1066, 1976.
6. Giangiacomo J, Danker DK, Adelstein E. The effect of preoperative subconjunctival triamcinolone administration on glaucoma filtration. Arch Ophthalmol 104:838, 1986.
7. Knapp A, Heuer DK, Stern GA, Driebe WT. Serious corneal complications of glaucoma filtering surgery with postoperative 5-fluorouracil. Am J Ophthalmol 103:183, 1987.
8. Lee DA, Hersh P, Kersten D, Melaned S. Complications of subconjunctival 5-fluorouracil following glaucoma filtering surgery. Ophthalmic Surg 18:187, 1987.
9. Teng CC, Chi HH, Katzin HM. Histology and mechanism of filtering operations. Am J Ophthalmol 47:16, 1959.
10. Addicks EM, Quigley HA, Green WR, Robin AL. Histologic characteristics of filtering blebs in glaucomatous eyes. Arch Ophthalmol 101:795, 1983.
11. Blumenkranz MS, Clafin A, Hajek AS. Selection of therapeutic agents for intraocular proliferative disease: cell culture evaluation. Arch Ophthalmol 102:598, 1984.
12. Kwong EM, Litin BS, Jones MA, Hershler J. Effect of antineoplastic drugs on fibroblast proliferation in rabbit aqueous humor. Ophthalmic Surg 15:847, 1984.
13. Key JS, Litin BS, Jones MA, Herschler J. Delivery of antifibrolastic agents as adjuncts to filtration surgery— Part II: Delivery of 5-fluorouracil and bleomycin in a collagen implant: Polit study in the rabbit. Ophthalmic Surg 17:796, 1986.
14. Gressel MG, Parrish RK, Folbert R. 5-fluorouracil and glaucoma filtering surgery I: an animal model. Ophthalmology 91:378, 1984.

15. Heuer DK, Parrish RK, Gressel MG, et al. 5-fluorouracil and glaucoma filtering surgery II: a pilot study. Ophthalmology 91:384, 1984.
16. Heuer DK, Parrish RK, Gressel MG, et al. 5-fluorouracil and glaucoma surgery III: intermediate follow-up of a pilot study. Ophthalmology. In press.
17. Weinreb R. Titrating the dose of 5-fluorouracil after filtration surgery. Ophthalmology (suppl) 93:80, 1986.
18. Rockwood EJ: Flourouracil for filtration surgery. Audio Digest Ophthalmol 24(17), 1986.
19. Fishman P, Peyman G, Hendrick R. Intravitreal and subconjunctival liposome-encapsulated 5-fluorouracil in a rabbit model. Invest Ophthalmol Vis Sci. (Suppl) ARVO abstracts 27:348, 1986.
20. Simmons ST, Sherwood MB, Nichols DA, et al. Pharmacokinetics of a 5-fluorouracil liposomal delivery system. Br J Ophthalmol 72:688, 1988.
21. Skuta GL, Assil K, Parrish RK, Folbert R, Weinreb RN. Filtering surgery in owl monkeys treated with the antimetabolite 5-flourouridine 5-monophosphate entrapped in multioescular liposomes. Am J Ophthalmol 103:714, 1987.
22. Goodman PF, Alvarado JA, Stern W, Heath T, Kraner S. Liposomal incorporated following posterior lip sclerectomy in the primate. Invest Ophthalmol Vis Sci. (Suppl) ARVO abstracts 28:271, 1987.
23. Winter DF, Jones MA, Simmons ST, Smith RS. A histologic analysis of a 5-fluorouracil liposomal delivery system following subconjunctival injection in rabbits. Invest Ophthalmol Vis Sci. (Suppl) ARVO abstracts. 28:271, 1987.
24. Lee DA, Flores RA, Anderson PJ, Leong K. Filtration surgery in rabbits using slow release polymers and 5-FU. Invest Ophthalmol Vis Sci. (Suppl) ARVO abstracts 27:212, 1986.
25. Portugal L, Davis J, Parel JM, Parrish R. Biodegradable polymer development for ophthalmic applications. Invest Ophthalmol and Vis Sci. (Suppl) ARVO abstracts 29:82, 1988.
26. Smith TJ, Maurin MB, Milosovich SM, Hussain, A. A membrane based sustained released ocular delivery system for 5- flourouracil Investigative. Invest Ophthalmol Vis Sci. (Suppl) ARVO abstracts. 28:271, 1987.
27. Moorhead LC, Smith J, Stewart R, Kimbrough R. Effects of Beta-Aminopropionitrile after glaucoma filtration surgery; Pilot human study. Ann Ophthalmol 19:223-225, 1987.
28. McGuigan LJB, Cook DJ, Yablonski ME. Dexamethasone, D- Penicillamine, and glaucoma filtering surgery in rabbits. Invest Ophthalmol Vis Sci 27:1755, 1986.
29. Molteno ACB. Use of Molteno implants to treat secondary glaucoma. In Glaucoma (ed). Carins JG, New York: Grune and Stratton, 1986, p. 220.
30. Lemor M, Yeo JH, Glaser B. Oral cholchicine for the treatment of experimental traction retinal detachment. Arch Ophthalmol 104:1226, 1986.
31. de Bustros S, Lemor M, Sato M, Glaser B. Low-dose cholchicine inhibits astrocyte, fibroblast retinal pigment epithelial cell migration and proliferation. Arch Ophthalmol 104:1223, 1986.

32. Isernhagen R, Glaser B, Lemor M, Guedener X, Scherrman JM. Cholchicine levels in human blood and vitreous fluid following oral administration. Invest Ophthalmol Vis Sci. (Suppl) ARVO abstracts. 28:116, 1987.
33. Goodman AG, Gillman LS. The pharmacological basis of therapeutics. MacMillan 1985, p. 701.
34. Migdal C, Hitchings R. The developing bleb: effect of topical antiprostaglandins on the outcome of glaucoma fistalising surgery. Br J Ophthalmol 67:655, 1983.

The Use of the Simmons Shell Tamponade Technique and Attendant Complications

Richard P. Wilson, MD

Patients with advanced glaucoma or low-tension glaucoma who evidenced progressive damage at intraocular pressures considered a success for trabeculectomies continue to require full-thickness filtration procedures. In an effort to obtain the necessary low intraocular pressures but limit attendant adverse effects, Drs. Richard Simmons, Paul Chandler, and Morton Grant developed the tamponade technique.[1] After investigating a variety of materials, they settled on a methylmethacrylate shell (Fig. 13-8) which conformed to the limbal scleral contour and vaulted over the cornea. A thickened footplate, outlined in black to facilitate positioning, put external pressure over the filtration site (Fig. 13-9).

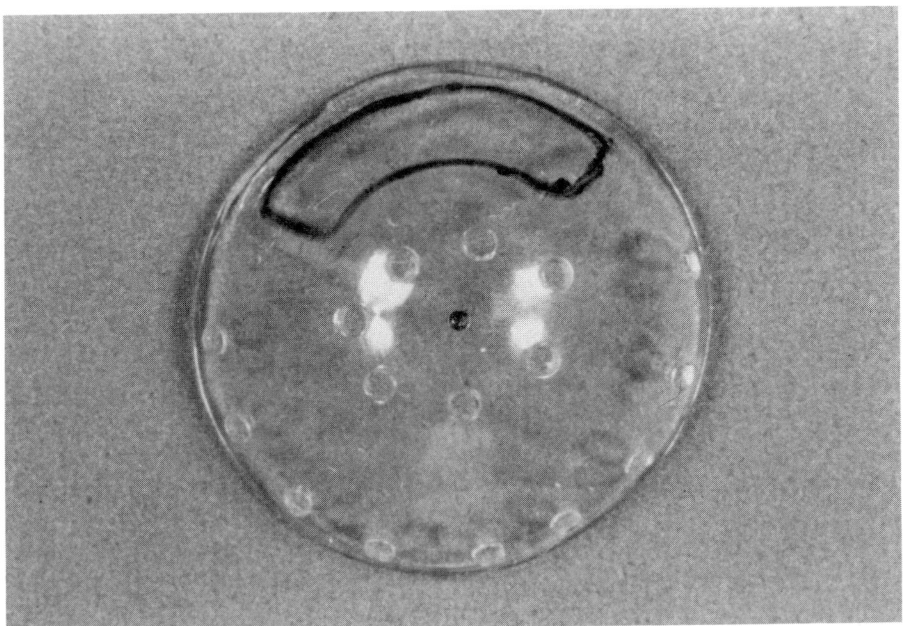

Figure 13-8. Methylmethacrylate shell with thickened footplate outlined in black to tamponade area of filtration. The center holes allow tears to circulate and ointment to be instilled under the shell. The outer holes are used for fixation sutures.

The aim of the technique was to increase early postoperative resistance to aqueous outflow, thereby reducing markedly the incidence of adverse effects. By forcing the filtered aqueous to spread out under the conjunctiva, a broad filtration area could be developed. This they hoped would lead to an increased capacity for aqueous transport, and a low final intraocular pressure without the development of a localized cystic bleb prone to later infection or rupture. Other uses proposed included reversing a flat chamber in the early postoperative period after filtering surgery, allowing buttonholes and late leaking filtration blebs to heal by inhibiting the flow through the fistula and providing support for the damaged area.

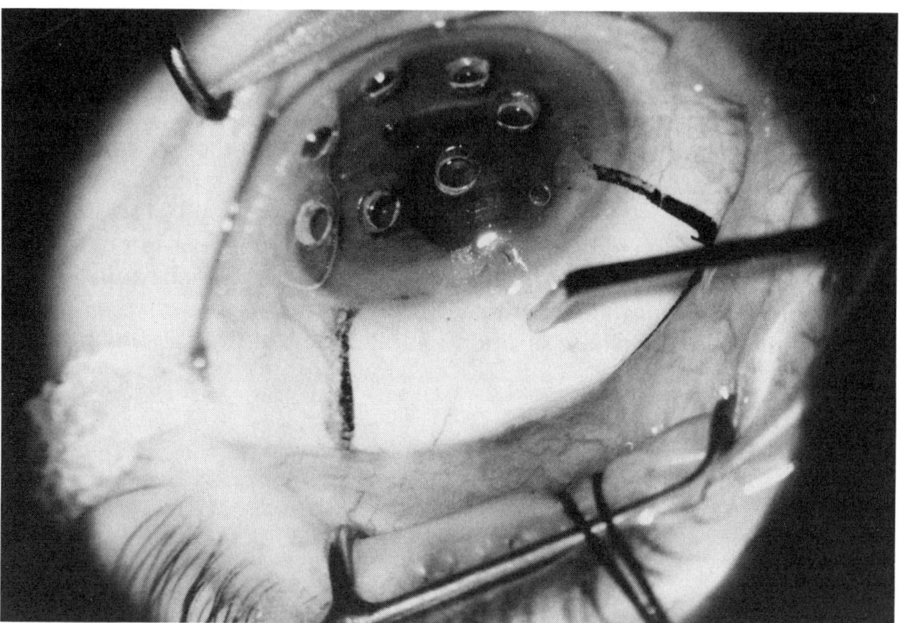

Figure 13-9. Area of tamponade shown with external pressure blanching conjunctival vessels.

The Shell

The tamponade shells are made of methylmethacrylate for a variety of reasons: the material is clear, permitting a view of the anterior chamber; rigid enough to hold its shape under pressure patch; and biologically inert with a long medical history. A slightly more flexible and oxygen-permeable material such as silicone would be more ideal and was tried but federal restrictions prevented their utilization.[1] The thickness of the shell is approximately 0.75 to 1 mm thick and conforms to the surface of the eye. A thicker area superiorly exerts the tamponade effect over the filtration site and is outlined in black to aid accurate placement. Two styles are made. Both have peripheral holes to permit an easy point for forceps fixation and suturing to the eye. One style has no central holes and the inherent suction in this design helps the lens center over the cornea. Adversely, however, there is less corneal wetting and more epithelial problems with this style, which is usually used without suturing to the globe. Situations for its use include tamponading the bleb in the early postoperative period to allow flat chambers to form, and tamponading buttonholes and late-leaking blebs. The other style has six to nine holes drilled in the central vault that allows better tear circulation and corneal wetting. This style is sutured to the sclera at the time of surgery to inhibit aqueous egress through the fistula, converting an unguarded sclerostomy to a guarded one.

Technique

The compression shell is placed on the eye with the footplate over the proposed filtering site. A broken or sharpened applicator stick moistened with methlene blue is used to mark the conjunctiva where the two fixation sutures will be placed. The shell is removed and stored in saline on the surgical tray. Two 9-0 nylon sutures are passed through episclera or sclera in the two inferior quadrants and placed to the side. Alternately, conjunctival sutures of 9-0 silk can be used to anchor the shell in place. The first way allows more imobilization of the shell but greater chance of subconjunctival bleeding. Conjunctival fixation has proven adequate and considerably easier but is this author's second choice.

A limbal-based conjunctival and Tenon's flap is elevated in conventional manner. A paracentesis track is made prior to entering the eye, and topical atropine is started to relax the ciliary muscle, easing any pressure on the anterior chamber. A full-thickness sclerostomy is made with punch or cautery and an iridectomy made. Hyaluronic acid is used to reform the anterior chamber, flush blood and debris from the eye, and promote hemostasis. Tenon's and conjunctiva are now closed with thin absorbable suture or, if desired, nylon. The compression shell is then placed on the eye, and the preplaced sutures pulled through the proper holes and tied loosely. This small leeway allows the shell to center better. Subconjunctival steroids are injected, and atropine ointment squeezed through one of the central holes in the shell to cushion its ride on the cornea. Antibiotic and steroid ointments, or a combination, are also applied prior to a compression dressing.

Recently, this author has been using a slightly myopic disposable extended wear contact lens to cushion the shell on the cornea. This greatly cuts down on the corneal erosions and makes the shell more comfortable for the 2 to 3 days it is in place. With a lens in place, however, ointments should not be placed under the shell.

The dressing is unique and essential to the effectiveness of the tamponade procedure. It consists of two molded cotton cylinders, the larger one 1 cm in diameter and tapered toward the ends for an overall length of 5 cm; the smaller about two-thirds the size of the other. The larger spindle is fitted into the hollow over the upper lid with the eye fixated straight ahead, compressing the footplate of the shell directly onto the filtration area. The smaller spindle fits over the lower lid, between the edge of the shell and the orbital rim. This acts to hold the shell in position. Oval eye patches are placed over the cotton spindles and taped tightly to maximize the pressure on the sclerostomy site.[1]

The early postoperative period is important if complications are to be minimized and the shell to be effective. The patient is warned to avoid eye movements as much as possible. The compression shell lags behind saccades and adds to the abuse that the cornea is sustaining from decreased wetting and friction with the rigid shell. Keeping both eyes closed, watching television, and one-on-one conversation are the most helpful activities in this regard.

Even with the best patient compliance with instructions, a corneal abrasion is generally inevitable if the shell is left on 3 days or more.

Daily examination at the slit-lamp is useful in assessing progress. A 360 degree bleb is usually present along with hypotony, evidenced by folds in Descemet's. Rarely will the shell tamponade technique not be able to maintain at least a three-quarters normal depth chamber. If the chamber is shallow, suspicion is directed at the fit of the shell, or the possibility of a suprachoroidal hemorrhage or aqueous misdirection. A finger-tension over the edge of the shell on downward gaze will sort out the first from the latter two causes, which should evidence a normal or elevated tension. If the shell is fitting poorly, its tethering sutures might need to be cut, and the eye carefully dressed to maintain the footplate superiorly. In this case, bilateral patches might be necessary to prevent undue scuffing of the cornea with eye movements. If the IOP is higher than expected and the chamber flat, a recent history of sudden pain should be elicited, indicative of a suprachoroidal hemorrhage. If preoperatively the patient had an element of angle closure glaucoma, aqueous misdirection syndrome becomes the most likely diagnosis in a patient with intact posterior capsule, pupillary block in a patient who is intracapsularly aphakic. For these latter conditions, shell removal and laser or surgical intervention is usually necessary if medical treatment fails. Management of these complications is discussed in Chapter 14.

The pressure dressing including the two cotton spindles is changed once a day[2] with liberal use of atropine ointment squeezed through the central holes under the shell. Steroid and antibiotic ointment is also used. If the patient is uncomfortable, then the cushion of ointment should be replaced more frequently. The shell is removed 4 to 7 days postoperatively at the surgeon's judgment. The decision is based primarily on the apparent stability of the anterior chamber and the extent of the bleb. A 360 degree bleb with deep anterior chamber at 4 days usually allows safe removal of the shell. The anterior chamber might shallow soon after removal, but reforms spontaneously in most cases. If the anterior chamber has not reformed after several hours, the shell can be reapplied and left on an additional 1 to 3 days. A minimal bleb and shallow chamber signals a choroidal detachment and decreased aqueous production. The shell should be left on longer unless the eye becomes too irritated. In that case, removal of the shell and surgical drainage of the choroidal detachment and reformation of the anterior chamber will result in better long-term filtration.

Care in shell removal is important to avoid further damage to the cornea and irritation to the area of filtration. The shell is grasped by two of the interior holes with forceps and the inferior pole lifted gently over the lower lid. The superior pole can be slid down from under the upper lid without friction on the cornea. A corneal abrasion is almost invariably present if a cushioning extended wear contact lens was not employed, and is treated with a pressure patch over antibiotic and atropine ointment. Steroids are used in moderation until the abrasion heals. The patient is observed to ensure maintenance of anterior chamber depth and healing of any corneal defect.

Results and Complications

The Simmons group has been fairly successful in their primary purpose of obtaining a low IOP with fewer side effects. Their experience with 171 patients reveals that 70% had an IOP less than 15 mm Hg at 18 months. Of these, only 13% developed a shallow or flat anterior chamber compared to 67% of a group with the same filtering surgery without the use of the compression shell. When the tamponade technique was used in conjunction with trabeculectomy, there was no improvement in the final IOP or decrease in the already low complication rate compared to trabeculectomy alone.[1]

If the shell tamponade technique is this successful, why is it so rarely used outside of Boston? The main disadvantage of the technique is the inconvenience to the patient and physician. In this era of DRGs and early discharge, a 6- to 9-day stay postoperatively puts a strain not only on the patient-doctor relationship, but also the doctor-hospital relationship. The postoperative care is time-consuming for the surgeon, and the shell-corneal friction and resultant abrasion uncomfortable for the patient. This discomfort increases with the length of time the shell is in use. In an effort to promote healing of the abrasion, steroids are not used for the first day or two after the shell is removed, although this seems to be the period when ocular inflammation is greatest. If steroids are started before the corneal epithelium has covered the defect, the abrasion might not heal for some time. This results in a subepithelial haze that is permanent, and if centrally located, can cloud vision noticeably.

Two patterns of corneal epithelial defect are noted.[1] One is the defect present before shell removal and which stains immediately. The second pattern is for there to be epithelial irregularity but no staining at the time of shell removal. Epithelial loss and staining present during the first day. The first pattern is often associated with peripheral abrasion and is usually because of shell movement related to poor fit, inadequate positioning, or fixation. Because there is only one size compression shell, any cornea or eye outside the usual dimensions will not conform to the shape of the shell. Abrasions generally result. Patients with congenital glaucoma often do less well with the shell tamponade technique because the large eye prevents a good fit of the shell to the limbus. The sclerectomy is inadequately tamponaded, and the poor conformity of the shell to the cornea causes peripheral abrasions, often superiorly, which cause more inflammation and inhibit the success of the procedure.

The vault of the compression shell over the central cornea prevents friction as the cause of central abrasions. Corneal dryness and poor epithelial nutrition are the likely causes of central defects of both patterns, especially the second. This is why every effort is made to place the ointment under the shell at the time of dressing changes. The ointment can be squeezed through the central holes, or in shells without central holes, under the edge of the shell.

Simmons and Singh mention sealing of the filtration area and infection as other possible complications.[1] However, both they and this author have had little problem with either. In order of importance, the main complications would have to be the ubiquitous corneal abrasion, choroidal detachment secondary to hypotony with resultant flat chamber, and late closure of the filtering fistula. The added discomfort, inability to use steroids in the early postoperative period, and prolonged patching make the corneal defects the most troublesome complication. Choroidal detachments with secondary flat anterior chambers appear with approximately the same frequency as with trabeculectomy. Scarring of the filtration site is augmented by the inflammation engendered by the shell, the lack of steroids at the height of inflammation, and any decrease in aqueous output secondary to choroidal detachment. This is counterbalanced by the size of the sclerostomy possible with this technique and the IOP results corroborate this as an infrequent problem.

Modifications

In an effort to shorten hospitalization and patient inconvenience without sacrificing results, a variety of modifications have been tried. Two have proved quite beneficial. As mentioned previously, the use of a soft, extended wear contact lens to cushion the shell in the post operative period has reduced corneal abrasions by 75% and allowed earlier discharge with less discomfort. Additionally, the author has developed a trapdoor procedure in which a routine trabeculectomy (Fig. 13-10) is performed but the scleral flap is not sutured. This unsutured flap under pressure from the compression shell effectively changes the procedure from an unguarded sclerostomy to a guarded one similar to a trabeculectomy (Fig. 13-11). This allows the maintenance of a deeper anterior chamber in the early postoperative period than possible with a full-thickness filtration procedure and the compression shell. In turn, this permits an earlier removal of the shell without decreasing its benefit. When the shell is removed, the bleb elevates and Tenon's attachments between scleral flap and conjunctiva lift the trapdoor, that is, scleral flap, converting the procedure to a full-thickness filter (Fig. 13-12A and B).

Using this technique on a consecutive 33 eyes of 25 patients, the author obtained an average IOP of 12.5 mm Hg at 8.7 months. 100% of the patients had an IOP under 20 mm Hg, 67% were under 14 mm Hg, and 33% were under 10 mm Hg. At the time of the final tonometry, 18% of the patients were on dipivefrin HC1 only, 3% were on dipivefrin and pilocarpine, and 6% were on these two medications plus timolol to maintain a low enough pressure to prevent progression of their advanced glaucoma. Importantly only one patient (3%) required reformation of the anterior chamber. In two cases, the compression shell was left on for four days secondary to a shallow chamber.

These results are quite similar to the reported results of Simmons et al, who had 70% of their patients at pressures less than 15 mm Hg, though at a longer follow-up. The trap-door modification of their technique therefore allows the surgeon to shorten the required hospitalization—as well as the time that the compression shell is a source of discomfort and inflammation to the patient without sacrificing effectiveness. The shell tamponade technique,

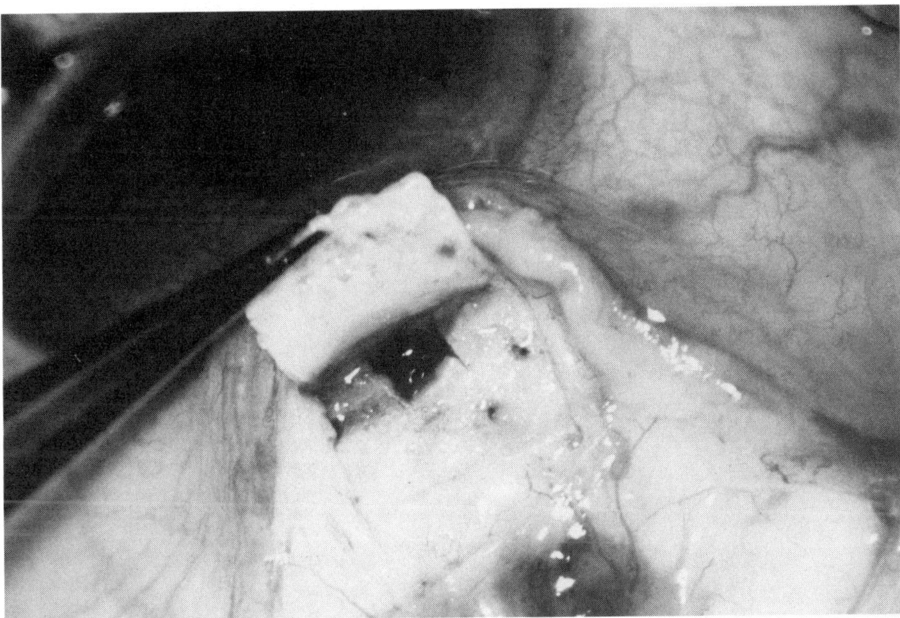

Figure 13-10. A large (4 X 4 mm) scleral flap covers a small (1.5 X 1.5 mm) trabeculectomy block.

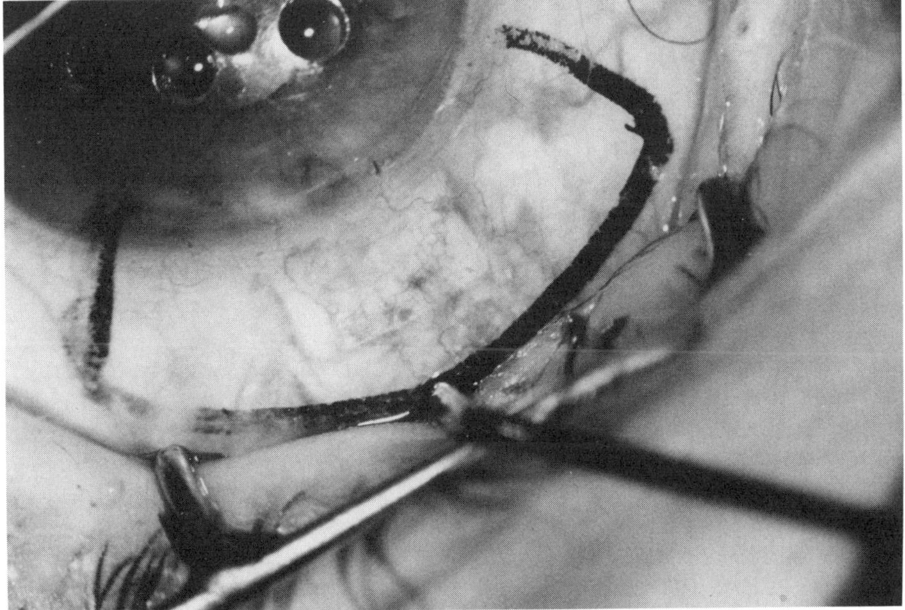

Figure 13-11. The shell, by tamponading the scleral flap down over the excised block, converts the full-thickness procedure to a guarded sclerostomy.

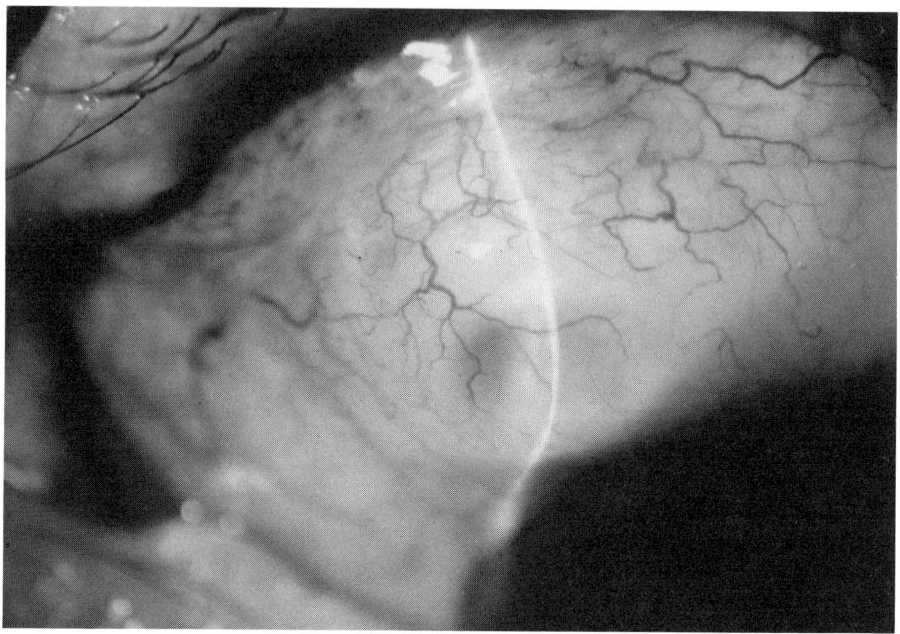

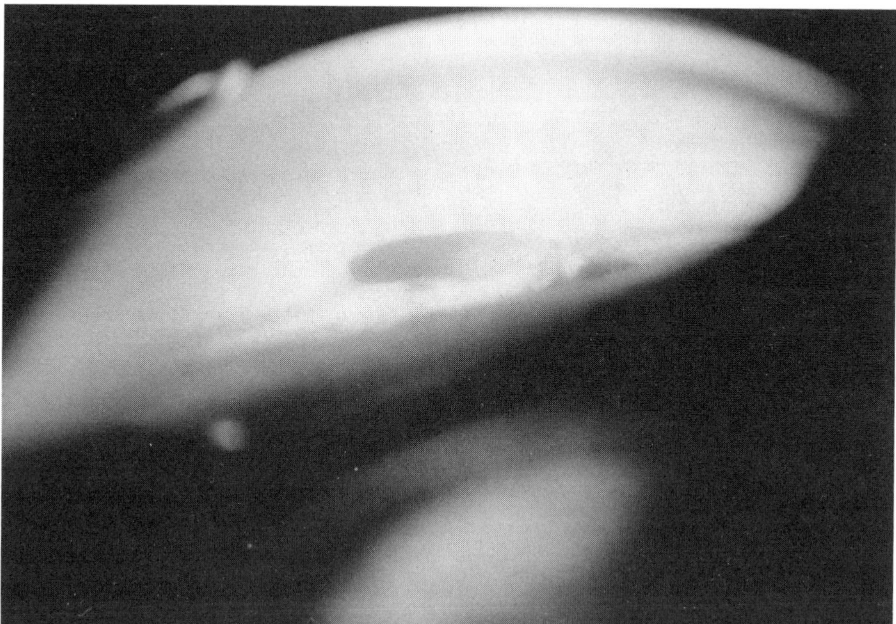

Figure 13-12. A. After the shell is removed, the scleral flap rotates up under the conjunctiva, removing the resistance to filtration. **B.** A large, full-thickness fistula results.

with or without this minor modification, is to the author's knowledge the safest and most effective procedure to obtain intraocular pressures in the 7 to 14 mm Hg range.

References

1. Simmons Richard J, Omah SS: "Shell Tamponade Technique in Glaucoma Surgery." Symposium On Glaucoma, Transactions of the New Orleans Academy of Ophthalmology, C.V. Mosby, St. Louis: 1981, pp. 266-267.
2. Simmons RJ, personal communication.

Releasable Sutures in Filtration Surgery

Richard P. Wilson, MD

The use of a releasable suture in filtration surgery to this author's knowledge originated with Robert Schaffer.[1] He used a subconjunctival horizontal mattress suture starting behind a thermal sclerostomy and exteriorized through clear cornea to cut down on the rapid postoperative egress of aqueous humor characteristic of these procedures. This suture was either released and removed after several days, or if a bow knot had been used, adjusted during the postoperative period to regulate aqueous outflow. The success of this technique in preventing flat chambers and choroidal detachments was limited by the gross nature of the filtering wound. Marked striae formation and induced astigmatism (Fig. 13-13) was necessary to produce a sufficient decrease in early postoperative outflow to avoid hypotony. If a slip or bow knot was used, patient discomfort was also a factor in the limited popularity of this technique. With the advent of guarded filtration procedures, releasable or adjustable sutures have been considered unnecessary. Yet, the variety of situations where releasable sutures would prove helpful has caused this author to develop a technique for use with trabeculectomy.

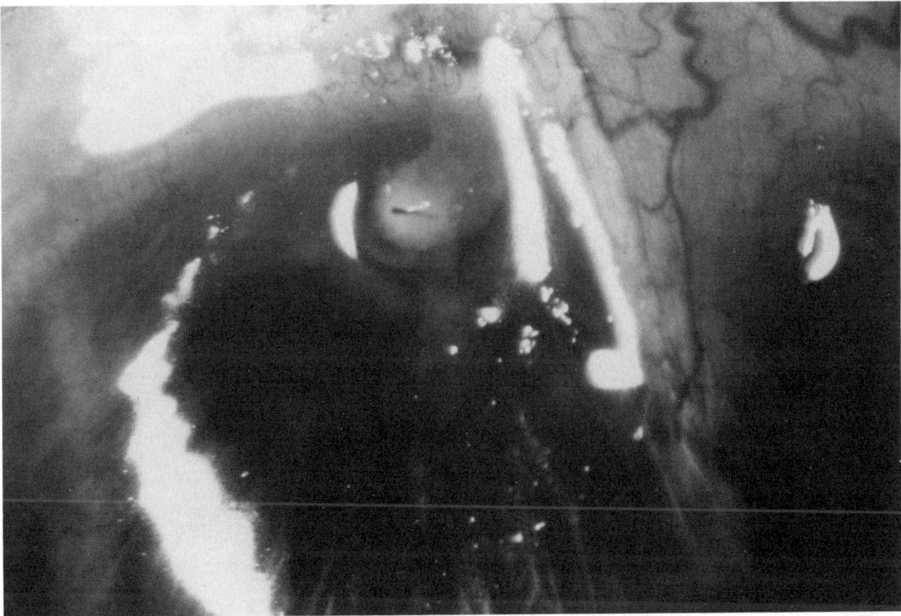

Figure 13-13. Externalized horizontal mattress of 10-0 nylon limiting outflow through thermal sclerostomy. Striae in cornea secondary to tension needed to partially close sclerostomy and ocular hypotony. This is easily reversible with removal of suture.

Procedure

A limbus or fornix-based conjunctival and Tenon's flap can be used, although the author has almost exclusively used a limbus-based flap when gross filtration is required. A paracentesis track is made prior to opening the eye. The scleral flap is approximately one-third scleral thickness and can be either triangular or rectangular. The most important variable is the amount of overlap of scleral flap over scleral block, i.e., how close the edge of the scleral block comes to the edge of the scleral flap. A large overlap with more and tighter sutures will result in less filtration; little overlap with only a few loose sutures allows more.

Usually filtration from all sides of the trabeculectomy site will coalesce to the site of least resistance as the scleral flap heals in position. Therefore, the side with the least overlap and loosest scleral flap will determine the long-term filtration rate, and the overall amount of early filtration will determine the complication rate from hypotony. By aiming the majority of aqueous egress to one side, the surgeon can maximize the flow through the fistula and the chance for it to remain patent. With this in mind, the use of releasable sutures allows the surgeon to adjust the amount of filtration depending upon how the operated eye reacts to the drop in IOP postoperatively. If one makes the scleral block all the way to the edge of the scleral flap on one side but allows one-half millimeter of scleral flap overlap on the other, (Fig. 13-14) two releasable sutures allow the surgeon to choose the rate of aqueous egress and then alter it in the postoperative period by releasing one, the other, or both sutures. Alternatively, one suture can close the side with no overlap, and outflow on the other side can be adjusted by the width of the overlap and the tightness of the posterior suture (Fig. 13-15). After 3 to 8 days, the releasable suture is released allowing a small area of full-thickness filtration.

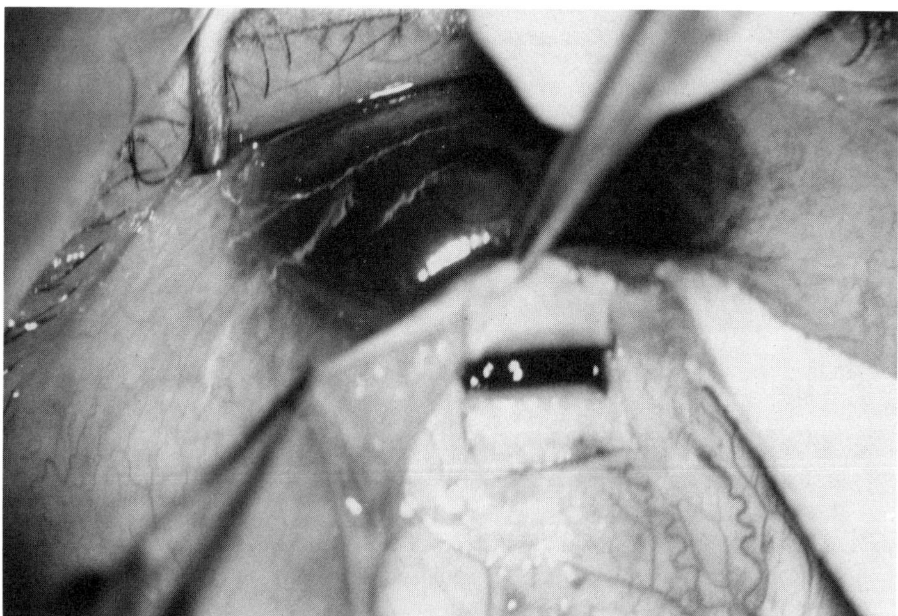

Figure 13-14. With the scleral block to the edge of the scleral flap on one side with no overlap, and on the other side with 1/2 mm of overlap, the surgeon can choose the rate of aqueous filtration in the postoperative period depending upon which releasable suture is cut.

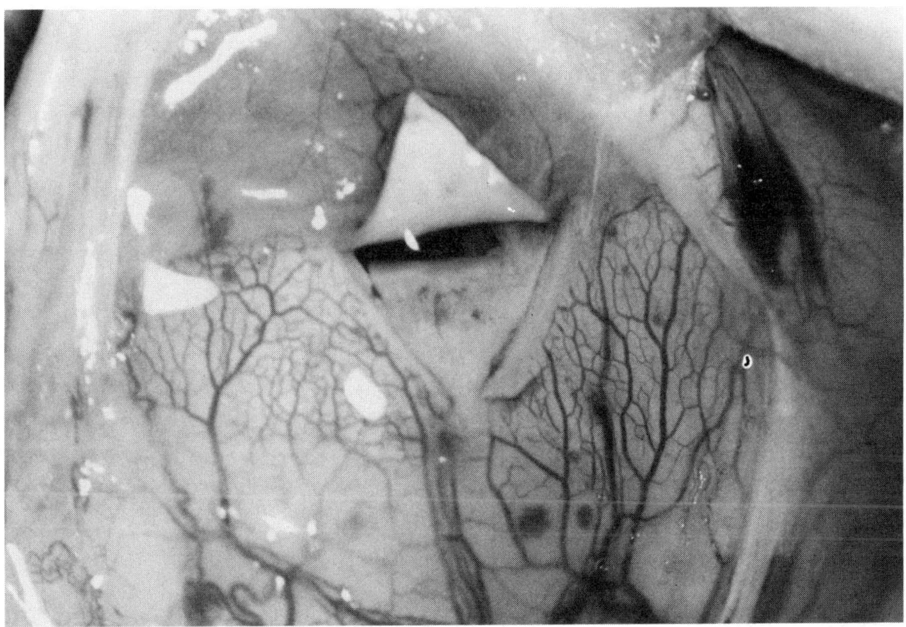

Figure 13-15. If only one releasable suture is to be used, no overlap of flap over block is left on one side of the trabeculectomy block, and more conservative than usual overlap is left on the other.

After the block is excised and an iridectomy done, the parameters varying to fit the patient's needs, one posterior suture for a triangle, two for a rectangle, are loosely placed to hold the flap in position. One or two releasable sutures are placed as needed. The needle is passed from anterior to the limbus in clear cornea (Fig. 13-16) to emerge from the sclera adjacent to the trabeculectomy site. (Fig. 13-17) A suture through the scleral flap and sclera is then taken as usual. (Fig. 13-18) On the third bite the needle enters the sclera behind the limbus and exits through clear cornea completing the exteriorization. (Fig. 13-19A) It is important to have the entrance and exit wounds in clear cornea far enough apart so that when the suture is later cut, the ends will not retract out of reach and the whole suture can be removed (Fig. 13-19B).

If two releasable sutures are to be used, both are placed before either is tied. As they are tied (Fig. 13-20), the anterior chamber is filled with balanced salt solution through the paracentesis and the tension on the sutures adjusted to allow the requisite amount of outflow. The amount of tension is generally greater than usual and the outflow more conservative as the aim of the procedure is to decrease postoperative complications yet allow greater filtration than would normally be obtained long-term by a staged release of flap sutures. While the suture can be made adjustable by tying a small bow knot and keeping the eye patched, any additional benefit seems to be offset by increased inflammation and discomfort. The author prefers to adjust postoperative outflow by cutting sutures at the correct time after the eye has become adjusted to the change in IOP. This allows the suture ends to be cut at the knot during surgery. The cornea usually epithelializes over the suture and the patients have little or no discomfort, although astigmatism is induced until the suture is cut.

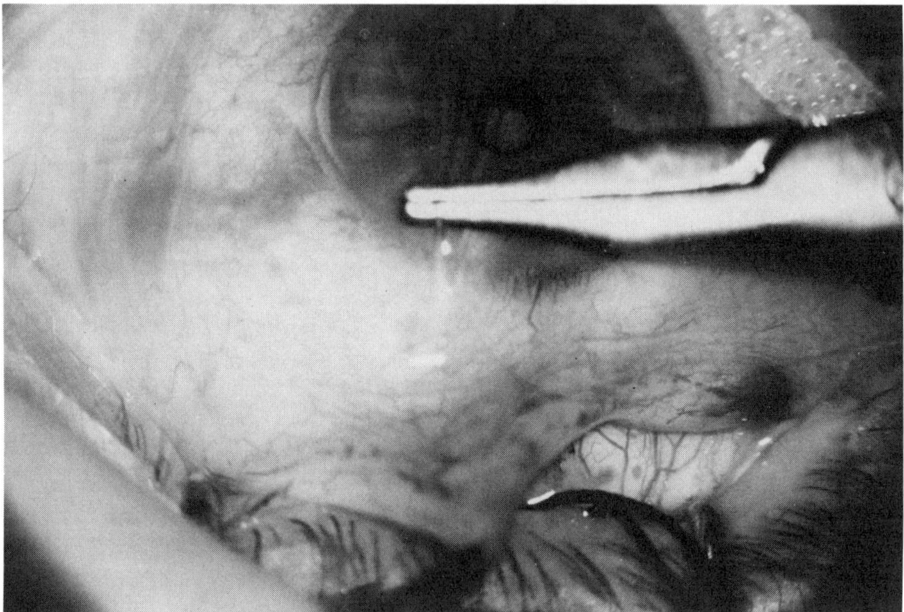

Figure 13-16. A 10-0 nylon suture is directed into clear cornea 1 mm anterior to the limbus and passes under it at approximately half corneal depth.

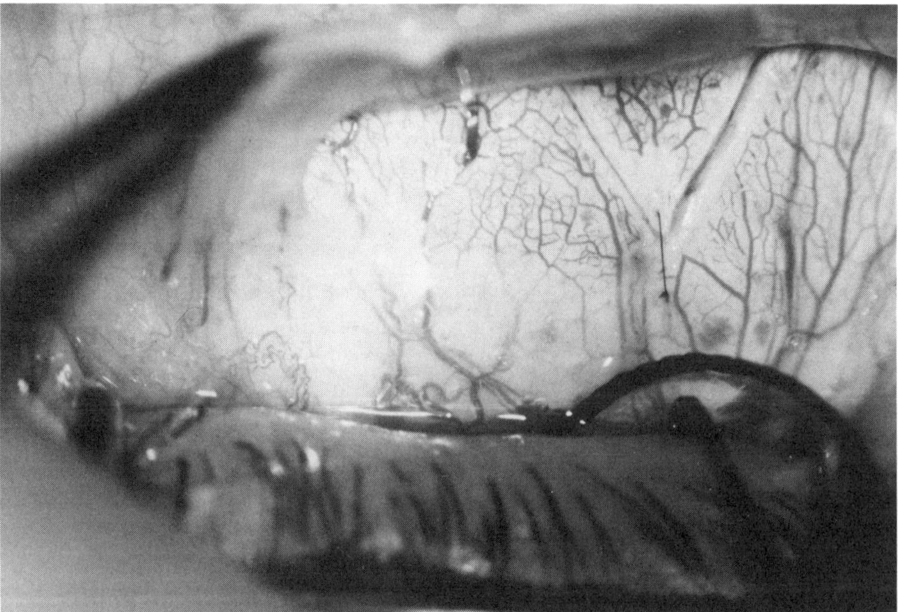

Figure 13-17. The needle emerges adjacent to the trabeculectomy flap.

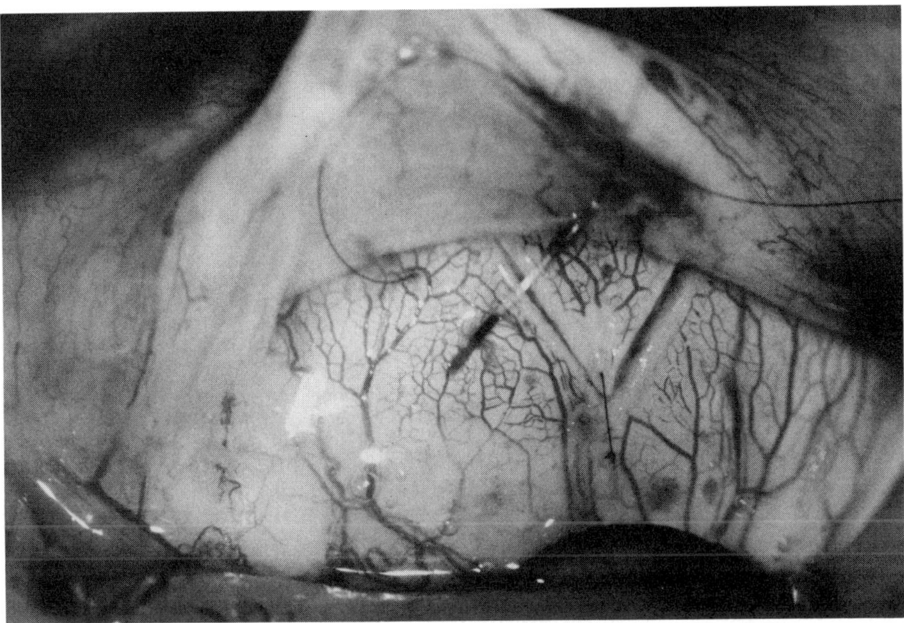

Figure 13-18. A bite through partial-thickness flap and opposing scleral wall is taken as usual.

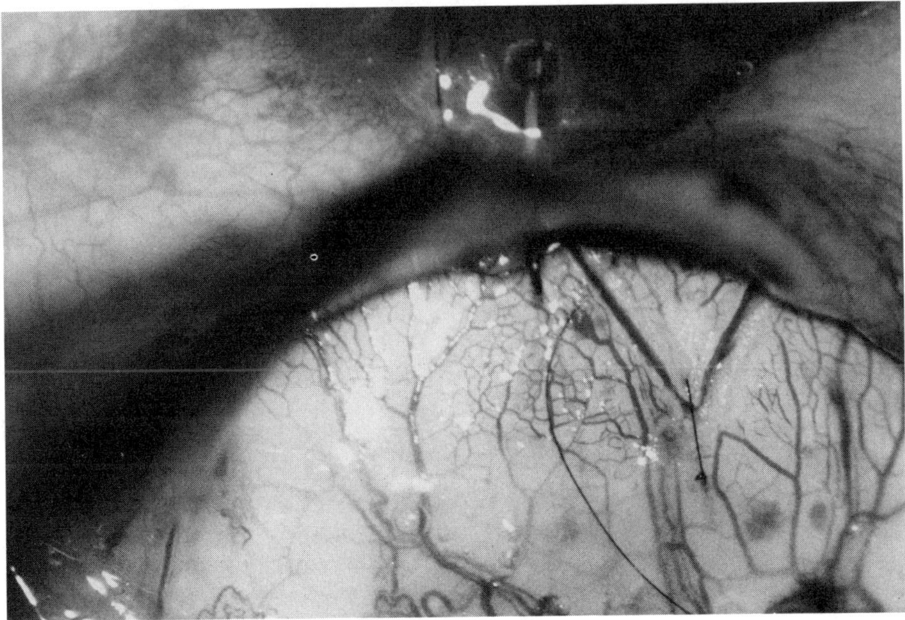

Figure 13-19. A. The needle is shown from its entrance into the sclera behind the limbus emerging through clear cornea anterior to the limbus.

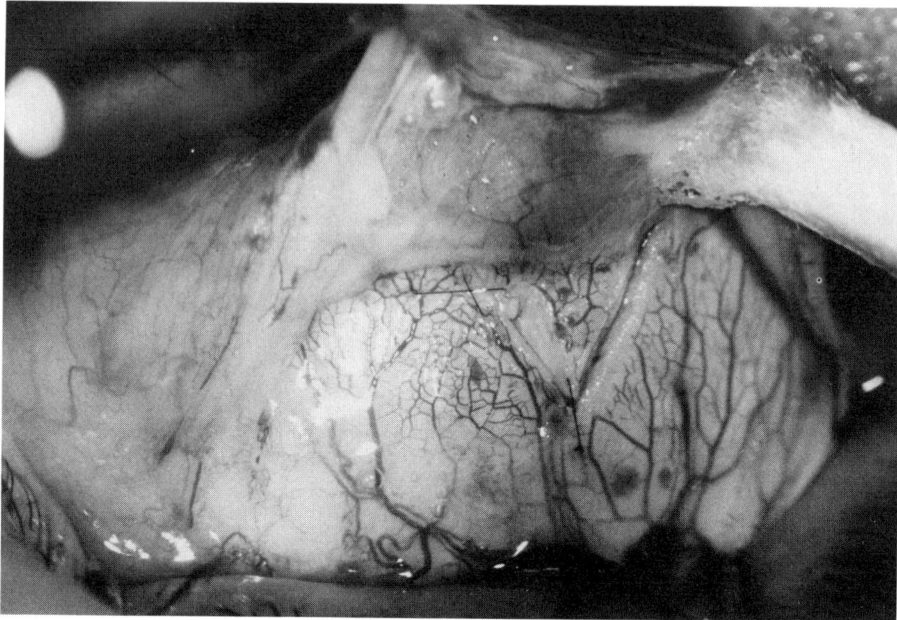

Figure 13-19. B. With both ends of the releasable suture exteriorized, the position of the suture securing the site of gross filtration is shown.

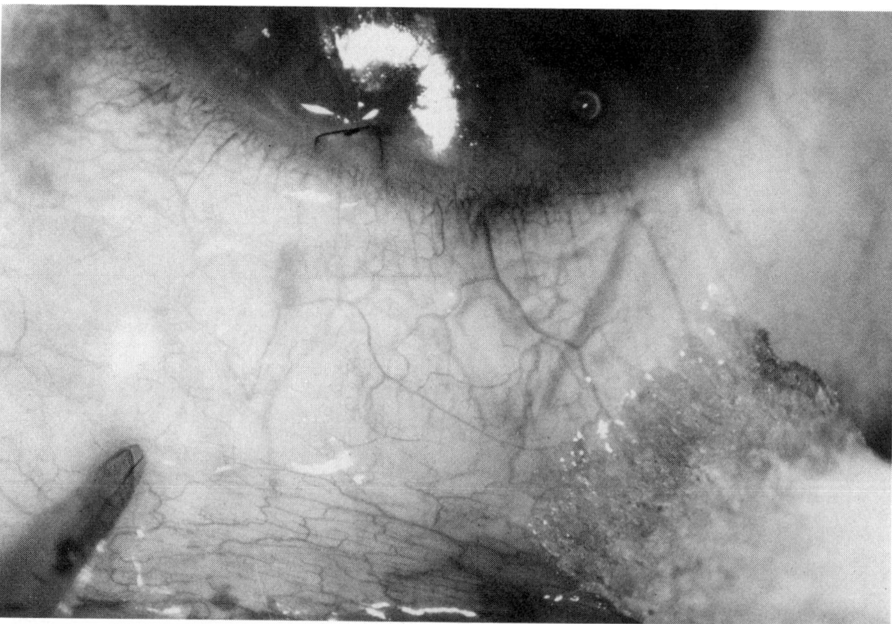

Figure 13-20. The ends of the releasable suture are tied with four throws on the first knot so the anterior chamber can be filled and the suture tightness adjusted for the correct amount of aqueous egress before the locking knots are added.

If the postoperative ocular tension is in the desired range, usually 6 to 14 depending upon the situation, the sutures are not cut until 2 weeks or more. If the tension is slightly higher than desired, the suture on the side with moderate scleral flap overlap is cut, and if more filtration required, removed. If more of an IOP drop is necessary, the suture on the side with no overlap is cut and, if necessary, removed. If filtration is still inadequate, inward pressure alongside the trabeculectomy site exerted with a cotton tipped applicator (Traverso maneuver).[2]

The Simmons Shell Tamponade Technique in this author's hands has been the only consistent method of achieving low pressures (8 to 14 mm Hg) with a low incidence of anterior chamber reformation.[2] The use of releasable sutures offers another method that requires less hospitalization and less patient discomfort. With this technique, a conservative trabeculectomy (generous overlap of scleral flap over trabeculectomy block on all sides) is performed (Fig. 13-21). Two releasable sutures are led with an extra scleral bite to the posterior corners of a rectangular scleral flap to secure this down as per a usual trabeculectomy (Fig. 13-22). During the first week after surgery these sutures are released, allowing the scleral flap to fly up and converting the guarded sclerostomy to an unguarded procedure (Fig. 13-23). This technique allows results in the low teens—but not into the single digits—as is often seen with the shell tamponade technique. The pressure of the shell on the conjunctiva overlying the fistula encourages a 360 degree bleb, with greater area of resorption than a trabeculectomy with fly-away flap (posterior releasable sutures) and therefore a lower pressure.

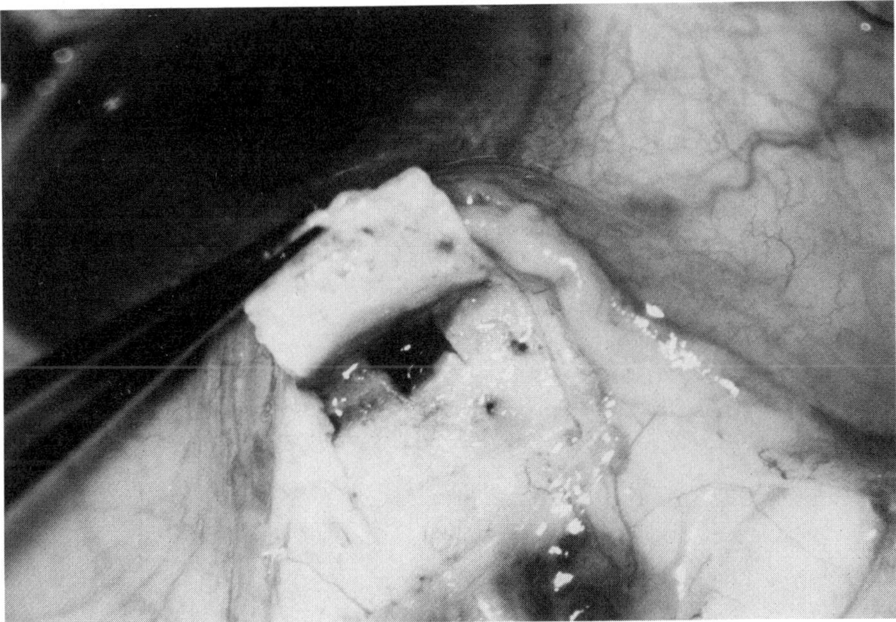

Figure 13-21. A small (1.5 X 1.5 mm) block is excised under a large (4 X 4 mm) flap, offering resistance to outflow with just two posterior sutures.

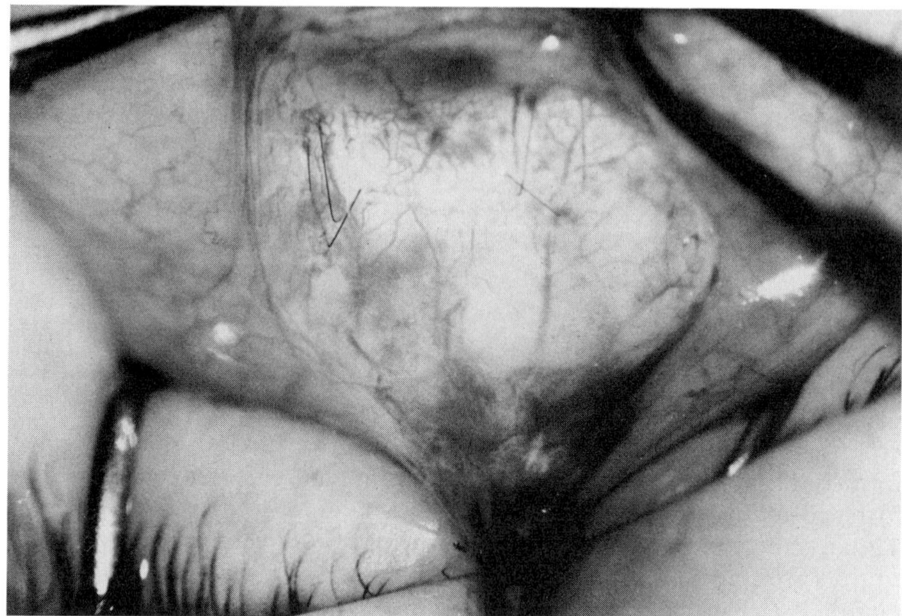

Figure 13-22. Two releasable sutures are led to the back corners of the trabeculectomy by an additional scleral bite. When both are released, the scleral flap flies up converting the protected filter to a full thickness one.

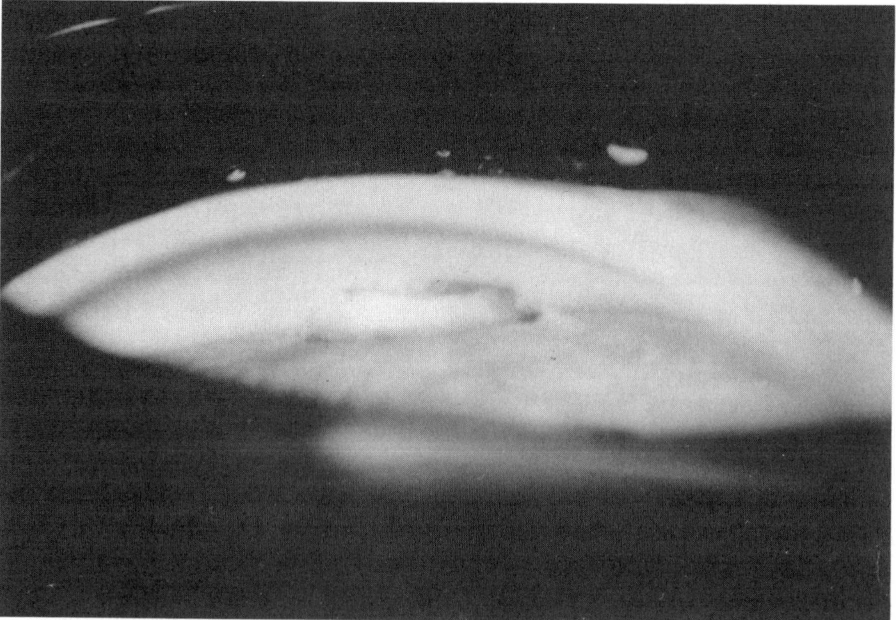

Figure 13-23. Gonioscopic view of sclerectomy with fly-away flap after release of exteriorized sutures.

Clearly the crucial aspect of releasable suture surgery as opposed to using the sutures in an adjustable fashion, is the timing on releasing them. The aim is to gradually lower the IOP and prevent the sudden drop associated with choroidal detachment formation. This is mainly accomplished in three ways:

1. The suture chosen to be removed first is cut but not pulled from its track. Although the suture is then under less tension, it still loosely tethers the scleral flap over the excised block. After ten to fifteen minutes, if the drop in IOP is insufficient, the suture is removed, allowing the flap to rise and permitting more aqueous egress.
2. The overlap on one side is greater than the other; therefore, the side with more overlap should be released first and several hours allowed to judge the pressure drop before considering release of the other suture.
3. With time the scleral flap becomes more adherent to its bed. The more time elapsed since surgery, the less will be the effect of suture cutting and/or removal. In cases where the surgeon guesses wrong and the amount of filtration is just right or too much, the sutures are not removed for 10 to 14 days. At that time there is little or no increase in filtration if 5-fluorouracil has not been used. If gross filtration is required and more risk must be taken to obtain an adequate tension, then suture cutting begins on the second to fifth days.

Unfortunately, experience is the best teacher of when to remove sutures and patients vary as to the time required for their scleral flaps to become adherent to the bed. On the other hand, less experience is required to obtain good results with this method than to guess at the time of surgery how much filtration to allow. This author uses releasable sutures routinely; however, the technique has proved most valuable in the following situations:

1. **Chronic angle closure glaucoma.** Normally the surgeon cannot be very aggressive without risking flat chambers and aqueous misdirection syndrome. This is especially a problem in far advanced disease where gross filtration and a low intraocular pressure are needed. Releasable sutures maintain anterior chamber depth and prevent hypotony until graded suture release allows aggressive filtration.
2. **Far advanced chronic open angle glaucoma.** Again gross filtration is required without increased complications. A fly-away flap will deliver results just short of the shell tamponade technique described by Simmons.[2]
3. **In combined trabeculectomy/extracapsular cataract extraction with or without an intraocular lens.** A deeper chamber and better titration of postoperative pressure is possible.
4. **In positive pressure eyes at surgery.** Usually this happens as the trabeculectomy block is being excised or with the peripheral irridectomy. The anterior chamber shallows and the eye becomes firm. In the past, the author has closed the trabeculectomy flap as quickly as possible to prevent vitreous loss, administered a 50 to 100 cc bolus of intravenous 25% mannitol, and continued to add sutures until the anterior chamber could be kept formed with air or balanced salt solution. This has saved the eye but the final IOP result has been higher than desired because of

the extra sutures. Releasable sutures and sodium hyaluronate have allowed a good long-term pressure result in a borderline nanophthalmic eye with the same scenario.

5. Outpatient trabeculectomy in this era of diagnosis related groups is being aggressively urged by third party payers. Releasable sutures provide an additional measure of safety for the patient and security for the doctor in this setting.

Since the development of this technique, Dunbar Hoskins has invented a lens which makes possible the cutting of 10-0 nylon sutures with the argon laser.[3] (Fig. 13-24) This provides an alternative to releasable sutures in many patients. Obviously to make this technique feasible, an argon laser must be available and convenient to the surgeon throughout the postoperative course. If Tenon's capsule is overly thick, it must be thinned at the time of surgery to allow laser suture lysis later, and even a translucent layer of red blood cells overlying the suture to be cut will prevent light transmission and result in a localized burn or conjunctival perforation. With these provisos, staged augmentation of filtration by laser release of subconjunctival sutures appears as effective in the above applications as the use of releasable sutures. Both methods allow the glaucoma surgeon increased control of the postoperative course and, with experience, can result in safer and more effective filtering surgery.

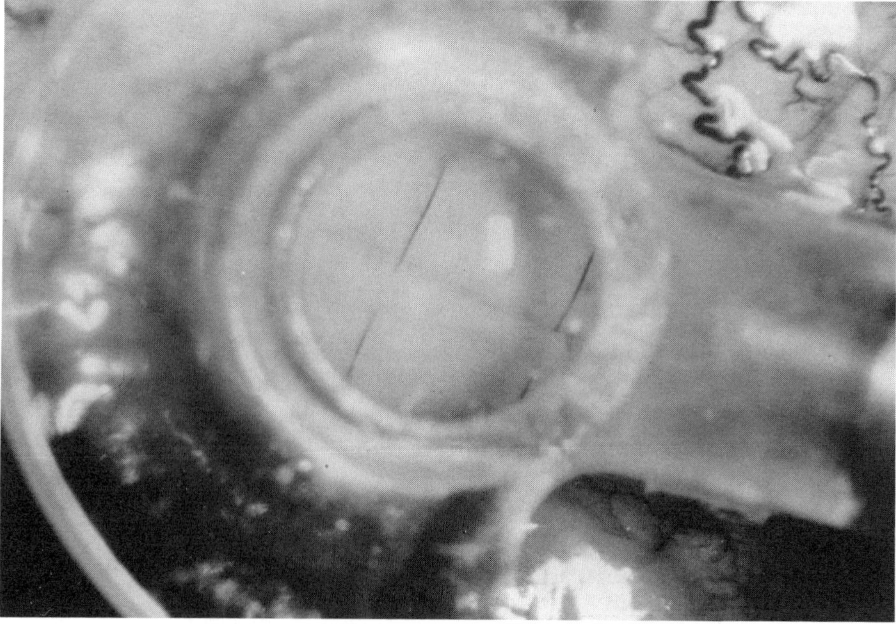

Figure 13-24. Two subconjunctival sutures cut with the argon laser. The Hoskins lens is still in place thinning the overlying conjunctiva.

References

1. Dunbar Hoskins, personal communication.
2. Simmons RJ, Omah SS. Shell Tamponade Technique in Glaucoma Surgery. C.V. Mosby Co., St. Louis: 1981, pp. 226-67.
3. Hoskins Jr, HD, Migliazzo C. Management of Failing Filtering Blebs with the Argon Laser. Ophthalmic Surgery 15:731-3, 1984.

CHAPTER 14

Specific Complications of Filtering Procedures

Management of Conjunctival Buttonholes

George L. Spaeth, MD

Tears, or "buttonholes" in the conjunctiva and Tenon's capsule are complications whose seriousness, when they occur during the performance of filtering procedures for glaucoma, is far greater than their size. They predispose to failure of the filtration procedure and to other more severe problems. They are often difficult to correct.[1-5] The first principle regarding buttonholes is: *avoid them*. The second principle is to make sure buttonholes that have occurred are recognized. The third is to take appropriate but not excessive steps after recognition.

The major reasons for tears in the conjunctiva associated with surgery are: 1) poor visualization and 2) use of instruments that penetrate the tissue. Conjunctiva and Tenon's capsule are tissues that withstand stretching very well. It is rare for them to be torn by traction. However, they are highly susceptible to penetration. Thus the usual cause for conjunctival buttonholes is penetration of the tissue by the tip of a needle, the point of a blade, the tip of a scissors, or the teeth of a forceps. If simple principles can be recalled and practiced, buttonholes almost always can be completely avoided. The surgeon should use an instrument such as Pierse-Hoskins forceps to hold conjunctiva (See Fig. 14-12) and should not employ Colibri, Bonn, or Castroviejo forceps; even serrated forceps such as the Wills Eye Hospital utility forceps can penetrate the tissue. When the conjunctiva is extraordinarily thin it is best handled with completely blunt forceps such as a McPherson or Harms tying forceps. Some prefer a moistened cellulose sponge. However, these too can tear tissue and if used must be employed with caution. Using proper instruments, the surgeon should not be reluctant to put the conjunctiva and Tenon's capsule on stretch. Indeed, failure to do so is a major cause for buttonholes; the loose tissue folds on itself in areas unnoticed by the surgeon, and the needle intended to penetrate merely one portion of the tissue penetrates another inadvertently.

An additional cause for a buttonhole is immediate or delayed necrosis of the conjunctival tissue where it has been cauterized. I am a strong advocate of cauterizing all bleeding on sclera, episclera, and Tenon's capsule, as well as the cut edge of conjunctiva. However, where conjunctiva covers the filtration area, which is virtually *everywhere* except at its intentionally cut edge, cautery on the thin conjunctiva carries with it a great risk of developing a full-thickness hole in the tissue.

One situation in which conjunctival buttonholes are especially likely to occur is in the process of dissecting conjunctiva adherent to episclera or sclera due to previous inflammation, trauma, or surgery. The surgeon should recognize the difficulty inherent in such dissections and plan the surgery accordingly. One helpful technique is to balloon up the tissue by injecting saline or anesthetic agent under the conjunctiva. The injection should be made at least 5 mm away from the area of maximum extent of the intended bleb, using a fine needle such as a #30 sharp. Where appropriate, the filtering procedure should be planned in a different area of the globe. However, it is not always possible to avoid dissections in scarred areas; in many cases the surgeon will have decided that the optimal position for the filtration procedure is at 12:00 o'clock, and that is the area which was previously involved in surgery for retinal detachment, cataract, glaucoma, etc.

There are two basic methods to avoid producing buttonholes in scarred conjunctiva. Both of them employ the principles mentioned already; specifically, handling the tissue with a non-toothed forceps and employing excellent visualization. In the first method the conjunctiva is incised away from the area of the scar and a free edge developed. Holding this edge with a toothless or Pierse-Hoskins forceps, the surgeon then tunnels under the conjunctiva utilizing a blunt-nosed scissors such as a Wescott. The scissors is advanced with the blade closed, and gently pushed between the conjunctiva and the underlying tissue. If resistance is marked, the technique is abandoned. However, in most instances, with gentleness, patience, and persistence it is possible to dissect conjunctival tissue bluntly in this fashion from the underlying tissue to which it is adherent. It is essential that the tips of the scissors are blunt, that they are never used for cutting but merely for blunt dissection by being spread, and that they are introduced into the tissue plane gently. Where it is apparent that the conjunctiva is so adherent to the underlying tissue that it cannot in fact be separated bluntly, then the surgeon is best advised not to separate the conjunctiva from the underlying tissue but to employ the second method.

This technique requires the surgeon to dissect a thin layer of the episclera along with the conjunctiva, so that the conjunctival flap consists of conjunctiva and episclera. This is done sharply, using a knife such as a #67 Beaver blade. This type of dissection is time-consuming and technically demanding. I find the most successful method of performing this sharp dissection is to hold the blade so that it is pulled across the tissue in a movement that is halfway between scraping and cutting. The blade is angled at 45 degrees in both planes. One disadvantage of the second sharp technique of dissecting a conjunctival flap is that it invariably results in significant bleeding.

Another situation in which buttonholes are likely to occur is when the surgeon is attempting to clear the conjunctival flap from the sclera where it terminates at the limbus. Again the usual cause for complication is inadequate visualization, or an attempt to dissect too far anteriorly. The problem usually occurs because the tissue is not being held in a way that permits the surgeon to see what he or she is actually doing.

Once the buttonholes have occurred, their management varies depending on the position of the tear, the nature of the eye, and the stage in the healing process.[1-6] The basic principle is that the buttonhole should be closed completely and tested to make sure that the closure is in fact watertight. If not possible, then the procedure probably needs to be altered to minimize or eliminate filtration occurring in the area of the buttonhole. The devastating effect on the surgical result of a leaking conjunctiva is so great that it is mandatory to examine the eye meticulously at the conclusion of *every* filtering procedure to rule out the presence of a buttonhole that might have occurred undetected during the surgical procedure. It is primarily to make possible the determination of the state of the eye at the end of a filtering procedure that I believe a paracentesis track is essential in every case. This permits the surgeon to fill the anterior chamber at the conclusion to determine how much filtration is occurring, how easily the chamber can be maintained, and if any leaks are present. Management of buttonholes at the time of the primary surgery is far easier than trying to handle the condition at a later stage. (Fig. 14-1)

Recognition of the presence of a buttonhole is essential. The use of a Seidel test is most helpful in this regard. The eye is anesthetized and then the area of the conjunctival flap is painted with fluorescein. The tissue, viewed under the cobalt blue light of the slit lamp, appears dark brown or black. The observer watches carefully to see if there is a change in color to a light green, which signals a leak as the fluorescein becomes diluted. If the test is initially negative, the observer, in most instances, will want to press on the eye in order to raise pressure and force aqueous through any hole present. This is the so-called "positive-pressure Seidel test." The observer cannot be completely assured that a leak is not present unless he or she has performed a positive-pressure Seidel test.

Wherever possible, tears in the conjunctiva are best closed with nonpenetrating sutures. That is, if the tear has gone through conjunctiva and Tenon's capsule, then the tissue should be reflected back so the conjunctival surface is against the globe, and the Tenon's capsule is directly visible. The suture closing the tear should be placed in Tenon's capsule; it should not penetrate completely through the tissue, as needle holes can later become microbuttonholes themselves. The most appropriate suture to employ is usually 10-0 nylon on the finest tapered needle available (a "vascular" needle).

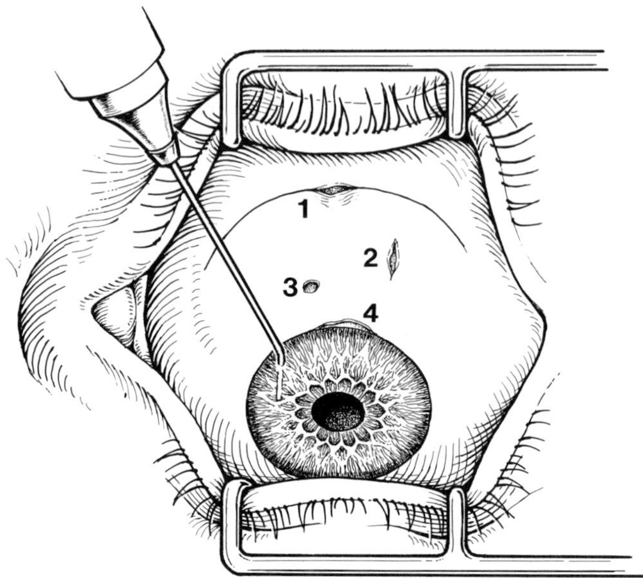

Figure 14-1. The various types of conjunctival buttonholes that are most characteristic are shown in this composite drawing. Filling the anterior chamber with balanced salt solution helps in detecting these buttonholes, and should be routinely performed at the conclusions of every filtration procedure.

Cutting needles can also be employed, but they are more likely to make a larger hole in the conjunctiva than is a needle such as the fine "vascular" needle swedged onto 10-0 nylon.

There is no advantage to using finer suture material. In actuality, a thicker suture, such as 8-0, would in many ways be preferable. It would distribute the pull on the tissue better and be less likely to cause a new tear. However, the needles on such larger sutures are themselves larger, and a major difficulty in closing buttonholes is the damage done to the tissue by the needle itself. Thus, the finest no-cutting *needle* is usually the most preferable, regardless of the type of suture material to which it is attached.

Vertical tears in the conjunctiva usually result from improper suturing of a limbus-based conjunctival flap. (see no. 2 in Fig. 14-1) They most frequently occur fairly far away from the limbus in an area in which Tenon's capsule is still copious. Where they are longer than 2 or 3 mm, they are best closed in one layer on the Tenon's side, by using a running nylon suture, tied at both ends, being sure that the needle does not penetrate through Tenon's capsule into the underlying conjunctiva. (Fig. 14-2)

Tears less than 2 mm long (see no. 3 in Fig. 14-1) are usually best closed by pursestring technique (Fig. 14-3). Here the conjunctival tissue is carefully put on stretch so that the full extent of the buttonhole is clearly visible. If the tear is full thickness (through Tenon's capsule and conjunctiva), the first bite is

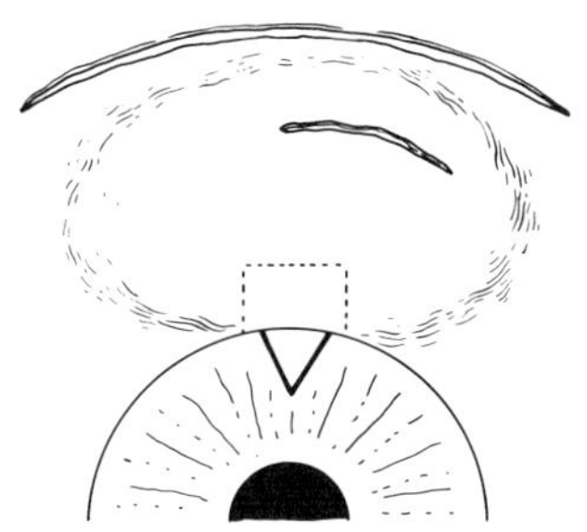
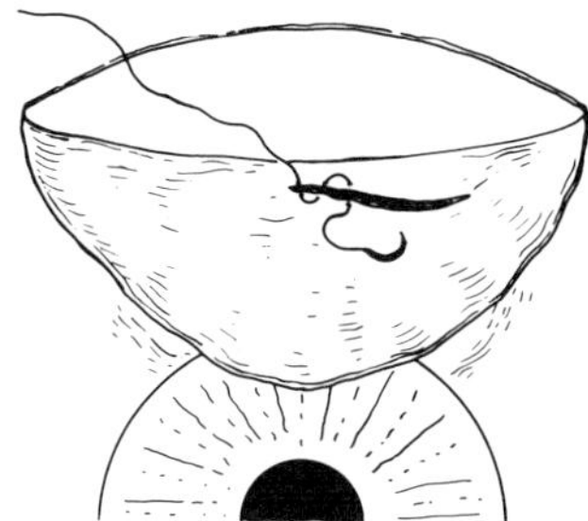

Figure 14-2. Longitudinal tears should be closed form the Tenon's side where possible.

placed in Tenon's capsule, entering the tissue about 0.5 mm outside one end of the tear. The needle is then meticulously threaded for the entire length of the buttonhole, exiting the tissue about 0.5 mm beyond to the other end. The needle is withdrawn and a similar pass made at right angles to the first, extending within Tenon's capsule for the entire length of the tear, not penetrating the conjunctiva. The needle is again withdrawn, and a third placement is made at right angles to the second, parallel to the first suture, though at the opposite side of the buttonhole, the needle proceeding in the opposite direction as the first pass. The final pass of the needle is made parallel to the second suture, so that the needle exits very close to the initial point of entry of the first suture placement. The two ends of the suture are tied so that three or even four loops are placed on the first throw. The two ends are pulled firmly and persistently, to assure that the tissue is firmly compressed upon itself, closing the buttonhole completely. Three additional single throws are then placed on the first throw to assure a completely secure knot. The ends of the knot are cut flush with the knot, using an extremely sharp knife and putting minimal traction on the tissue. When the tear is in conjunctiva and is noted after closure of the incision, the pursestring may be done from either the external or the internal surface of the conjunctiva, unlike the closure of Tenon's capsule, which is always done from the internal surface (Fig. 14-4).

When small buttonhole occurs in conjunctiva where there is no Tenon's capsule, the technique of suture placement is slightly different. The surgeon should zoom the microscope to high magnification. The conjunctiva should be reflected back, in a fashion similar to that just described. However, here there is no Tenon's capsule, so that the needle must be placed with exquisite delicacy, just into the deep layer of the conjunctiva, without penetrating the entire thickness of conjunctiva. The needle is then passed in conjunctiva, staying in the deep layer and being careful never to allow the needle to penetrate the full thickness of the conjunctiva. The pursestring is performed in the same way, and the suture carefully closed to eliminate the buttonhole.

When a conjunctival buttonhole occurs directly at the limbus, and when the tear is 2 mm or less (see no. 4 in Fig. 14-1), it is usually possible to close it with a horizontal mattress suture (Fig. 14-5). Closure is best done with

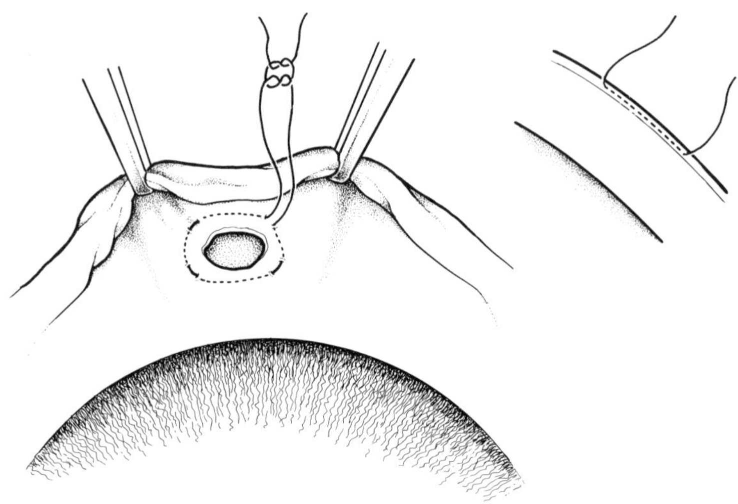

Figure 14-3. The pursestring technique of closure.

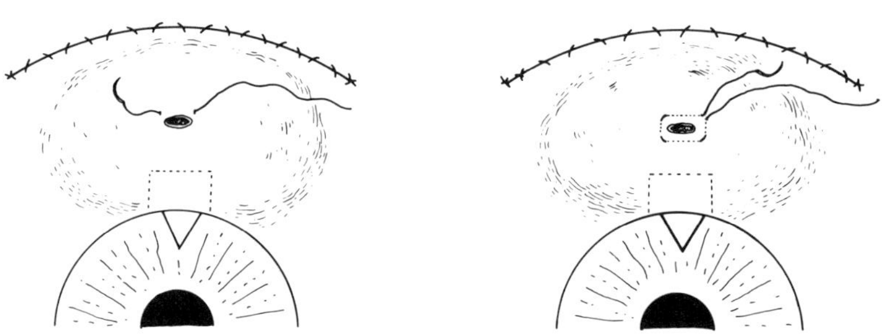

Figure 14-4. The pursestring technique of closure from the conjunctival side.

a double-armed suture. The cornea adjacent to the tear is de-epithelialized. The first bite is placed in the superficial portion of the conjunctiva, again being careful not to penetrate the thickness of the conjunctiva (Fig. 14-6). The needle then enters the cornea approximately a millimeter of two anterior to the limbus, well into the cornea. The second needle is then placed in a similar fashion at the other extremity of the buttonhole and the suture tied in clear cornea, pulling the conjunctiva well down over the area of the tear (Fig. 14-7).

If the buttonhole is longer than 2 mm, it can be closed with multiple mattress sutures or, probably more effectively, by using a running suture that pulls the conjunctiva well down over the limbus onto the cornea.

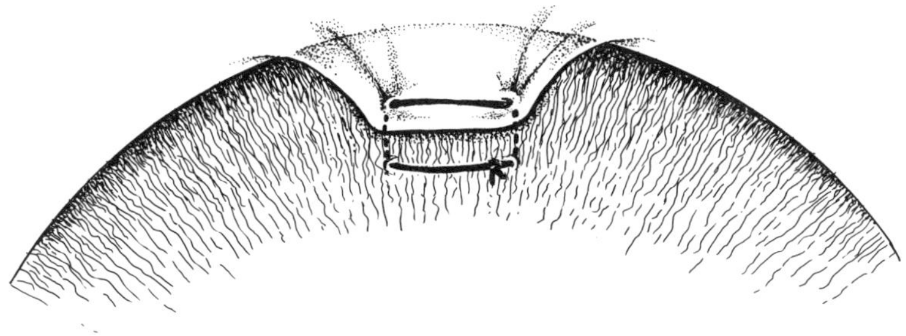

Figure 14-5. Buttonholes at the limbus can be closed with the mattress suture pulling the tissue well over cornea which has had its epithelium denuded.

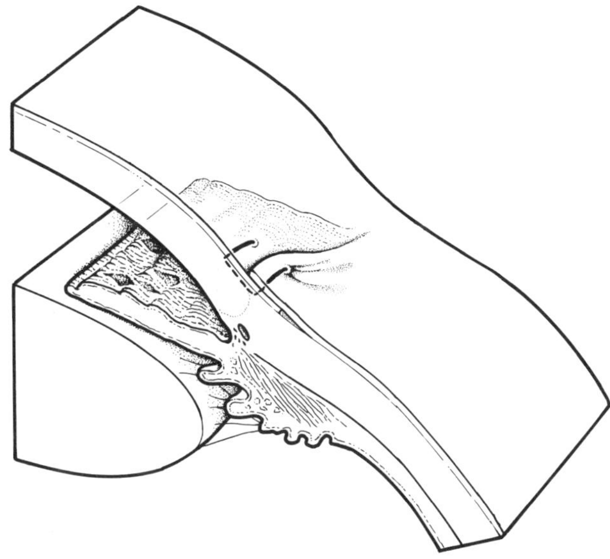

Figure 14-6. It is important there is significant overlap of conjunctiva onto clear cornea.

After buttonholes have been closed, the surgeon should test the area to make sure it is watertight. One way to do this is to grasp the incised edge of the conjunctiva at both its extremities, lift the conjunctival flap up towards the operating microscope, and put it on stretch both upwards and to both sides, thus causing it to take the shape of a vertical wall (Fig. 14-8). The conjunctival side is dried meticulously with sponges. Balanced salt solution is then directed forcibly against this wall from the Tenon's side; no wetting of the "other side" should occur.

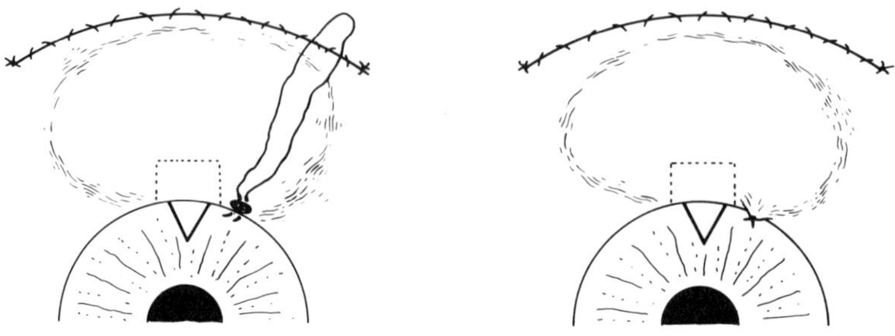

Figure 14-7. Method of placing sutures to repair a limbal buttonhole.

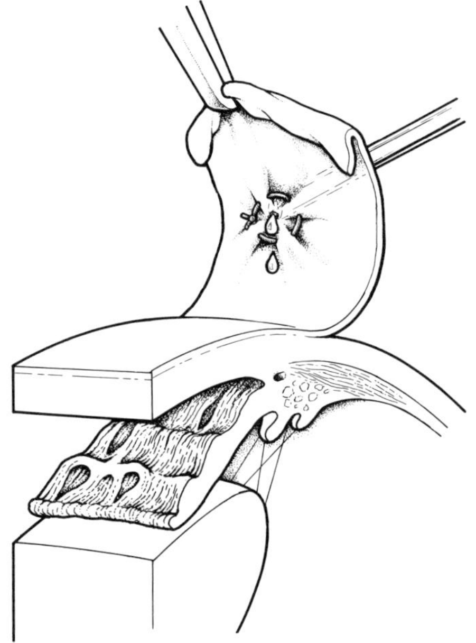

Figure 14-8. Buttonholes should be tested to make sure that no leakage is present.

When a buttonhole occurs within 1 or 2 mm of the incised edge of a limbal-based conjunctival flap (see no. 1 in Fig. 14-1) separate closure of the tear is usually unnecessary; the sutures used to close the conjunctival incision can simply be placed anterior to the tear, so that the buttonhole and conjunctival incision are included simultaneously in one row of sutures (Fig. 14-9).

Some buttonholes may not be noted until the anterior chamber is being filled with saline at the conclusion of the filtering procedure. It is usually best to take down the conjunctival flap completely and repair the buttonhole from the Tenon's capsule side, as described earlier. The exception would be those tears that occur directly at the limbus and which can be repaired by carefully pulling the conjunctiva tightly down onto the cornea, using 10-0 nylon, as mentioned above.

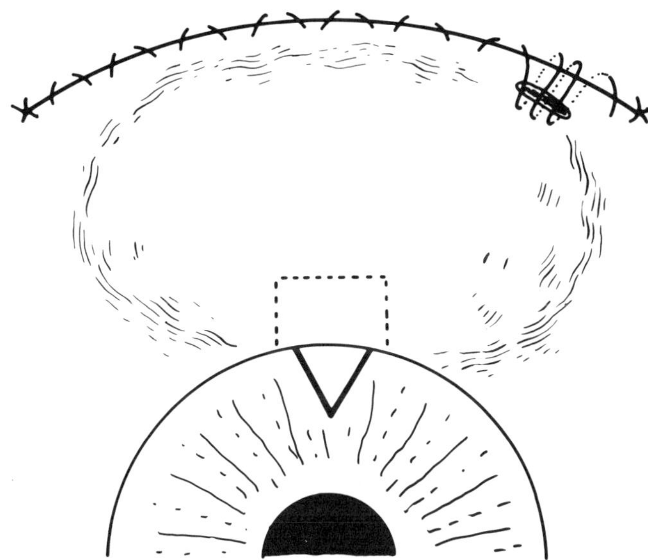

Figure 14-9. Tears near the incision can be incorporated into closure of the conjunctival incision.

In some cases leaks in the conjunctiva will not be noticed until the postoperative period. Because these are often so difficult to repair and their effects on the eye are often so serious, the surgeon should be sure that there are no leaks before concluding the surgical procedure.

If a dehiscence in the conjunctival incision is noted postoperatively, it is a relatively easy matter to suture together the open portion of the incision. The patient does not usually need to be taken back to the operating room to accomplish this. It can be done using an operating microscope in a minor surgery room. However, where the tear is in conjunctiva itself, away from the incision, repair is far more difficult. Placing sutures through inflammed conjuctiva all too frequently only results in more inflammation and a larger tear, and turns a serious situation into one which can become a catastrophe. Therefore, with the exception of dehisced conjunctival incisions, the first approach to the management of conjunctival tears that are first detected in the postoperative period is *medical*, surgery usually being resorted to only if medical therapy fails.

The basic principles are to try to preserve the bleb, avoid hypotony, and avoid circumstances that would discourage healing. As long as the aqueous continues to be manufactured copiously, and the conjunctival bleb remains elevated, the chance of a favorable outcome is still good. Agents such as 5-fluorouracil should be avoided, and topical ocular and systemic corticosteroids used cautiously or not at all. The instillation of atropine 1% every five minutes for four doses, followed by phenylephrine 2.5% every five minutes for four doses, helps assure adequate cycloplegia and mydriasis.

Motion of the lid over the tissue may theoretically hamper the development of an epithelial covering over the tear; therefore, a *light* patch that keeps the lid from moving will possibly be beneficial. A single eyepad is secured in place with tape and a shield placed over the eyepad. This is usually best left in place for twenty-four hours without the eye being distributed in the interim. This conservative mode of treatment is recommended wherever buttonholes are pinpoint, where the intraocular pressure is not low, and where the bleb is not collapsing. Firm pressure patches should not be applied as they can force the aqueous from the eye, causing hypotony and a flat anterior chamber. In most instances placing more than one eyepad on the closed eye results in excessive pressure.

If the tear occurs within several millimeters of the limbus, a large soft contact lens of wide enough circumference to cover the buttonhole can be placed. This can encourage epithelialization and closure.

Some buttonholes will close spontaneously. It is not merely a factor of their size or location. Often the further away it is from an area of aqueous flow, the more likely it is to close. However, tiny buttonholes do not always heal quickly, or even at all; when the buttonhole is over an area where aqueous humor collects, and the aqueous flows actively through the hole, the tear may remain patent for weeks. In some of these cases serious hypotony develops. (It should be remembered that the smaller the tear, the more rapid will be the rate of flow through the rent).

Where a conjunctival buttonhole is leaking so profusely that the bleb is flattening and the intraocular pressure is falling, the conjunctival tear should be repaired. This is especially important if the eye becomes hypotonous and develops a choroidal detachment with a flat anterior chamber. If the tear is close enough to the limbus that it can be covered with a contact lens, then cyanoacrylate glue can be tried. The tear is dried as completely as possible and a very small amount of glue is placed directly on the buttonhole (Fig. 14-10). It hardens immediately.

The resulting rough-edged protuberance is usually too uncomfortable for the patient to tolerate unless covered with a contact lens (Fig. 14-11). If the glue can be left in place until it falls off spontaneously a week or two later, it can assist in healing of the buttonhole. However, in some instances the glue will harden in the shape of a "collar button," and when this sloughs or is removed, leakage will be as copious as before.

Where surgical repair is necessary, it is usually best done in the operating room, often under general anesthesia. If the patient is cooperative and can be adequately sedated, then use of topical proparacaine, reinforced in some instances with topical cocaine, in conjunction with a facial nerve block usually provides adequate akinesia and anesthesia. Because a retrobulbar hemorrhage would be so unmanageable in a patient with a patent fistula, a retrobulbar block is not recommended.

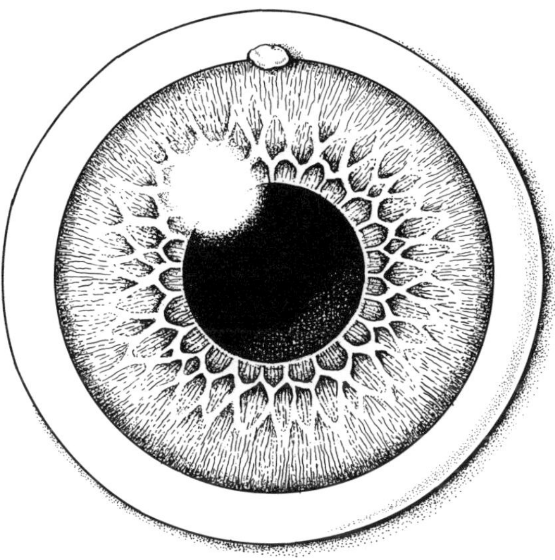

Figure 14-10. Postoperatively, lesions that continue to leak may frequently be covered satisfactorily by "glue."

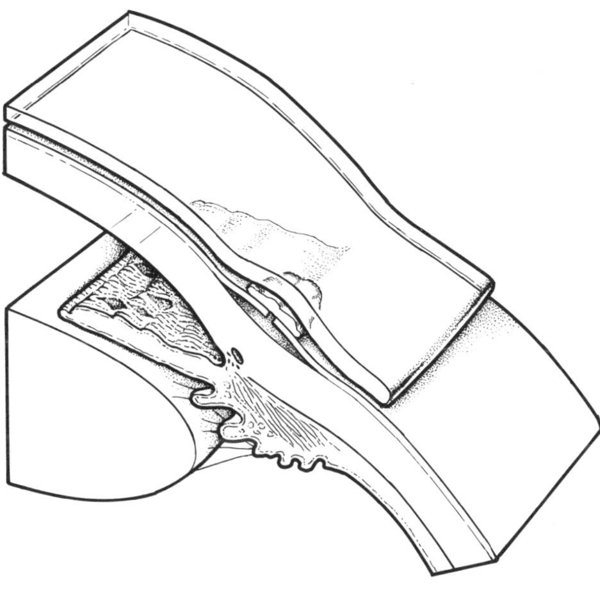

Figure 14-11. In order to relieve the symptoms of "glue" leaks, large contact lenses should be employed to cover the area of the "gluing."

In most instances it is preferable to take down the entire flap and then repair the buttonhole at the time of surgery, as described earlier in this chapter. The surgeon should not be misled into thinking that it will be easy to put sutures in the edge of the tear and pull the tissue together. In most instances the tissue is "cheesy" and the sutures pull through, enlarging the size of the rent. Some surgeons believe that using a larger suture such as 7-0 polygalactin (Vicryl) provides better holding, but the larger needles attached to such sutures cause more tearing of the tissue than is acceptable. In addition, the sutures themselves can cause further tissue necrosis. If conjunctiva cannot be easily approximated with a fine suture such as 10-0 nylon, it will not be able to be held with a larger suture. Where tissues are forcibly approximated, they will pull apart later in most instances.

In some cases a large area of sclera is exposed; this is especially likely to occur where multiple attempts to repair a leak have already been made. In these cases salvage of the eye takes precedence over development of filtration; the surgeon's primary goal is to restore the planes of the eye and correct the leak. This may require closing the sclerostomy. Less drastic is the technique of removing Tenon's capsule from a different portion of the eye and pulling this tautly over the leak, with sufficient firmness that restoration of the chamber is possible. This should then be covered with a large fornix-based flap pulled well over de-epithelialized cornea, and sutured firmly onto the cornea with multiple 10-0 nylon sutures. It is usually necessary to undermine the tissue extensively in order to free the conjunctiva adequately. If it is put on excessive stretch it will promptly pull off the cornea, leaving the eye worse than before.

References

1. Cohen JS, Shaffer RN, Hetherington J. Hoskins D. Revision of filtration surgery. Arch Ophthalmol 95:1612-1615, 1977.
2. Dellaporta A. Repairing filtering blebs (Letter). Am J Ophthalmol 94(2):269-271, 1982.
3. Galin MA, Hung PT. Surgical repair of leaking blebs. Am J Ophthalmol 83:328-333, 1977.
4. Grady FJ, Forbes M. Tissue adhesive for repair of conjunctival buttonhole in glaucoma surgery. Am J Ophthalmol 68:656-658, 1969.
5. Melamed S, Hersh P, Kerstein D, et al. The use of glaucoma shell tamponade in leaking filtration blebs. Ophthalmology 93:839-842, 1986.
6. Petursson GJ, Fraunfelder FT. Repair of an inadvertent buttonhole or leaking filtering bleb. Arch Ophthalmol 97:926-927, 1979.

Difficulties with the Scleral Flap in Trabeculectomy

George L. Spaeth, MD

The ideal type of scleral flap in trabeculectomy (or sclerotomy) has not been determined. One study has shown that the size of the scleral flap, size of the excised block, and position of the block (Cairns or Watson method) are unrelated to the final intraocular pressure.[1] However, the effect of varying thickness of the scleral flap or amount of overlap of the underlying bed has not been systematically studied. My clinical impression is that the thickness of the flap is related to the final result; where the flap is very thin, that is, approximately one-fifth or less the thickness of the sclera, filtration appears to be more copious. Complications, however, also appear to be more common. Where the flap is thick, flow is limited and the final pressure is higher. Additionally, the smaller the overlap between the radial edge of the scleral flap and the radial edge of the excised block the larger the amount of filtration. My preference generally is to make a "thin" flap (around one-quarter or slightly thicker if a very low pressure is desired) with a "large" overlap (slightly less than a half millimeter). If the scleral flap is too thick (half the thickness of the sclera or thicker), it tends to scar down, leading to failure of the procedure. If the scleral flap is too thin (less than a fifth the thickness of the normal sclera), leakage can be excessive, predisposing to flat anterior chamber, hypotony, and choroidal detachment.

The thinner the flap, the greater the care that must be taken in closing it. When the flap is one-fifth the thickness of the sclera, or thinner than that, cutting needles such as those typically swedged onto 10-0 nylon are usually the most appropriate. The surgeon must be careful not to penetrate the scleral flap completely when placing the sutures in the scleral flap. These sutures used to close the scleral flap should be extremely superficial. This can be accomplished by placing the tip of a very sharp needle on the surface of the scleral flap, about 1 mm from the edges to be closed, and then carefully advancing the needle, staying within the thickness of the scleral flap. If the needle penetrates through a thin flap, it quite frequently pulls through the scleral flap when the suture is tied, leaving a shredded edge without overlap; this makes adequate coverage of the sclerostomy very difficult.

One way to dissect a scleral flap of proper thickness is as follows. The magnification of the operating scope should be increased for this portion of the procedure. The size is approximately 3 × 3 mm. The dissection of the flap starts at one posterior corner, and the flap is made quite thick initially, cutting deep down into the sclera. The radial grooves are made about half the thickness of the sclera. Once the flap has been started, it is "easy" to make the flap thinner or thicker (Fig. 14-12). This demands meticulous visualization; the surgeon should insist that the assistant keep the field absolutely clean and dry. Both the deep and the superficial surfaces should be observed frequently

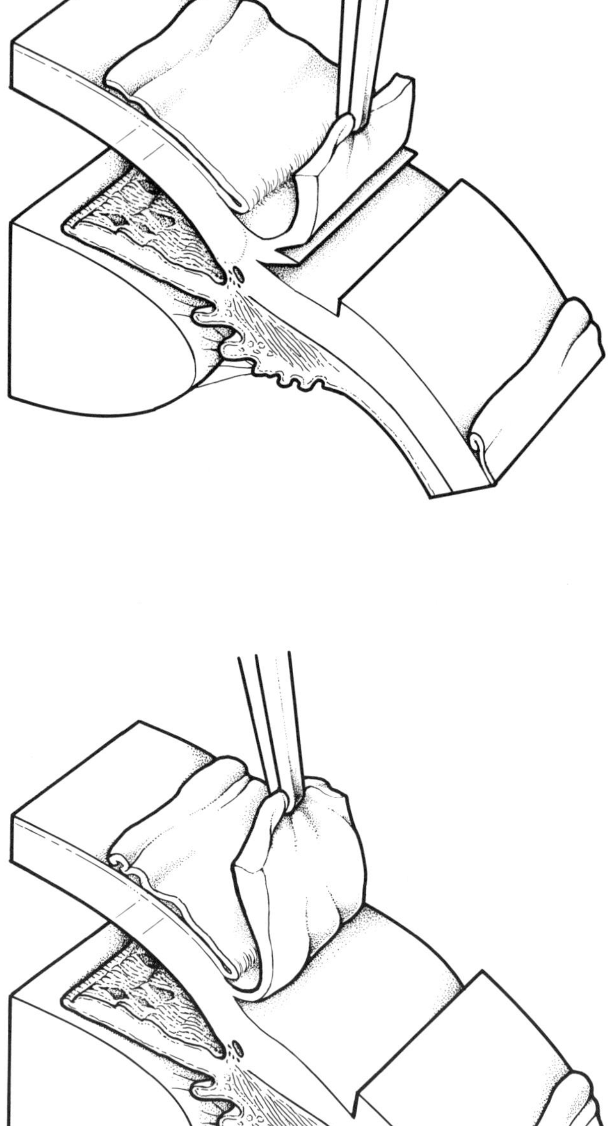

Figure 14-12. A. Holding a flap with a nontoothed forceps, the scleral flap is dissected, starting with thicker tissue, and then making the tissue thinner as it extends anteriorly. **B.** The thickness of the flap can easily be adjusted as the dissection proceeds.

(Fig. 14-13). Toothed forceps should be avoided, as they can penetrate the flap. The flap should be held with a toothless forceps such as a Pierse-Hoskins. If cautery is applied on the flap itself, it should be very minimal, so that it does not produce a hole that will later leak excessively.

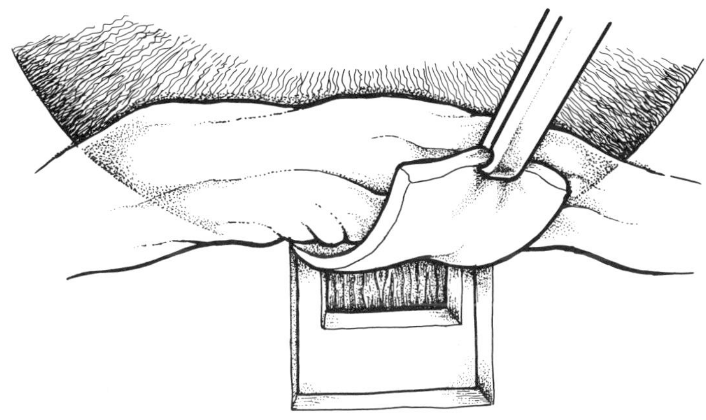

Figure 14-13. Good visibility is the central concern. The block of tissue removed internally should be anterior to the scleral spur.

If a tear or an excessive leak in the scleral flap is noted, the surgeon must decide whether or not the likelihood of a flat anterior chamber is great enough to take corrective steps. The most important clue is the ease with which the anterior chamber remains formed when filled at the time of surgery. Balanced salt solution is injected into the anterior chamber through the previously placed parencentesis track, and the surgeon monitors the intraocular pressure digitally (see Fig. 14-1). When the chamber is vigorously filled, the IOP should rise; indeed, the eye should become firm, with an IOP around 20 mm Hg or higher. After stopping injection of saline into the anterior chamber through the parencentesis track, the eye should soften. If it does not, it is unlikely that filtration will be adequate. If the chamber remains deep, even after the eye has become softer, the likelihood of a later flat anterior chamber is probably sufficiently small that the surgeon may wish to leave the tear in the scleral flap unrepaired, being especially careful, however, to close the Tenon's capsule tightly, and conjunctiva perfectly, so as to achieve a watertight closure.

Where leakage through the scleral flap is excessive, so that the chamber collapses, it is usually advisable to try to provide additional resistance to outflow (Fig. 14-14).

If the scleral flap is so thin that it has already been torn, or if it has been amputated from its base, closing it further is usually difficult or impossible. Rather than make such an attempt, provision of an additional covering over the scleral flap is usually wiser. This can be accomplished by transferring a piece of Tenon's capsule from the area of the incision in Tenon's capsule,

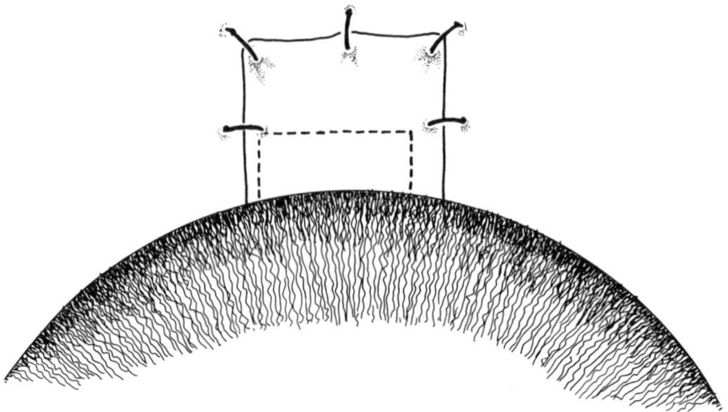

Figure 14-14. Sufficient sutures should be placed so that the anterior chamber can be well formed. Text describes the technique in detail.

choosing as thick a piece of tissue as is available. Tenon's capsule is usually present to the extent of marked redundancy about 8 to 10 mm posterior to the limbus in the superotemporal quadrant.

Once identified, a swatch approximately 4 × 4 mm, measured when the tissue is on stretch, is excised (Fig. 14-15). This will then be pulled down tightly over the area of the scleral flap. One corner of the tissue is sutured into the "cornea." Recall, the conjunctival flap is dissected to reveal a completely clean corneoscleral sulcus. This should reveal a clear corner, *immediately posterior to the conjunctiva,* as far anterior as possible and approximately 2 mm nasally to the nasal radial groove. 10-0 nylon is an appropriate material to employ.

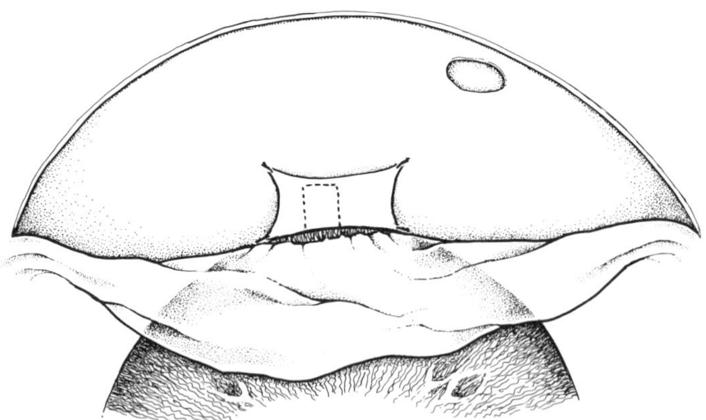

Figure 14-15. Placement of Tenon's "graft" over excessively filtering scleral flap.

The opposite edge of the excised piece of Tenon's capsule, that is, the corner on the temporal side, is then grasped and pulled temporally so that it is put on *tight* stretch. If this extends more than a millimeter or two beyond the temporal edge of the scleral flap, the excess tissue is excised. This anterior temporal corner is then sutured into the cornea as close to the posterior edge of the conjunctival reflection as possible; that is, the needle is inserted as close to the anterior extent of the conjunction as can be accomplished. The posterior nasal corner of the "Tenon's capsule graft" is then grasped and forcibly pulled posteriorly and nasally, again putting the tissue on firm stretch, and is secured firmly to the sclera with 10-0 nylon. The posterior temporal edge is then similarly pulled taut and sutured to the sclera.

At the conclusion the area of the trabeculectomy flap should be completely covered with the "Tenon's graft," which is on firm stretch (Fig. 14-15). As is recommended with all filtration procedures, the procedure concludes by filling the anterior chamber with balanced salt solution through a previously placed keratostomy. Whereas the amount of saline leaking through the torn scleral flap was previously excessive, following the repair just described, it is usually possible to form the chamber satisfactorily with minimal leakage underneath the cut edges of the Tenon's graft. If this cannot be accomplished, the surgeon must consider the relative risks of performing a full thickness procedure with the risk of not achieving a sufficiently lower IOP. If a very low IOP is the primary goal, the surgeon will conclude the procedure by closing the Tenon's-conjunctival flap carefully over the leaking sclera, instill 2.5% phenylephrine drops (four drops over four minutes) and atropine 1% ointment, and observe the patient especially carefully in the postoperative period. Use of a compression shell such as that described by Simmons may possibly decrease the chance of a flat anterior chamber. If the safety of the eye is the primary goal, an appropriately sized piece of partial-thickness sclera from an area immediately adjacent to the defect can be developed, hinged along one of the radial grooves of the scleral flap. This new, partial-thickness, still-connected flap can then be folded over the leaking area and sutured into full-thickness sclera. A donor sclera flap should *not* be used, as the inflammatory response will be so great as to cause failure of the procedure.

Reference

1. Starita FJ, Fellman FL, Spaeth GL, Poryzees EM. Effect of varying size of scleral flap and corneal block on trabeculectomy. Ophthalmic Surgery 15:484-487, 1984.

Flat Anterior Chamber

George L. Spaeth, MD

Probably the most common and irritating complication of filtering glaucoma surgery is the so-called "flat anterior chamber." Simply making a big hole in the eye is not the secret to successful surgery. The sequence of excessive filtration, hypotension, ciliochoroidal detachment, aqueous shutdown, failure of the bleb, scarring of the sclerostomy, resumption of aqueous flow, and uncontrollable glaucoma is all too familiar. In such a situation the patient has had a procedure of little or no benefit. The flat anterior chamber, however, is not just a common nuisance. It also can result in damage to the eye: more rapidly progressing cataract, peripheral anterior synechiae, posterior synechiae, and corneal decompensation.

As with most complications, the best treatment is avoidance. Flat anterior chamber, however, cannot be completely avoided because a leak is purposely made; inevitably there will be cases in which filtration is excessive. The frequency of flat anterior chamber, on the other hand, can be minimized. One important step is making sure that the anterior chamber is well formed at the close of surgery. It is rarely advisable for the surgeon to leave the operating room before the anterior chamber has been reformed and is maintaining itself satisfactorily.

Reformation of the anterior chamber at the time of surgery demands the presence of a patent keratostomy. For this as well as for other reasons the author believes a paracentesis with a sharp 25-gauge needle should be employed in *every* filtering glaucoma procedure. The keratostomy is performed so that the needle is *always* parallel to the iris and *never* angled toward the lens. If fixation is secure, the procedure is almost without risk. Prior to closing the conjunctiva the anterior chamber should be filled with balanced salt solution, through the previously placed keratostomy, with a 30-gauge blunt cannula. If the chamber does not remain formed, then additional sutures need to be placed in the scleral flap or other steps taken to determine why the chamber is flattening and what needs to be done to keep it formed.

Prevention of other causes for a flat anterior chamber, such as pupillary block and malignant glaucoma, is also important. This entails making sure the iridectomy is patent, and that the eye is maximally cyclopleged at the conclusion of the procedure. I instill atropine 1% repeatedly after the iridectomy is completed, and instill atropine ointment at the close.

Definition and Grading of a Flat Anterior Chamber

First, it is appropriate to define "flat anterior chamber." Literally, a flat anterior chamber means that there is contact between the corneal endothelium and some underlying tissue—iris, lens, intraocular lens, etc. There are, however, differing grades and significances of a flat anterior chamber. One workable system is that suggested by the author (Fig. 14-16). A Grade I anterior chamber describes contact which is *limited to the peripheral iris and cornea*.

In Grade II, the corneal endothelium is in contact with the iris in *all areas except over the pupil and immediately adjacent to the pupil*. Grade IIA has the additional problem of contact between the cornea and a structure underlying the peripheral iris, such as the lens in the area of a peripheral iridectomy. A Grade III flat anterior chamber describes the situation in which there is *no anterior chamber in any area* (that is, there is lens-endothelial touch centrally).

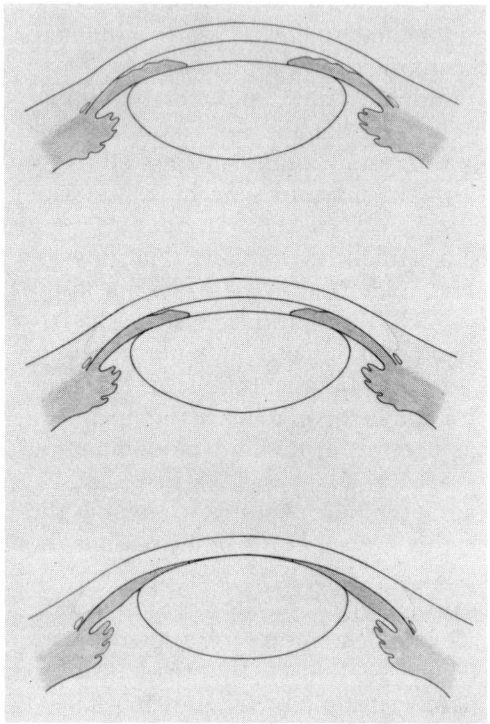

Figure 14-16. System for grading shallow or "flat" anterior chamber. **A.** Grade I. Peripheral iris-cornea contact. **B.** Grade II. Iris-cornea contact extends almost to pupil margin; there is no lens-cornea contact. **C.** Grade III. Contact is present between cornea and underlying lens (or vitreous or pseudo phakos).

Strictly speaking, only a Grade III flat anterior chamber is really a "flat" anterior chamber. All the others are gradations of "shallow" anterior chambers. The distinction is not merely academic. A Grade III flat anterior chamber virtually never clears up without surgical intervention. Additionally, when the corneal endothelium is in contact with the lens epithelium, the vitreous, the lens capsule, or an intraocular lens, the health of the eye is immediately in jeopardy. Surgical intervention is urgent. Within hours there can be permanent adhesion between the corneal endothelium and the lens epithelium (or other surface). If reformation of the anterior chamber occurs after such an adhesion has developed, it results in significant permanent damage to the cornea, and often to the lens as well. Thus the recognition of a Grade III flat anterior chamber and its accurate distinction from a Grade II anterior chamber is important.

Mechanism of Flat Anterior Chamber

Three major mechanisms are responsible for a shallowing of the anterior chamber following surgery: 1) imbalance between the pressure posterior to the iris and the pressure anterior to the iris; 2) inadequate aqueous formation (this is related to the first); and 3) anterior rotation of the ciliary body.

Abnormalities of aqueous flow account for the majority of flat anterior chambers following glaucoma surgery. Where there is excessive filtration, the anterior chamber simply collapses due to the higher pressure posterior to the iris. Factors influencing such a collapse are the magnitude of the pressure difference and the forces that tend to maintain the tissues in their proper planes. Healthy, strong, longitudinal muscles of the ciliary body pulling against well-anchored zonules of the normal lens form a potent force pulling the lens-iris diaphragm posteriorly, maintaining the anterior chamber even where there is a complete sclerostomy with no resistance whatsoever to aqueous outflow. However, with increasing age the ciliary body becomes atrophic. The absence of complete cycloplegia allows the sphincter of the ciliary body to overcome the longitudinal fibers, pulling the lens-iris diaphragm anteriorly. Zonules are weakened in eyes that have the exfoliation syndrome, have been traumatized, or are elderly. It thus is not surprising that the elderly patient with a mature lens and the exfoliation syndrome is far more likely to have a flat anterior chamber following glaucoma surgery than is the 15-year-old myope with juvenile glaucoma.

Imbalance of pressure can be the result of interference with the flow of aqueous from the posterior to the anterior chamber caused by lens-iris adhesions, excessively tight apposition of the iris to the lens or pseudophakos, excessive air in the anterior chamber, vitreous extruding through the pupil, etc. In such cases, especially where the adhesions are limited to the pupillary margin and where the iris is flaccid (as in the elderly or the blue-eyed), the interference with aqueous flow frequently results in an iris bombé. However, where the iris is thick, or where adhesions are extensive, iris bombé may be slight or even absent. One must not rely on the presence of an iris bombé to diagnose pupillary block glaucoma. It is a valuable sign when observed and should definitely be looked for, but its absence should not be considered proof of the absence of pupillary block.

One diagnostic sign of help in selected situations, especially where the eye is quiet and the distinction between pupillary block and aqueous misdirection glaucoma is difficult, is the use of intravenously administered fluorescein. Normally, fluorescein oozes from the posterior into the anterior chamber approximately 30 seconds following the injection of sodium fluorescein into the antecubital vein (using the same agent employed for routine fluorescein angiography). The fluorescein tinges the aqueous, making its flow visible when examining the patient at the slit-lamp. The room must be darkened, and I prefer using a thin white beam with the light intensity at its maximum. The use of the blue filter enhances the fluorescence, but is not as helpful as might be anticipated, as it reduces the intensity. In the normal eye, one can see the fluorescein seeping through the pupil, often in isolated streams, whereas in the affected eye, there is reduced or absent flow through the pupil. It is important to recall that in certain conditions the vessels of the iris leak fluorescein, and so fluorescein can appear in the anterior chamber even where there is total pupillary block. Fluorescein leakage at the blood vessels is especially common with rubeosis iridis, ocular inflammation, and the exfoliation syndrome. Thus the examiner does not look for fluorescein in the anterior chamber, but rather for the flow of fluorescein-tinged aqueous through the pupil.

In the aqueous misdirection syndrome, fluorescein-tinged aqueous humor is seen to pool in the posterior segment, posterior to the lens in the phakic patient, or to the vitreous face, inflammatory membrane, or pseudophakos in the aphakic patient.

The aqueous misdirection syndrome is probably far more common than is generally realized. In this entity aqueous humor is trapped in the posterior segment of the eye. The classical presentation is a combination of a Grade III or perhaps Grade II flat anterior chamber in association with a high intraocular pressure and pupillary block in an eye just having had intraocular surgery. The most frequently afflicted patient is the one with acute or chronic angle closure glaucoma having a filtration procedure. However, it is unlikely that it is the angle closure component which is the predisposing factor; rather it is probably the smallness of the anterior segment. Shaffer and coworkers have entitled the entity "ciliary block glaucoma," which appears appropriate. The lens moves anteriorly, pressing against the ciliary body, blocking the normal flow of aqueous humor from the posterior to the anterior chambers. And indeed, the most important aspect of treatment is the use of agents that will result in posterior movement of the lens-iris diaphragm.

Thus, maximum cycloplegia, as can be achieved with use of atropine 1% every five minutes for four doses (or perhaps even atropine 4% in most cases), combined with phenylephrine 2.5% every five minutes for four doses, constitutes the single most important aspect of therapy. The atropine paralyzes the sphincter muscle of the ciliary body, and the phenylephrine stimulates the longitudinal muscle of the ciliary body; this combination results in the lens being pulled posteriorly away from the ciliary ring, allowing the aqueous to pass normally into the area of the pupil. As the effect of the atropine and phenylephrine wears off, the lens can return to its abnormally anterior position with recurrence of the ciliary block glaucoma and the consequent aqueous misdirection.

The older name for the aqueous misdirection syndrome, malignant glaucoma, has much to commend it. Until the condition was better understood, and there were better pharmacologic agents, indeed the condition was malignant in the sense that the anticipated outcome was loss of the eye. This is not difficult to understand when one realizes that the process is a self-perpetuating one. The misdirection of aqueous into the posterior segment of the eye increases the pressure in the posterior segment, forcing the lens anteriorly; as just mentioned, this anterior position of the lens itself then blocks the flow of aqueous, misdirecting more aqueous humor back into the posterior segment. Thus, the condition feeds on itself, and unless the cycle is broken, the result is an extremely high intraocular pressure, total collapse of the anterior chamber, and loss of the eye.

I prefer the phrase *aqueous misdirection syndrome* rather than *ciliary block glaucoma* or *malignant glaucoma* as it appears to reflect more accurately the actual process that is occurring. In some individuals, ciliary block is not present; the condition can occur in patients with relatively deep anterior chambers in whom there is an impervious vitreous face or a membrane in the plane of the lens, blocking the aqueous flow into the anterior chamber. Here the basic pathological process appears to be a blockage of flow unrelated to the ciliary body.

Treatment of Aqueous Misdirection Syndrome

The goal of treatment is to eliminate the faulty direction of aqueous flow and to restore normal flow into the anterior chamber. In the phakic patient, this is best accomplished by administration of topical atropine and phenylephrine. Atropine 1% four times daily is usually adequate to produce maximal cycloplegia, reducing the tone of the circular muscle of the ciliary body, as a consequence of which the zonules are put on stretch and the lens tends to be flattened and filled posteriorly. In addition receptors for adrenergic agents are also present in the longitudinal muscle of the ciliary body, and phenylephrine serves to stimulate these, both dilating the ciliary ring in the same way the conjoint use of a cycloplegic and a mydriatic agent dilate the pupil more effectively than either the cycloplegic or mydriatic alone. Thus, these agents should be used in conjunction in the treatment of malignant glaucoma. Phenylephrine 2.5% four times daily is also near maximal treatment. In some individuals atropine 4% or phenylephrine 10% or both are also justified. The atropine and phenylephrine should be used acutely and then be continued. In fact, the use of atropine may be necessary for many weeks, or even months, or in some cases indefinitely to prevent the recurrence of malignant glaucoma.

In addition, agents designed to reduce aqueous flow are especially helpful in the acute stages of the syndrome. Thus topical beta blockers and systemic carbonic anhydrase inhibitors in full doses are appropriate. These agents are not always advised. But the author has seen cases in which they definitely appeared to "turn the tide" and transform an apparently resistant aqueous misdirection syndrome into one in which the chamber deepened nicely and the pressure fell satisfactorily. Once the chamber has deepened, one of the mechanisms for the malignant glaucoma may have been correct, specifically ciliary block. Thus after deepening of the chamber has been observed, it is frequently possible to reduce or even stop the aqueous suppressants. The atropine and phenylephrine will maintain the lens-iris diaphragm in a more posterior position, allowing continued normal circulation of aqueous. The atropine, however, as mentioned above, should not be stopped in such cases, but rather should be tapered very gradually.

In resistant cases additional help can be obtained by shrinking the vitreous with isosorbide, glycerine or intravenous mannitol. Again, once the lens has been restored to its proper plane, these agents can usually be discontinued.

Reformation of the anterior chamber can be assisted in some cases by the injection of an agent such as hyaluronic acid (Healon) through a paracentesis into the anterior chamber. This is usually not appropriate in patients with a high intraocular pressure but, as discussed later, can be especially beneficial in patients with excessive filtration and ciliary block glaucoma related to collapse of the anterior chamber.

In the type of aqueous misdirection syndrome where there is a membrane of some sort, such as hyaloid face or inflammatory membrane, cycloplegics and mydriatics are helpful, but the aqueous suppressants and osmotic agents are essential to lower the pressure acutely. It is usual, however, for the condition to recur unless there is a rupture of the membrane. This can be done with neodymium:YAG laser, with a transpupillary discussion, or other similar methods in the aphakic patient. Indeed, some authors have even recommended using the neodymium:YAG laser through a clear lens in order to rupture the vitreous. However, this is still experimental and carries obvious hazards with it. In the phakic patient it may be necessary to introduce an instrument through the pars plana into the vitreous, disrupting the vitreous, breaking down the aqueous pockets. It is probably best to use a vitreous cutting machine for this, but where such instruments are not available, use of an 18-gauge needle is often adequate.

I believe that aqueous misdirection plays a role far more frequently in the development of angle closure and flat anterior chamber than is generally recognized. In fact, I believe that some cases of what appears to be classic primary angle closure glaucoma are probably manifestations of the aqueous misdirection syndrome; here the pathogenesis is a pupillary block that is sufficiently strong that aqueous is secreted back into the vitreous, moving the lens-iris diaphragm anteriorly, flattening the anterior chamber, and transforming a narrow angle into a closed angle. Iridectomy is effective in such cases because it eliminates pupillary block, and in so doing eliminates the gradient of pressure that causes the misdirection of aqueous flow into the posterior chamber. This theory is *completely speculative*, but it seems to fit with clinical experience.

In cases in which excessive filtration following the filtration procedure leads to collapse of the anterior chamber, the surgeon may note the presence of an extremely high bleb, a flat anterior chamber, and an intraocular pressure of 5 to 15 mm Hg. It would be hard to explain this constellation of findings solely on the basis of excessive filtration. I postulate that the natural history of such a condition is excessive filtration, lower pressure in the anterior chamber than in the posterior chamber, collapse of the anterior chamber, blockage of aqueous flow anteriorly by lenticular opposition to the ciliary body (ciliary block glaucoma), and consequent aqueous misdirection. If in these situations the anterior chamber remains flat, the aqueous misdirection continues. The excess filtration lessens, because of the lack of flow into the anterior chamber; as this occurs the pressure rises precipitously due to full-fledged "malignant glaucoma." If the anterior chamber reforms—due to partial flow into the anterior chamber meeting adequate resistance at the sclera or underneath the conjunctival-Tenon's capsule flap, or due to reformation of the anterior chamber with saline or sodium hyaluronate—the lens-diaphragm is pushed posteriorly, which in most cases eliminates the ciliary block, correcting the aqueous misdirection and allowing aqueous once again to flow into the anterior chamber. In such cases one can see the paradoxical combination of a *deepening of the anterior chamber with a fall in its intraocular pressure and an increased height of the filtering bleb.*

If the eye fails to make aqueous humor, the intraocular pressure can also fall while there is persistence of the flat anterior chamber. In such cases the bleb collapses, the intraocular pressure remains low, and the chamber remains flat. The surgeon may incorrectly conclude that the basic problem is solely excessive filtration. However, when the ciliary body again resumes production of aqueous humor, a full-blown malignant glaucoma ensues.

Suggested Readings

Buschmann W, Linnert D. Echography of the vitreous: case of aphakia and malignant aphakic glaucoma. Klin Mbl Augenheilk 168:453-461, 1976.

Chandler PA, Grant WM. Lectures on Glaucoma. Philadelphia, Lea & Febiger, 1965, pp. 393-407.

Chandler PA, Simmons RJ, Grant WM. Malignant glaucoma—medical and surgical treatment. Am J Ophthalmol 66-495-501, 1968.

Ellis PP. Malignant glaucoma occurring 16 years after successful filtering surgery. Ann Ophthalmol 16(2):177-179, 1984.

Epstein DL, Steinert RJ, Puliafito CA. Neodymium-YAG laser therapy to the anterior hyaloid in aphakic malignant (ciliovitreal block) glaucoma. Am J Ophthalmol 98(2):137-143, 1984.

Fanous S, Brouilette G. Ciliary block glaucoma: Malignant glaucoma in the absence of a history of surgery and miotic therapy. Can J Ophthalmol 18(6):302-303, 1983.

Frezzotti R, Gentili MC. Medical therapy attempts in malignant glaucoma. Am J Ophthalmol 57:402-406, 1964.

Henry C. Traitement de glaucome malin. Une methode de decompression retrolenticulaire. Bull Soc Ophthal Franc 66:674- 676, 1966.

Levene R. A new concept of malignant glaucoma. Arch Ophthalmol 87:497-506, 1972.

Macoul KL. Residual glaucoma and miotics. Arch Ophthalmol 88:210- 211, 1972.

Merritt JC. Malignant glaucoma induced by miotics postoperatively in open-angle glaucoma. Arch Ophthalmol 95:1988-1989, 1977.

Momoeda S, Hayashi H, Oshima K. Anterior pars plana vitrectomy for phakic malignant glaucoma. Jpn J Ophthalmol 27:73-79, 1983.

Rieser JC, Schwartz B. Miotic-induced malignant glaucoma. Arch Ophthalmol 87:706-712;1972.

Rochels R, Hackelbusch R. Echographische Befunde bein Aderhautabhebung. Klin Monatsbl Augenh 182(1):54-56, 1983.

Romanchuk KG. Seidel's test using 10% fluorescein. Can J Ophthalmol 14:253-256, 1979.

Sampaolesi R. Postoperative flat anterior chamber after glaucoma surgery. La atalamia postoperatoria en el glaucoma. An Inst Barraquer 10(1-2):124-150, 1972.

Scheie H, Morse H. Shallow anterior chamber as a sign of nonsurgical choroidal detachment. Ann Ophthalmol 6:317-319, 1974.

Schwartz AL, Anderson DR. Malignant glaucoma in an eye with no antecedent operation or miotics. Arch Ophthalmol 93:379-381, 1975.

Scott AS, Smith VH. Retrolental decompression for malignant glaucoma. Brit J Ophthalmol 45:654-661, 1961.

Shaffer RN, Hoskins HD: Ciliary block (malignant) glaucoma. Ophthalmology 85:215-221, 1978.

Simmons RJ. Malignant glaucoma. Brit J Ophthalmol 56:263-272, 1972.

Stewart RH, Kimbrough RL. A method of managing flat anterior chamber following trabeculectomy. Ophthalmic Surg 11:382-383, 1980.

Strasser G. Neodymium-YAG laser therapy to the anterior hyaloid in aphakic malignant (ciliovitreal block) glaucoma. Am J Ophthalmol 99:368, 1985.

Sugar HS. Registry of interesting cases: Bilateral aphakic malignant glaucoma. Arch Ophthalmol 87:347-351, 1972.

Malignant Glaucoma

Dan A. Nichols, MD

Malignant glaucoma is an unusual term for an uncommon complication of glaucoma therapy. The term was first used by von Graefe in 1869 to describe a type of glaucoma that occurred following ocular surgery—particularly glaucoma surgery—that he called malignant glaucoma because it was so resistant to treatment.[1] Modern estimates are that this complication occurs in 0.6[2] to 4%[3-5] of surgical procedures for angle closure glaucoma.

An apparently identical clinical picture has been reported following cataract surgery in patients without antecedent glaucoma,[6] following treatment with miotics,[7,8] and in association with trauma[9] and inflammation.[9-11] There have even been reports of malignant glaucoma occurring spontaneously.[12-14] The greatest risk, however, appears to be in patients undergoing peripheral iridectomy or trabeculectomy following angle closure glaucoma.

Despite the fact that malignant glaucoma has been recognized for more than 100 years, there are still unresolved problems with regard to its diagnosis, pathophysiology, classification, and treatment. The diagnosis of malignant glaucoma can be difficult in its earliest stages and in nonclassical settings. A full understanding of the pathophysiology of this disorder is lacking, especially the role of ciliolenticular or ciliovitreal block and the role of the anterior hyaloid. Lacking this understanding, it is difficult to know whether certain nonclassical presentations are truly the same disorder or not. Finally, advances in vitreous surgery and the advent of Nd:YAG therapy to the anterior hyaloid have made the choice of treatment for patients failing medical management increasingly complex.

Diagnosis

Traditionally, the diagnosis of malignant glaucoma has been made on the basis of the setting in which it occurs, the physical signs present, and the response to treatment.

Setting

- Occurring in eye with acute or chronic angle closure glaucoma.
- Following peripheral iridectomy or trabeculectomy.

Signs

- IOP elevation.
- Marked anterior displacement of the lens-iris diaphragm.
- Flat or shallow peripheral *and* central anterior chamber.

Response to Treatment

- Unrelieved by peripheral iridectomy (usually occurring in the presence of a patent iridectomy).
- Unresponsive to or exacerbated by miotics.
- Relieved by mydriatic-cycloplegics.

Levene[15] has contrasted this classical definition with a modern definition that includes cases with the same physical signs and response to treatment but that occur in a different clinical setting. This modern definition encompasses those cases cited here that are associated with trauma, inflammation, and miotics, as well as certain cases of the classical type in which the same pathophysiology is present unrecognized before surgery. If we accept this broader definition the diagnosis becomes more difficult and malignant glaucoma might be more easily confused with other types of acute glaucoma—particularly acute pupillary block glaucoma.

Pupillary block glaucoma is unlikely to be confused with malignant glaucoma in the classical setting. Outside of this setting, however, other diagnostic features must be considered (Table 14-1). The anterior chamber configuration is one of the most important distinguishing diagnostic features (Fig. 14-17).

Table 14-1. Malignant Glaucoma vs. Pupillary Block Glaucoma

	Malignant Glaucoma	Pupillary Block Glaucoma
Setting	Usually following surgery	Usually spontaneous
IOP	Usually elevated	Usually elevated
Anterior Chamber	Flat or shallow centrally and peripherally	Flat or shallow peripherally only
	No bombé	Iris bombé
Response to Iridectomy	Not relieved, may precipitate	Relieved
Response to Miotics	Exacerbated or precipitated	Often relieved
Response to Cycloplegics	Often relieved	May precipitate

In pupillary block glaucoma aqueous is trapped within the posterior chamber, usually causing the iris to bow forward into a bombe configuration. The central anterior chamber is characteristically deeper than the peripheral chamber, and might be as deep as in the fellow eye. In malignant glaucoma the block is more posterior, forcing the entire lens-iris diaphragm forward, shallowing both the central and peripheral anterior chamber. Levene[9,15] feels that pupillary block and malignant glaucoma can coexist and that shallowing of the central chamber in acute pupillary block glaucoma should alert the ophthalmologist that the chain of events leading to classical malignant glaucoma has begun.

The distinction between the anterior chamber configurations of pupillary block and malignant glaucoma can be difficult or impossible to make in aphakic or pseudophakic eyes (and even in some phakic eyes). In this situation, the presence of one or more patent iridectomies is necessary to make the appropriate diagnosis. A diagnosis of pupillary block is suspect if a patent iridectomy is present. If there is uncertainty, another iridectomy should be performed. If the chamber deepens, some degree of pupillary block must have been present.

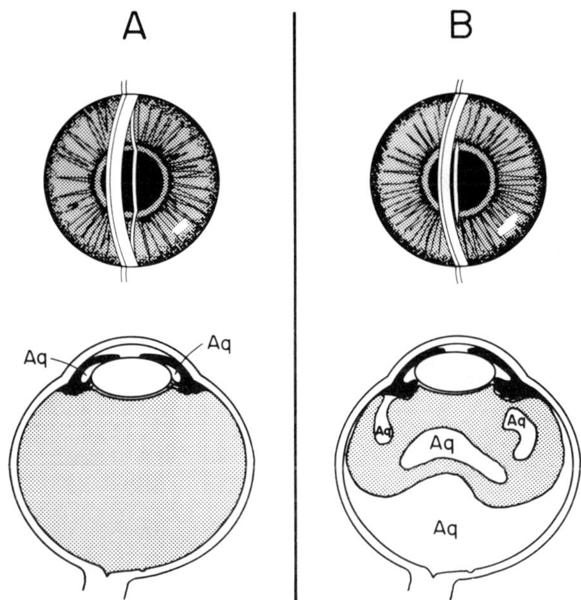

Figure 14-17. A. In pupillary block glaucoma the block is at the pupillary margin. Aqueous is trapped in the posterior chamber causing anterior bowing of the peripheral iris. The central chamber remains moderately deep. **B.** In malignant glaucoma the block is in the region of ciliary-lenticular-hyaloidal apposition. Aqueous is trapped within or behind the vitreous body. Forward displacement of the lens-iris diaphragm causes uniform shallowing of the anterior chamber. (After Shields.[27])

Another situation in which prompt diagnosis of malignant glaucoma might prove difficult is in the postoperative flat anterior chamber (Table 14-2; see also previous section of this chapter). The anterior chamber also can be uniformly shallow in the other important conditions in the differential diagnosis. In excessive filtration or choroidal effusion, however, the IOP is usually lower than it is in cases of malignant glaucoma. The pressure might be elevated with a flat chamber in the case of suprachoroidal hemorrhage; choroidal elevation and ocular pain might help to distinguish this entity. Whenever the chamber is shallow and the IOP higher than expected, the diagnosis of malignant glaucoma should be entertained. Treatment with mydriatic-cycloplegic and osmotic agents might be appropriate. Unfortunately, there is little in the way of ancillary testing to help with the diagnosis. It has been reported that localized pools of aqueous humor can be seen within the vitreous on ultrasonography.[6] But many now feel that aqueous is generally more homogenously dispersed throughout the vitreous.[17] One technique of help in selected situations, especially where the eye is quiet and the distinction between pupillary block and malignant glaucoma is difficult, is the use of intravenously administered fluorescein.[18] Normally fluorescein oozes from the posterior into the anterior chamber approximately 30 seconds following the injection of sodium fluorescein into the antecubital vein. Fluorescein tinges the aqueous, making its flow visible when examining the patient at the slit lamp. In the normal eye, one can see fluorescein seeping through the pupil, often in isolated streams; in the affected eye, there is reduced or absent flow through the pupil. The examiner does not look for fluorescein in the anterior chamber, which might leak from iris vessels, but rather for the flow of fluorescein-tinged aqueous through the pupil. In malignant glaucoma, fluorescein tinged aqueous is seen to pool in the posterior segment, posterior to the lens in the phakic patient, or to the vitreous face, inflammatory membrane, or pseudophakos in the aphakic patient.

Table 14-2. Differential Diagnosis of Flat Anterior Chamber After Trabeculectomy

	Malignant Glaucoma	Excessive Filtration	Choroidal Effusion	Suprachoroidal Hemorrhage
IOP	Higher than expected	Lower than expected	Low	High or low
Anterior Chamber	Uniformly shallow	Uniformly shallow	Uniformly shallow	Uniformly shallow
Bleb Appearance	Lower than expected	High	High or low	High or low
Fundus	Normal	Normal or elevated	Choroidal elevation	Choroidal elevation

Pathophysiology

Although many advances have been made in the understanding of this disease, its pathophysiology is still not completely understood. Shaffer[19] recognized the importance of the vitreous in the pathophysiology of malignant glaucoma. He proposed that posteriorly directed aqueous accumulated behind a posterior vitreous detachment leading to anterior displacement of the lens-iris diaphragm and closure of the anterior chamber angle. While most authorities accept that posterior accumulation of aqueous—either behind or within the vitreous—is involved in this disease, the question of what causes and maintains the posterior diversion has been more difficult to answer. Weiss and Shaffer[20] postulate that the tips of the ciliary processes come into apposition with the lens equator or anterior hyaloid leading to a ciliolenticular block, or in the case of aphakia a ciliovitreal block. This could occur only in small shallow-chambered eyes with little separation between the lens equator and the anterior ciliary body. Shallowing of the anterior chamber at the time of surgery could precipitate the block, leading to posterior aqueous flow, further anterior displacement of the lens-iris diaphragm, and reinforcement of the block, setting up a vicious cycle.

Levene[9] believes that in many cases this cycle is begun preoperatively with anterior displacement of the lens and that the process is only exacerbated by surgery. He reports a case and cites others from the literature in which spontaneous malignant glaucoma occurred in a fellow eye after peripheral iridectomy in an eye with angle closure. He proposed that certain small narrow angle eyes susceptible to angle closure are also susceptible to malignant or "direct lens block" glaucoma, and that the latter is caused by a more exaggerated shallowing of the chamber and forward movement of the lens.

Anterior displacement of the lens-iris diaphragm might also be caused by abnormal laxity of the zonules and this was the initial concept behind mydriatic-cycloplegic therapy for this disease.[21] The laxity might be caused by inflammation and prolonged angle closure.[2] Others have reported cases in which anterior displacement appears to be caused by ciliary body inflammation and swelling with anterior rotation of the ciliary body.[10,11] This mechanism might be especially important in nonclassical malignant glaucoma occurring in eyes without prior surgery.

Another potential site of abnormality is the anterior hyaloid face. Shaffer[18] observed that when lens extraction and posterior sclerotomy were performed for malignant glaucoma, the anterior chamber would not always deepen and the eye might remain hard unless incisions were made through the anterior hyaloid and into the vitreous. Shaffer and Hoskins[22] noted that the anterior hyaloid appeared abnormally thickened at the time of surgery. They reasoned that small tears or breaks in this dense anterior hyaloid might permit posterior aqueous flow but act as a ball-valve preventing forward flow.

The anterior hyaloid and vitreous provide little resistance to fluid flow under normal conditions.[23] With increased posterior pressure, however, significant resistance to flow develops.[24] Therefore, once aqueous flow is diverted posteriorly, the increased posterior pressure would cause an increased resistance to anterior aqueous flow.[25] Eventually the vitreous body is forced forward into apposition with the ciliary body, lens, and iris. In this position there might be reduced hyaloid surface available for fluid transfer, further increasing the resistance to aqueous flow.[17,24]

Treatment

Medical

Prior to 1962 the medical therapy of malignant glaucoma was almost uniformly ineffective.[3] In that year Chandler and Grant[21] introduced the use of mydriatic-cycloplegic agents, arguing that the customary treatment with miotic agents was not only ineffective but actually served to precipitate or exacerbate the condition. The purpose of the treatment was to tighten the zonules, which they believed to be slack, thus pulling the lens- iris diaphragm posteriorly. In Shaffer and Hoskins'[22] interpretation this widened the ciliary ring, breaking the ciliolenticular block.

In 1963 Weiss and coworkers recommended the use of intravenous mannitol.[26] Mannitol and other hyperosmotic agents are apparently effective by removing posteriorly trapped aqueous, allowing deepening of the anterior chamber and resolution of the block to anterior flow.

Some authors have recommended the use of topical or systemic steroids.[11,15] Some types of malignant glaucoma might involve ciliary body inflammation and swelling with anterior rotation of the ciliary processes, steroids might help to reverse the process by reducing this inflammation.

CAIs are generally added, both for IOP reduction and to reduce posterior pooling of aqueous. The addition of CAIs has been reported to be effective when mydriatic-cycloplegic therapy has failed.[3] Topical beta blockers also can be used in addition to or in place of CAIs.[5,27]

Thus an effective medical regimen might include atropine 1% and phenylephrine 2.5% four times daily, prednisolone acetate every two hours, timolol 0.5% twice daily, acetazolamide 250 mg orally four times daily, and intravenous mannitol 1.5 to 2 gm/kg or oral isosorbide 1.5 gm/kg once or twice daily. Medical treatment will bring about resolution in 50% of cases within five days.[5,27] At that point therapy is gradually reduced, maintaining the atropine indefinitely. It might be appropriate to taper the dose of atropine slowly, decreasing it over a period of months. It might need to be continued once or twice weekly for the duration of the patient's life.

Surgical therapy is indicated as soon as it is apparent that medical treatment will not succeed. This might be early in the course of the disease, for example in a case where the eye cannot withstand the continued elevated pressure for a period of several days. In other cases, it might be appropriate to delay surgery until a full course of medical treatment has been attempted. One must consider both the condition of the eye and the effectiveness of therapy when deciding to move on to surgical intervention.

Surgical

Prior to the relatively recent advent of successful medical therapy, surgical intervention held the only hope for effective treatment of malignant glaucoma. Perhaps the earliest technique was posterior sclerotomy. Chandler[3] credits its first use to Weber in 1877. Weber made a sclerotomy 8 to 10 mm posterior to the limbus relieving a case of malignant glaucoma. More recent descriptions involve aspiration of vitreous and posteriorly collected aqueous through a pars plana sclerotomy site.[3,28] The original intention of this procedure was to relieve trapped aqueous within or behind the vitreous body. It might be effective, however, only when the incision is anterior enough that it also disrupts the anterior hyaloid.[22]

Lens extraction is also a longstanding surgical treatment for malignant glaucoma.[29] When this technique is successful, vitreous is usually lost at the time of surgery. Shaffer[19] found that when lens extraction followed posterior sclerotomy and vitreous was not lost with the lens extraction, the glaucoma did not resolve. However, the chamber would deepen and the glaucoma would resolve if incisions were made through the anterior hyaloid and deep into the anterior vitreous.

The techniques of posterior sclerotomy with aspiration and anterior hyaloid incision were developed prior to the era of modern vitreous surgery. Many surgeons now prefer pars plana vitrectomy with automated vitrectomy instrumentation.[30] This technique has been used to treat pseudophakic malignant glaucoma by core vitrectomy with excision of portions of the posterior capsule and zonules, leaving the intraocular lens in place.[31] Interestingly, these authors state that when core vitrectomy alone was carried out the anterior chamber did not deepen. However, after excision of a local area of zonules and posterior capsule with the victrectomy instrument, the anterior chamber deepened spontaneously.

Laser Therapy

Herschler[32] reported successful treatment of malignant glaucoma in five of six patients by using the argon laser to shrink ciliary processes. Others have reported similar results, even in lieu of mydriatic-cycloplegic therapy.[33] It has been suggested that argon laser treatment of the ciliary processes might work by disturbing the adjacent anterior hyaloid, rather than by causing withdrawal of the ciliary processes.[17,34]

More recently, disruption of the anterior hyaloid has been achieved by use of the Nd:YAG laser. Epstein and colleagues[17] first reported success with the procedure in three aphakic eyes and two eyes with intraocular lenses. Later Brown and coworkers[35] described treatment of one pseudophakic and one phakic patient. In aphakic and pseudophakic eyes the hyaloid can be disrupted either peripherally, through a peripheral iridectomy, or centrally, through the pupil. Although transpupillary treatment in phakic eyes is theoretically possible, it risks damage to the crystalline lens. A large peripheral iridectomy might provide an adequate view of the anterior hyaloid, but laser iridectomies might not be adequate for this purpose.

Discussion

The term *malignant glaucoma* is unsatisfactory in several respects. It conveys nothing about the pathophysiology of the disorder. Perhaps worse, it carries the implication of a neoplastic process. Furthermore, it leaves unclear whether the more recently described cases of glaucoma with a similar appearance and behavior ought to also be called "malignant." Though more recent terms such as *ciliary block glaucoma*[20] and *direct lens block glaucoma*[9] have been advocated, it is not clear that they adequately describe the pathophysiology either and they have not displaced the traditional term.

If we consider the various theories of the pathophysiology of malignant glaucoma, it is clear that they are not mutually exclusive. Rather each can contribute to an ongoing process or cycle of malignant glaucoma (Fig. 14-18). The cycle can be set into motion at any of several starting points. For example, the primary event might be anterior displacement of the lens-iris diaphragm. This could be because of anterior rotation of the ciliary body from inflammation or swelling or from miotics; or, it could be because of loss of the anterior chamber at the time of surgery or postoperatively. Whatever the cause, this anterior displacement would bring the ciliary processes and lens or vitreous into closer apposition leading to ciliary block.

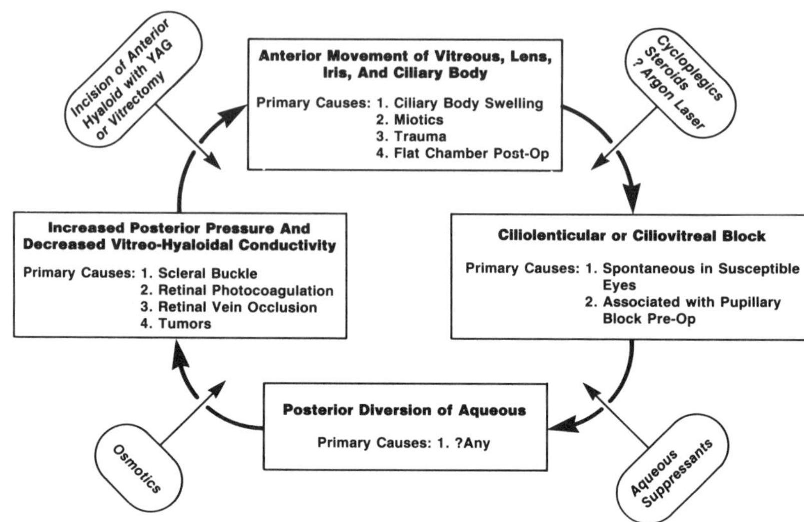

Figure 14-18. Malignant glaucoma can be conceived of as a cycle that can begin with any of several events. Once set into motion the cycle will continue unless interrupted by some external force. (Full discussion in text.)

Ciliary block was originally intended to denote a water-tight seal between the ciliary processes and lens,[20] but this need not be the case. Closer apposition between the ciliary processes and lens could lead to a *relative* ciliolenticular block by reducing the area of hyaloid available to transmit fluid[17,24] and increasing the resistance to the anterior flow of aqueous. (In somewhat the same way that a relative pupillary block can divert the flow of aqueous and precipitate angle closure glaucoma.)

With increased resistance to flow, aqueous would be diverted posteriorly. The increasing posterior pressure would lead to decreased vitreo-hyaloidal conductivity, eventually leading to further anterior movement of the vitreous, lens, iris, and ciliary body.[24,25] Once set into motion, the cycle would continue unless broken by some external force.

The cycle could begin at other points as well. For example, ciliary block might be the primary event in certain small narrow angle eyes.[9,20] Increased posterior pressure might be the cause of the angle closure that is unresponsive to iridectomy following retinal detachment surgery,[36] retinal photocoagulation,[37] central retinal vein occlusion,[38] and with malignant tumors.[39,40] It would seem unlikely that posterior diversion of aqueous could be a primary cause without something resisting its normal anterior flow.

It is not difficult to see why the greatest risk for malignant glaucoma follows surgery for angle closure glaucoma. Here we have multiple potential causes with inflammation and swelling, treatment with miotics, and flat anterior chambers after surgery—all occurring in a small-chambered eye that is particularly susceptible.

Within this scheme, the various treatments of malignant glaucoma can be seen as intervening in the cycle at certain critical points. Cycloplegics and sometimes steroids would prevent anterior movement of the lens-iris diaphragm from leading to ciliary block. Argon laser treatment of the ciliary processes might also reverse this process. Aqueous suppressants prevent posterior diversion. Osmotic agents remove trapped aqueous from the vitreous lessening the drop in vitreal-hyaloidal conductivity. Incision of the hyaloidal face by Nd:YAG or surgical treatment prevents the increasing posterior pressure from moving the vitreous body forward and breaks the cycle.

Thus, there is no single site of pathology in the clinical picture of malignant glaucoma. Early cases in which the full cycle of pathology has not yet developed can be reversed by treatment directed at the initiating event. More full-blown cases might require multiple treatments. The full cycle can be decisively interrupted by incision of the hyaloid and anterior vitreous. The progression from a single initiating event to the full-blown cycle represents the broad spectrum of disease that we recognize as malignant glaucoma.

References

1. von Graefe A. Beitrage zur pathologie und therapie des glaucoma. Arch Fur Ophthalmol 15:108-252, 1869.
2. Lowe RF. Malignant glaucoma related to primary angle-closure glaucoma. Aust J Ophthalmol 7:11-18, 1979.
3. Chandler PA, Simmons RJ, Grant WM. Malignant glaucoma. Medical and surgical treatment. Am J Ophthalmol 66:495-502, 1968.
4. Simmons RJ. Malignant glaucoma. Br J Ophthalmol 56:263-272, 1972.
5. Simmons RJ, Thomas JV Malignant glaucoma. In Ritch R and Shields MB (eds): *The Secondary Glaucomas*. St. Louis: CV Mosby, 1982, p. 331-343.
6. Hanish SJ, Lamberg RL, Gordon JM. Malignant glaucoma following cataract extraction and intraocular lens implant. Ophthalmic Surg 13:713-714, 1982.
7. Rieser JC, Schwartz B. Miotic-induced malignant glaucoma. Arch Ophthalmol 87:706-712, 1972.
8. Merritt JC. Malignant glaucoma induced by miotics postoperatively in open-angle glaucoma. Arch Ophthalmol 95:1988- 1989, 1977.
9. Levene R: A new concept of malignant glaucoma. Arch Ophthalmol 87:497-506, 1972.
10. Phelps CD. Angle-closure glaucoma secondary to ciliary body swelling. Arch Ophthalmol 92:287-290, 1974.
11. Beckman H, Blau RP. Oral steroid therapy for ciliary (pseudomalignant) glaucoma. Glaucoma 3:169-175, 1981.
12. Schwartz AL, Anderson DR. "Malignant glaucoma" in an eye with no antecendent operation or miotics. Arch Ophthalmol 93:379-381, 1975.
13. Manku MS. Spontaneous bilateral malignant glaucoma. Aust NZ J Opthalmology 13(3):249-259, 1985.

14. Fanous S, Brouillette G. Ciliary block glaucoma: Malignant glaucoma in the absence of a history of surgery and of miotic therapy. Can J Ophthalmol 18(6):302-303, 1983.
15. Levene RZ. Current concepts of malignant glaucoma. Ophthalmic Surg 17:515-520, 1986.
16. Perrone S, Steindler P, D'Ermo F, Doro D. Preoperative echographic localization of aqueous humor deposits in malignant glaucoma; an experimental and clinical study. In Henkind P (ed): ACTA XXIV International Congress Ophthalmol, Vol 1, San Francisco, California, New York: JB Lippincott, 1982, p.119-121.
17. Epstein DL, Steinert RF, Puliafito CA. Neodymium-YAG laser therapy to the anterior hyaloid in aphakic malignant (ciliovitreal block) glaucoma. Am J Ophthalmol 98:137-143, 1984.
18. Ray RR, Binkhorst RD. The diagnosis of pupillary block by intravenous injection of fluorescein. Am J Ophthalmol 61:481-483, 1966.
19. Shaffer RN. The role of vitreous detachment on aphakic and malignant glaucoma. Trans Am Acad Ophthalmol Otol 58:217-231, 1954.
20. Weiss DI, Shaffer RN. Ciliary block (malignant) glaucoma. Trans Am Acad Ophthalmol Otol 76:450-461, 1972.
21. Chandler PA, Grant WM. Mydriatic-cycloplegic treatment in malignant glaucoma. Arch Ophthalmol 68:353-359, 1962.
22. Shaffer RN, Hoskins HD Jr. Ciliary block (malignant) glaucoma. Opthalmology 85:215-221, 1978.
23. Grant WM. Experimental aqueous perfusion in enucleated human eyes. Arch Ophthalmol 69:783-801, 1963.
24. Epstein DL, Hashimoto JM, Anderson PJ, Grant WM. Experimental perfusions through the anterior and vitreous chambers with possible relationships to malignant glaucoma. Am J Ophthalmol 88:1078-1086, 1979.
25. Quigley HA. Malignant glaucoma and fluid flow rate. Am J Ophthalmol 89:879-880, 1980.
26. Weiss DI, Shaffer RN, Harrington DO. Treatment of malignant glaucoma with intravenous mannitol infusion. Medical reformation of the anterior chamber by means of an osmotic agent: a preliminary report. Arch Ophthalmol 69:154-158, 1963.
27. Shields, MB. Glaucomas following ocular surgery. In Shields MB: Textbook of Glaucoma, 2nd edition. Baltimore: Williams & Wilkins, 1987, p. 334-358.
28. Chandler PA. A new operation for malignant glaucoma. A preliminary report. Trans Am Ophthalmol Soc 62:408-424, 1964.
29. Chandler PA. Malignant glaucoma. Trans Am Ophthalmol Soc 48:128-143, 1950.
30. Weiss H, Shin DH, Kollarits CR. Vitrectomy for malignant (ciliary block) glaucomas. Int Ophthalmol Clinics 21:113-119, 1981.
31. Lynch MG, Brown RH, Michels RG, et al. Surgical vitrectomy for pseudophakic malignant glaucoma. Am J Ophthalmol 102:149-153, 1986.

32. Herschler J. Laser shrinkage of the ciliary processes. A treatment for malignant (ciliary block) glaucoma. Ophthalmol 87:1155-1159, 1980.
33. Weber PA, Henry MA, Kapetansky FM. Argon laser treatment of the ciliary processes in aphakic glaucoma with flat anterior chamber. Am J Ophthamol 97:82-85, 1984.
34. Simmons RJ, in discussion, Herschler J. Laser shrinkage of ciliary processes. A treatment for malignant (ciliary block) glaucoma. Ophthalmol 87:1158-1159, 1980.
35. Brown RH, Lynch MG, Tearse JE, et al. Neodymium-YAG vitreous surgery for phakic and pseudophakic malignant glaucoma. Arch Ophthalmol 104:1464-1466, 1986.
36. Perez RN, Phelps CD, Burton TC. Angle-closure glaucoma following scleral buckling operations. Trans Am Acad Ophthalmol Otol 81:247-252, 1976.
37. Phelps CD. Glaucoma associated with retinal disorders. In Ritch R and Shields MB (eds): The Secondary Glaucomas. St. Louis: CV Mosby, 1982, p. 150-161.
38. Grant WM. Shallowing of the anterior chamber following occlusion of the central retinal vein. Am J Ophthalmol 75:384- 389, 1973.
39. Shields MB, Klintworth GK. Anterior uveal melanomas and intraocular pressure. Ophthalmology 87:503-517, 1980.
40. Yanoff M. Glaucoma mechanisms in ocular malignant melanomas. Am J Ophthalmol 70:898-904, 1970.

Suprachoroidal Hemorrhage

Louis B. Cantor, MD

Incidence

Suprachoroidal hemorrhage is a serious complication that can be seen with any intraocular surgery. The incidence of this complication in the general population undergoing cataract extractions has been reported to be between 0.05% and 0.4% with an average of approximately 0.2% in retrospective studies.[1,2] It has long been thought that glaucoma is a major predisposing factor for suprachoroidal hemorrhage. The incidence of suprachoroidal hemorrhage in glaucoma patients undergoing various types of intraocular surgery has been reported to be 0.73%, which is significantly greater than the incidence reported in the general population undergoing cataract extractions.[1] The incidence following filtering alone has also been reported to be quite high.[3]

Pathogenesis

The pathogenesis of suprachoroidal hemorrhage has been described anatomically by Manshot.[4,5] The source of the hemorrhage is usually one of the short or long posterior ciliary arteries. In 9 of Manshot's 10 cases, the hemorrhage was localized to have originated from one or more ruptured necrotic posterior ciliary arteries. In the tenth, a markedly sclerotic and dilated choroidal artery was implicated.

Muller reported on the pathologic findings of eight eyes with suprachoroidal hemorrhage.[6] His findings also showed that the site of predilection for the hemorrhage was the short posterior ciliary vessels, particularly at their point of entrance into the suprachoroidal space from their scleral canals. A similar necrosis of vessel walls was noted in branches of the long posterior ciliary artery and in retrograde branches from the anterior ciliary artery. The vascular necrosis was also noted in choroidal vessels, but to a much lesser extent, and was rarely seen in retinal vessels.

The fact that patients with glaucoma have a particularly high incidence of suprachoroidal hemorrhage was also suggested by Samuels in 1931.[7] He described seven cases of suprachoroidal hemorrhage following glaucoma surgery. All seven of these eyes were enucleated for relief of pain. The abnormalities of those specimens supported the idea that a necrotic posterior ciliary artery was a reason for the bleeding.

The factors that might contribute to vascular necrosis and subsequent rupture of the vascular wall are not fully understood. The nutritional supply to a vascular wall is provided by penetration of plasma constituents through the endothelium, the vasa vasorum, and penetration of extravascular fluid into the vascular wall. Since arterioles do not possess vasa vasorum the nutrition of the arteriolar wall is only by passive diffusion of fluid from inside and outside the vessel wall. Any factor that might impede this transmural flow can predis pose to ischemic vascular necrosis or degeneration. The primary factors that are thought to impair transmural flow are: arteriosclerosis (either secondary to hypertension or age-related factors) or elevated IOP.

Essential hypertension accounts for 90% of individuals with hypertension. Essential hypertension causes a hyaline degeneration of the vascular wall secondary to a hyperpermeable or injured endothelium that leads to narrowing of the vascular lumen and decreased elasticity of the vessel wall. Similar, although milder changes might be present in a majority of patients over the age of 60, just as a result of the aging process.

Elevated IOP can interfere with nutrition of the vascular wall in many ways. The elevated extravascular pressure can interfere with the outflow of fluid through the vessel wall by reducing the hydrostatic pressure difference across the vessel wall. Also, if the IOP exceeds the diastolic intraarteriole pressure the vessel might actually collapse during diastole. If arteriolosclerosis, which can further decrease flow and intravascular pressure within the vessel, were further imposed upon this situation, the vessel might remain collapsed during systole, resulting in ischemic necrosis. In almost all cases studied, the necrosis of the vascular wall was localized to that area of the vessel just inside the globe in the suprachoroidal space. Within the scleral canals the penetrating vessels are fixed and not subjected to the elevated IOP. Immediately upon entering the globe, however, the vessels might be prone to collapse when exposed to elevated pressure and are likely to rupture when the glaucomatous eye is surgically decompressed, if the vessel wall is weakened. The importance of elevated IOP to suprachoroidal hemorrhage is also emphasized by the fact that spontaneous suprachoroidal hemorrhage is rarely reported in the absence of glaucoma. It usually follows cases of sudden spontaneous hypotony, such as spontaneous corneal perforations from corneal ulcers, in glaucomatous eyes.[8-10] Decompression of the globe that occurs during intraocular surgery can also lead to anterior displacement of the retina and choroid, placing traction on already weakened posterior ciliary arteries at their point of emergence from their intrascleral canals. This effect, along with the profound change in pressure across the vessel wall, can result in a blowout in the vessel wall with hemorrhage. It can also be speculated that the higher the pressure in the eye prior to surgical decompression, the more apt it is for hemorrhage to occur.

While these factors are probably responsible for most suprachoroidal hemorrhages, they are not applicable to all. Suprachoroidal hemorrhage has been reported in young patients undergoing cataract extraction without apparent vascular disease or glaucoma.[11,12] The incidence of suprachoroidal hemorrhage has also been reported to be particularly high in glaucoma patients who were aphakic or highly myopic, suggesting that other factors are also important.[3] The incidence of suprachoroidal hemorrhage is particularly high in aphakic eyes that have had a vitrectomy performed at the time of glaucoma filtration surgery.[13] Theoretically, any condition that predisposes to vascular fragility and forward displacement of the retina and choroid can also play a role in cases of suprachoroidal hemorrhage.

The exact reasons why myopia is a risk factor are not understood, but the association appears real. Myopia has been reported to be associated with choroidal vasculopathy that might predispose to bleeding after intraocular surgery.[14] Also, myopic eyes have a larger intraocular area in which to form effusions, and also have decreased scleral and vitreal support for vulnerable vessels. Myopia's role in predisposing to suprachoroidal hemorrhage has also been reported in the milder entity of limited choroidal hemorrhage. Limited suprachoroidal hemorrhage was noted in 14.5% of highly myopic eyes undergoing lens extraction.[17,18]

It has been reported that prolonged hypotony can increase the risk of postoperative suprachoroidal hemorrhage.[3] The more prolonged the hypotony, the greater the likelihood of choroidal effusions and inflammation. Hypotonia alone does not produce experimental choroidal detachment.[19,20] Hypotony plus inflammation or venous congestion can produce an effusion into the ciliochoroidal space. In the hypotonous eye, venous pressure is dependent upon the venous pressure outside the eye as opposed to the normal eye where the transmural venous pressure is primarily dependent upon the IOP. In the hypotonous eye, transmural pressure across choroidal vessels is higher than in the normal eye. Furthermore, the pressure gradient is much more sensitive to transient elevations of venous pressure, such as those produced by valsalva.

It has been postulated that choroidal effusion is a precursor to suprachoroidal effusion in most cases. A recent clinicopathologic study of a typical ciliochoroidal effusion was identified as causing traction on stretched posterior ciliary arteries causing early hemorrhage into the suprachoroidal space.[15,16] Based on these and other studies it appears logical to establish normal IOP relationships within the eye as quickly as possible, and to be especially cautious in patients with glaucoma, myopia, cardiovascular disease, or advanced age.[21]

Other factors thought to be associated with this complication include diabetes, periarteritis, and vitreous loss. In addition, intraoperative hemorrhage can be more common in patients with blood dyscrasias, such as thrombocytopenia, polycythemia, or hemophilia. Patients on anticoagulant therapy (such as Coumadin) should, with the consent of their internist, have anticoagulant medication discontinued prior to intraocular surgery. Prothrombin levels should be corrected to at least 50% of normal prior to surgery, if possible. Increasing numbers of patients are using low dose aspirin to reduce the risk of thrombosis and in patients at high risk for suprachoroidal hemorrhage it would probably be advisable to stop aspirin therapy at least two weeks prior to surgery, again with the approval of their internist. (Table 14-3)

Management

Prompt recognition and action are necessary once a suprachoroidal hemorrhage has been identified. The clinical appearance of the suprachoroidal hemorrhage within the pupil is probably directly related to the size of the ruptured vessel and the pressure within that vessel. If the process is gradual, a dark mass can be observed through the pupil to evolve slowly. With a larger or more high pressure vessel rupture, the hemorrhage might be more expulsive and the patient will experience ocular pain, often even despite local anesthesia.

Table 14-3. Risk Factors for Suprachoroidal Hemorrhage

Systemic	Ocular
Advanced age	Aphakia
Arteriosclerosis	Choroidal effusion
Blood dyscrasias	Glaucoma
Carotid-cavernous fistula	High myopia
Chronic cough	Hypotony
Sturge-Weber Syndrome	Inflammation
Valsalva	5-fluorouracil

It is generally agreed by all that prompt, secure closure of the incision is the first goal in treatment of a suprachoroidal hemorrhage that occurs at the time of surgery.[1,22] Beyond this point there are some differences of opinion as to how a suprachoroidal hemorrhage should be managed. A posterior sclerotomy was first successfully used to treat a suprachoroidal hemorrhage by Verhoeff in 1915 and was subsequently also reported by others.[23,24,25] Some authors have advised immediate drainage of the hemorrhage through a sclerostomy, and at times also combined with a vitrectomy in aphakic patients especially if the hemorrhage is large.[26,27] Support for this approach generally comes from published reports in the past that reflect a poor prognosis following suprachoroidal hemorrhage, especially if the hemorrhage is massive.[3,28,29] Other reports do not necessarily support a poor prognosis and aggressive intervention.[1] Upon close inspection of those publications that reflect a poor outcome it still remains unclear what the prognosis following suprachoroidal hemorrhage actually is, even in cases where the hemorrhage is large.

The use of antimetabolites and previous surgical procedures, especially cyclocryotherapy, might have contributed to the poor prognosis in some cases. In other series, the poor outcome was still seen despite very aggressive intervention, perhaps suggesting that intervention itself was associated with the poor result. Therefore, a conservative approach to treatment of a suprachoroidal hemorrhage is probably appropriate. If the hemorrhage occurs at the time of surgery, the first priority is secure closure of the incision and repositing prolapsed uvea. Preplaced sutures of sufficient tensile strength (8-0 or thicker) to withstand a high pressure should already be in place and can be quickly pulled up. If not, the surgeon's finger can be used to tamponade the incision site temporarily while sutures are placed. The uvea should be gently reposited with irrigation and blunt instruments and additional sutures placed. If the IOP is high and there is discomfort the pressure can be lowered with intravenous acetazolamide and/or osmotic agents.

Once the eye has been stabilized, the anterior chamber can be reformed through the incision or a paracentesis tract. If the eye is aphakic, and vitreous has extruded an anterior vitrectomy can be performed, though this might be safely delayed until later. The vitrectomy should be performed anteriorly either through the incision or clear cornea as the pars plana region is likely to be detached secondary to the hemorrhage. A constant infusion through a separate site is probably advisable to maintain a firm globe and decrease the chance of further hemorrhage if a vitrectomy is to be attempted.

Treatment for postoperative suprachoroidal hemorrhage is directed toward control of the IOP and relief of pain. The suprachoroidal space is not drained unless there is intolerable pain, a persistent flat anterior chamber, or other specific indication such as persistent "kissing" choroidal detachments. Occasionally, draining the suprachoroidal hemorrhage might precipitate further bleeding because hypotony might be again induced. If drainage is attempted, every effort should be made to maintain a relatively stable pressure inside the eye either by utilizing frequent injections into the anterior chamber or a constant infusion system through clear cornea (such as a 25-gauge butterfly needle connected by an intravenous infusion line to a bottle of balanced salt solution placed approximately 18 inches above the patient's eye).[26]

The majority of these eyes will do well with conservative management and useful vision will be recovered.[1] Occasionally a fibrous reaction can occur within the vitreous that will not allow the retina to settle and retinal detachments will develop, particularly if there has been some breakthrough bleeding into the vitreous cavity at the time of the hemorrhage, and surgical intervention to remove the vitreous and reattach the retina might become necessary. If the initial hemorrhage was not contained and there was extensive loss of intraocular contents, particularly retina, then the prognosis is grim.

The wide variations in techniques with which people approach suprachoroidal hemorrhage probably stems in most part from the fact that few, if any, individuals ever see enough cases of suprachoroidal hemorrhage during their lifetime to be able to objectively evaluate various approaches. It will probably require a large, multicenter, controlled, and randomized study to fully explore the various treatment options and decide to whom they are best applied. There are perhaps certain circumstances where more aggressive intervention is indicated based upon factors other than the mere size of the hemorrhage and other circumstances where even a very massive type hemorrhage should not be aggressively approached. We need the answers to these questions, and hopefully with time we will begin to understand this dreaded complication better.

References

1. Cantor LB, Katz LJ, Spaeth GL. Complications of surgery in glaucoma: suprachoroidal expulsive hemorrhage in glaucoma patients undergoing intraocular surgery. Ophthalmology 92:1266-1270, 1985.

2. Payne JW, Kameen AJ, Jensen AD, et al. Expulsive hemorrhage: its incidence in cataract surgery and a report of four bilateral cases. Trans Am Ophthalmol Soc 83:181-204, 1985.
3. Ruderman JM, Harbin TS Jr, Campbell DG. Postoperative suprachoroidal hemorrhage following filtering procedures. Arch Ophthalmol. 104:201-205, 1986.
4. Manshot WA. Glaucoma-vascular necrosis-expulsive hemorrhage. Acta Ophthalmol 23:309-342, 1945.
5. Manshot WA. The pathology of expulsive hemorrhage. Am J Ophthalmol 40:15-24, 1955.
6. Muller H. Expulsive hemorrhage. Trans Ophthalmol Soc UK 79:621-634, 1959.
7. Samuels B. Postoperative non-expulsive suprachoroidal hemorrhage. Arch Ophthalmol 6:843-851, 1931.
8. Pe'er J, Weiner A, Vidaurri L. Clinicopathologic report of spontaneous expulsive hemorrhage. Ann Ophthalmology 19:139-141, 1987.
9. Williams K, Rentiers PK. Spontaneous expulsive choroidal hemorrhage. Arch Ophthalmol 83:191-194, 1970.
10. Winslow RL, Stevenson W III, Yanoff M. Spontaneous expulsive choroidal hemorrhage. Arch Ophthalmol 92:33-36, 1971.
11. Cordes FC. Linear extraction in congenital cataract surgery. Am J Ophthalmol 52:355-360, 1961.
12. Francois P, Wannebroucq C, Guilbert-Legrand. Les hemorrhages expulsives. A propos de 6 cas. Bull Soc Ophthalmol Fr 66:579-585, 1966.
13. Givens K, Shields MB. Suprachoroidal hemorrhage after glaucoma filtering surgery. Am J Ophthalmol 103:689-694, 1987.
14. Duke-Elder S. Ophthalmic optics and refraction, Duke-Elder, S. (ed): System of Ophthalmology. London, Henry Kimpton, 5:301- 362, 1970.
15. Maumenee AE, Schwartz MF. Acute intraoperative choroidal effusion. Am. J. Ophthalmol 100:147-154, 1985.
16. Wolter RJ, Garfinkel RA. Ciliochoroidal effusion as a precursor of suprachoroidal hemorrhage: A pathologic study. Ophthalmic Surg 19:344-349, 1988.
17. Hoffman P, Pollack A, Moshe O. Limited choroidal hemorrhage associated with intracapsular cataract extraction. Arch Ophthalmol 102:1761-1765, 1984.
18. Bukelman A, Hoffman P, Oliver M. Limited choroidal hemorrhage associated with extracapsular cataract extraction. Arch Ophthalmol 105:338-341, 1987.
19. Capper, et al. Mechanism of serous choroidal detachment. Arch Ophthalmol 55:101-113, 1956.
20. Collins ET. Intraocular tension: I. An experimental investigation as to some of the effects of hypotony in rabbit eyes. Trans Ophthalmol Soc UK, 38:217-277, 1918.
21. Brubaker RF. Intraocular surgery and choroidal hemorrhage. Arch Ophthalmol 102:1753-1754, 1984.

22. Haynes JH, Payne JW, Green WR. Clinicopathologic study of eyes obtained from a patient 6 and 2 years after operative choroidal hemorrhage. Ophthalmic Surg. 18: 667-671, 1987.
23. Duehr PA, Hogensen CD. Treatment of subchoroidal hemorrhage by posterior sclerotomy. Arch Ophthalmol 38:365-367, 1947.
24. Vail D. Posterior sclerotomy as a form of treatment in subchoroidal expulsive hemorrhage. Am J Ophthalmol 21:256-260, 1938.
25. Verhoeff FH. Scleral puncture for expulsive subchoroidal hemorrhage following sclerotomy/scleral puncture for postoperative separation of the choroid. Ophthalmol Res 24:55-59, 1915.
26. Abrams GW, Thomas MA, Williams GA, et al. Management of postoperative suprachoroidal hemorrhage with continuous-infusion air pump. Arch Ophthalmol 104:1455-1458, 1986.
27. Frenkel REP, Shin DH. Prevention and management of delayed suprachoroidal hemorrhage after filtration surgery. Arch Ophthalmol 104:1459-1463, 1986.
28. Gressel MG, Parrish RK, Heuer DK. Delayed nonexpulsive suprachoroidal hemorrhage. Arch Ophthalmol 102:1757-1760, 1984.
29. Tarakji MS, Matta CS. Expulsive hemorrhage: Report of five cases. Ann Ophthalmol 10:1269-1271, 1978.

Hyphema

Louis B. Cantor, MD

Hyphema is a common postoperative occurrence in glaucomatous eyes following intraocular surgery. In general, the causes and complications of hyphema following anterior segment surgery in glaucomatous and nonglaucomatous eyes are similar. In glaucomatous eyes undergoing filtering surgery—either alone or combined with cataract extraction—bleeding most commonly arises from the ciliary body or cut ends of Schlemm's canal, though it might also arise from the corneoscleral incision or iris. In general, hyphema presents at surgery or within the first two or three days following surgery, though it might occur later. In most cases, the hyphema is limited and no specific therapy is indicated.[1,2,3,4]

Predisposing Factors

In the majority of cases there are no predisposing factors for the development of a hyphema. Blood dyscrasias, such as hemophilia, thrombocytopenia, and polycythemia might predispose to hyphema. These disorders can be managed preoperatively with the help of a hematologist. Anticoagulant therapy might also predispose to hyphema and patients who are on warfarin (Coumadin) should have preoperative correction of their prothrombin time to at least 50% of normal. If possible, it also might be helpful to avoid aspirin products for at least two weeks prior to surgery, because of its effects on platelets.

Site of Bleeding

Bleeding from Schlemm's canal is likely to occur following filtering surgery, especially if a posterior block of tissue has been removed and Schlemm's canal has been cut across. Removing a posterior block might not only lead to reflux of blood from Schlemm's canal, but is also more likely to result in trauma to the ciliary body. The cut edges of Schlemm's canal can be difficult to cauterize because of their being fixed within the sclera. If minimal cautery is not effective, application of a cotton tip applicator or sponge to the site and applying gentle pressure is usually effective.

Damage to the ciliary body is a common cause of hyphema, either because of a direct injury from instrumentation or indirectly from pulling on the iris. The ciliary body is especially prone to injury while performing a peripheral iridectomy. Bleeding from the ciliary body might at times be quite extensive, especially if the annular artery has been injured. Gentle cautery or direct pressure is usually sufficient to stop the bleeding. Care must be taken when cauterizing or manipulating the ciliary body to avoid damage to the lens, zonules, or hyaloid face. It also might be helpful to fill the anterior chamber with a viscoelastic agent to direct the blood out the incision, rather than allowing it to drain into the anterior chamber.

Bleeding can result from a scleral incision, especially with placement of deep sutures. Incomplete healing of the incision (a desirable outcome in most glaucoma surgeries) might predispose to bleeding because of highly vascularized granulation tissue that might be present in the incompletely opposed edges of the incision. Hyphema also can be a late complication because of vascularization of the incision, as has been reported following cataract extraction and filtering surgery.[5,6]

Bleeding from the iris is relatively uncommon and usually minor. If the iris is abnormal, such as in rubeosis, heterochromic iridocyclitis, anterior iridocyclitis, congenital glaucoma, or anterior chamber cleavage defects, bleeding is more likely. It is difficult—if not impossible—to cauterize the iris and generally no treatment is required. If the bleeding is persistent, instillation of a viscoelastic agent into the anterior chamber usually is helpful.

Complications

Blood in the anterior chamber is usually of no consequence, but at times might be a problem, even a potentially serious problem. Blood in the anterior chamber might have a deleterious effect on the corneal endothelium, especially if the endothelial cells are already compromised. Blood staining of the cornea can occur, especially if there is repeated bleeding into the anterior chamber and the IOP is elevated. Increased IOP is a recognized complication of hyphema, particularly if a functioning filter is not present or if the filtering site is obstructed by a blood clot. The trabecular meshwork can become obstructed by red blood cells directly or by a macrophage response elicited by blood breakdown products, leading to a secondary hemolytic open angle glaucoma.[7] Rarely, the blood can persist in the anterior chamber, resulting in granulomatous masses in the anterior chamber, particularly on the iris and the filtration angle.[8] Occasionally, an extensive or "eightball" hyphema can occur. These extensive hemorrhages are particularly prone to complications of increased IOP and corneal bloodstaining.

Management

The best treatment for hyphema is prevention and the best prevention is meticulous handling of the tissues and appropriate use of cautery. Hyphemas will still occur, but in the vast majority of cases no treatment is necessary and the blood will be absorbed within a brief period of time. The use of cycloplegics, corticosteroids, patching, and bed rest are of unproven value. Treatment of increased IOP should be undertaken if necessary and the preferred agents in most cases are aqueous suppressants (beta blockers and CAIs), though these agents can inhibit the ability of the eye to rapidly wash the blood out. In acute or short-term situations, osmotic agents also can be useful. In black patients it is essential to assess whether the patient has sickle trait or sickle cell anemia because CAIs, which cause a metabolic acidosis, and osmotic agents, which cause an increase in serum osmolarity, might lead to increased sickling, which can have widespread systemic complications as well as further increasing the IOP.

If recurrent bleeding is noted, a bleeding site sometimes can be located by gonioscopy and argon laser can be used to coagulate the bleeding site.[6] If the hyphema is persistent or very large, it might become necessary to wash out the anterior chamber. Hyphema of greater than 50% of the anterior chamber are especially prone to complications and probably should be removed. Hyphema of this magnitude will often lead to failure of any filtration bleb in addition to other previously mentioned problems related to the blood. Elevating the head of the bed 20 to 30 degrees might prevent blood from obstructing a superior sclerotomy site (or other positions if the sclerotomy was performed nasally or temporally) to help prevent IOP elevations might be all that is necessary in some cases to prevent having to wash out the hyphema.

Deciding when to intervene is not always an easy decision. When there is known severe optic nerve damage even a mildly elevated IOP might not be acceptable for more than a few days. Corneal bloodstaining can occur early if there are signs of corneal endothelial cell dysfunction. Removal of the hyphema or clot can be associated with damage to the iris and lens or lead to conjunctival buttonholing or other complications related to any intraocular surgery, such as suprachoroidal hemorrhage or endophthalmitis. In a healthy cornea it is generally felt that corneal bloodstaining is unlikely to occur in less than 4 to 5 days at an IOP less than 40 mm Hg or 2 to 3 days at an IOP of 50 mm Hg. What IOP is tolerable and for how long in an eye with glaucomatous optic nerve damage depends upon one's knowledge of the individual patient. Of special concern, however, are those patients with sickle trait or sickle cell anemia where infarction of the optic nerve can occur at relatively low IOP. In these individual patients, the IOP probably should not be allowed to exceed 25 to 30 mm Hg for any extended period of time.

Liquid blood can easily be removed with irrigation. The irrigation can be allowed to "wash-out" the blood back through a single incision into the anterior chamber or a second site can be utilized for expression of the blood and irrigant. If a clot has formed and requires evacuation it can be removed by one of several techniques. The primary precaution in removing a clot is to not grasp the clot with forceps and remove it because other intraocular tissues can be adherent or incorporated in the clot. It is generally best to "express" the clot gently through a corneal or corneoscleral incision of sufficient size to allow the clot to evacuate itself. If this proves unsuccessful, a vitrectomy instrument set at low vacuum can be used to debulk and remove most of the clot.

Summary

Hyphema following glaucoma surgery is relatively common, but is apparently rarely of significant consequence. Unfortunately, there are no long-term series that assess the effects of hyphema with regard to IOP control. Patience is the hallmark of therapy and the vast majority of these eyes will do extremely well and a good surgical result will not be compromised by the presence of the blood in the anterior chamber. When indicated, removal of the hyphema can be accomplished safely without compromise of the surgical goals in most cases.

References

1. Luntz MH. Surgical therapy-filtering surgery for glaucoma. In Cairns, J (ed): Glaucoma Vol. II. Orlando: Grune & Stratton, 1986, pp 621.
2. Ilif N. Complications in ophthalmic surgery. New York: Churchhill Livingstone, 1983, pp 54-55, 148.
3. Jaffe N. Cataract surgery and its complications. Third Ed., St. Louis: C.V. Mosby. 1981, pp. 409-414.
4. Krupin T, Waltman S. Complications in ophthalmic surgery. Second Ed., Philadelphia: J.B. Lippincott, 1984, pp. 74, 184.
5. Swan, KC. Hyphema due to wound vascularization after cataract extraction. Arch Ophthalmol, 89:87-90, 1973.
6. Wilensky JT. Late hyphema after filtering surgery for glaucoma. Ophthalmol Surg 14:227-228, 1983.
7. Fenton RH, Zimmerman LE. Hemolytic glaucoma. An unusual cause of acute open-angle secondary glaucoma. Arch Ophthalmol 70:236-239, 1963.
8. Appelmans M, Michiels J. Xantho-chromic aqueous humour. Acta XVI Int Congr Ophthalmol, London 1:202-706, 1950.

Vitreous Loss During Glaucoma Surgery

Louis B. Cantor, MD

Vitreous loss during glaucoma surgery is an uncommon complication. It is important, however, that the operating surgeon understand this complication and the various factors that might predispose to vitreous loss in both the phakic and aphakic eye. If there is impending vitreous loss or if vitreous loss has occurred, an understanding of when and how to manage this complication is necessary.

Predisposing Factors

In general, the factors that predispose to vitreous loss are the same in glaucomatous and nonglaucomatous eyes, though there are some differences.[1,2,3] Preoperative evaluation is important. The factors to consider are summarized in Table 14-4. A history of vitreous loss during surgery of the fellow eye might alert one to look for vitreous loss at the time of operation in the second eye. A history of pulmonary problems that predispose to valsalva, such as bronchitis or emphysema, should alert the surgeon that vitreous loss is likely. Patients with short, thick necks might have increased venous pressure, with increased pressure on the globe when placed in the supine position.

Table 14-4. Factors That Increase the Risk of Vitreous Loss

Ocular Factors:	Systemic Factors:
Aphakia	Chronic cough
Conjunctival scarring	Chronic obstructive pulmonary disease
Dislocated or subluxated lens	Emphysema
High myopia	Increased venous pressure
History of previous intraocular surgery	Obesity
History of vitreous loss in fellow eye	Short, thick neck
Increased orbital resistance	
Proptosis	

Ocular findings that might increase the likelihood of vitreous loss include proptosis, high myopia, previous intraocular surgery or trauma, and a subluxated or dislocated lens. Surgery in the aphakic or pseudophakic eye (especially where a posterior capsulotomy has been performed) carries an increased risk of vitreous loss.

Prevention

Several precautions can be taken to reduce the risk of vitreous loss including: providing adequate preoperative sedation and analgesia; assuring careful draping and support of the lids; tilting of the table in a reverse trandelenberg position; and obtaining maximal ocular hypotension prior to surgery, either by ocular massage, acetazolamide, or hyperosmotic agents. Adequate preoperative sedation and analgesia can be accomplished by several methods. In general, a well-informed patient is less apprehensive and will require less medication when local anesthesia with intravenous sedation is chosen. In some individuals, adequate sedation only can be accomplished with general anesthesia. Therefore, the anesthesia must be tapered to the individual and monitored so that anesthesia can be given or withheld when appropriate. It is important to avoid excess sedation because the patient might become disoriented or move at an inopportune time. Positioning of the drapes and lid speculum to avoid pressure on the globe and maximize exposure will lessen the risk of vitreous loss. The type of lid speculum depends upon experience and preferences, but in general a wire speculum works well. Placing the patient in a comfortable position with the head elevated in a reverse trandelenberg will decrease venous pressure and the risk of complications. Lowering the IOP, by digital massage or by use of osmotic agents, will lessen the likelihood of vitreous loss.

The surgeon must recognize impending vitreous loss, because prompt recognition and proper management can minimize or even prevent this complication. Signs of elevated posterior segment pressure and impending vitreous loss include: iris prolapse through the incision, forward displacement of the lens iris diaphragm, gaping of the wound, shallowing of the anterior chamber, and tension lines in the cornea. Frequently, however, the anterior chamber will shallow and iris might prolapse when a sclerotomy is performed. Without high posterior segment pressure the anterior chamber should be easily deepened with saline solution or the iris reposited following an iridectomy. If this proves difficult, the possibility of impending vitreous loss is high.

Management

Vitreous loss at the time of trabeculectomy in phakic eyes is rare (less than 0.5%).[4] Vitreous loss primarily occurs when there has been rupture of the lens zonules or the hyaloid face, which usually results from excessive manipulation or previous trauma. The vitreous should be removed from the surgical site with sponges, scissors, or a vitrectomy instrument. If an adequate vitrectomy can be done without trauma to the lens, the filtration site might function well. If an adequate vitrectomy cannot be performed, it is probably best to close the scleral flap with 10-0 nylon sutures and perform another trabeculectomy at another site. Lens injury, if present, can remain limited to the surgical site if it is small, while larger injuries can cause gradual wide spread extension, or acute cataract formation, occasionally with severe uveitis.[5] Loss of vitreous can also lead to bullous keratopathy, epithelial and fibrous downgrowth, iris prolapse, uveitis, retinal detachment, cystoid macular edema, vitreous fibrosis and opacification, vitreous contraction bands, and pupillary membrane formation. Endophthalmitis also can result if vitreous is incarcerated in the incision and prevents complete healing. Therefore, it is better to extract the vitreous once it has been disturbed, rather than allow it to cause these potentially avoidable complications (Table 14-5).

Table 14-5. Complications of Vitreous Loss	
Astigmatism	Fibrous downgrowth
Bullous keratopathy	Fibrous traction bands
Cataract	Iris prolapse
Chronic inflammation	Pupillary distortion
Cystoid macular edema	Pupillary membranes
Disc edema	Retinal detachment
Endophthalmitis	Secondary glaucoma
Epithelial downgrowth	Suprachoroidal hemorrhage
Fibrous condensation of vitreous	Vitreous hemorrhage

In the aphakic eye, vitreous loss is a more common occurrence and actually can be expected in many cases. If vitreous is filling the anterior chamber, a vitrectomy can be planned as part of the primary procedure through a separate clear corneal incision or through the filtration site itself. Extensive vitrectomy is not indicated because this does not improve the overall success of the filtering surgery. The anterior chamber should be debulked of vitreous using a cutting vitrectomy instrument to prevent postoperative complications of vitreous incarceration into the incision.

In any case in which vitreous loss has occurred, the surgical procedure should be interrupted and the cause of the vitreous loss identified. If the vitreous loss occurs during a cataract procedure or combined filtration and cataract surgery, preplaced sutures, which are highly recommended, can be used to close the incision. It is essential that a suprachoroidal hemorrhage be suspected and ruled out whenever vitreous loss occurs. Failure to quickly diagnose a suprachoroidal hemorrhage can lead to a disastrous result. External ocular pressure can be diagnosed quickly by adjusting the lid retractors and superior rectus suture. A tight lateral canthal ligament with pressure on the globe can be eliminated. Residual ocular motility or orbicularis oculi function can be relieved with additional local anesthesia, though further retrobulbar or peribulbar anesthesia should be avoided once the eye has been opened. A Van Lint approach for local anesthesia should be avoided in favor of an O'Brien or Atkinson technique because the eyelid edema can increase pressure on the globe.

Ocular motility problems are probably best treated by small injections of anesthetic agent over the muscles or by increased sedation. If the patient is restless, the anesthesiologist or surgeon might need to assist or reassure the patient. Intravenous hyperosmotic agents might be administered to reduce the vitreous volume if necessary. If there has been scleral collapse, such as might occur in aphakic or highly myopic eyes, scleral support can be provided with superficial traction sutures, or with a scleral ring if the surgical procedure allows. A subclinical retrobulbar hemorrhage also might be a cause of external pressure on the globe and can be recognized by noting a firm orbit or by an expanding subconjunctival hemorrhage.

Cataract surgery in glaucomatous eyes, either combined with a filtering procedure or alone, is particularly predisposed to the complication of vitreous loss because of many factors. If a limbus-based conjunctival flap is used, visualization can be difficult when performing the cataract extraction. Careful handling of the conjunctiva by the assistant to maximize visualization when a limbus-based flap is used, or using a fornix-based conjunctival flap might be helpful. Small fixed pupils, secondary to chronic miotic therapy or posterior synechiae, are common and limit visualization when attempting to perform the anterior capsulotomy. It is, therefore, not uncommon to see anterior capsular flaps or other problems with the capsulotomy that make rupture of the posterior capsule or zonular rupture with subsequent vitreous loss more likely events. A small pupil also makes expression of the nucleus difficult in planned extracapsular cataract extractions. Phacoemulsification is extremely difficult to perform in a patient with a small pupil. Performing a sector iridectomy might prove very helpful in these cases. This will improve visualization greatly and allow for the performance of a better anterior capsulotomy and make nucleus expression easier in extracapsular surgery. If desired, the sector iridectomy can be closed at the end of the procedure for cosmetic purposes.

Though relatively uncommon, vitreous loss can occur during glaucoma surgery. The possibility of vitreous loss exists with any intraocular surgery, but can be particularly likely in certain situations. Measures to lessen the likelihood of vitreous loss should be considered in all cases (Table 14-6). With modern instrumentation and surgical techniques our ability to manage vitreous loss when it occurs and preserve a good surgical result has been greatly improved.

Table 14-6. Measures to Prevent Vitreous Loss Prior to Surgery

Analgesia	Proper positioning on operation table
Antiemesis	Sedation
Local anesthesia	Softening the eye

References

1. Jaffe NS. Cataract surgery and its complications. 3rd Ed. St. Louis: C.V. Mosby, 1981, p. 252.
2. Krupin T, Waltman SR. Complications in ophthalmic surgery. 2nd Ed. Philadelphia: J.B. Lippincott, 1984, p. 49.
3. Spaeth GL. Ophthalmic Surgery: principles and practices. Philadelphia: W.B. Saunders 1982, p. 162.
4. Cairns JE. Glaucoma. Orlando: Grune & Stratton, 1986, p. 593.
5. Swann KD, Lindgren TW. Unintentional lens injury in glaucoma surgery. Trans Am Ophthalmol Soc 78:55-69, 1980.

Endophthalmitis

L. Jay Katz, MD

Endophthalmitis

Incidence

Intraocular infection can follow any surgical procedure whenever the globe is incised. With filtering surgery, where the wound is intentionally left open for IOP control, the risk of endophthalmitis persists long after the completion of surgery. The incidence of infection following cataract extraction has been reported from 0.05% to 0.3% with the former figure more indicative of modern era surgical techniques in the operating room.[1-6] Since the aim of glaucoma surgery is to create a direct communication for aqueous flow from the anterior chamber into the subconjunctival space, with only conjunctiva and perhaps Tenon's capsule covering the fistula, it is not surprising that endophthalmitis following filtering surgery has a higher incidence than cataract surgery, being 0.1 to 2%.[8-18] The evaluation, management, and clinical implications of endophthalmitis for eyes with filtering blebs are in some ways distinctly different than postcataract extraction eyes.

Endophthalmitis can occur many years after filtration surgery and the clinician and patient must be constantly aware of this possibility. When treating the intraocular infection, not only is the integrity of the eye in terms of vision at stake, but also the functional ability of the filtration bleb to continue controlling the IOP.

Clinical Features

In the presence of filtration blebs, three potential compartments might be involved: the subconjunctival space, the anterior and posterior chambers (anterior segment), and the vitreous cavity. Usually, the spread of infection proceeds in that order with an infected bleb progressing to anterior, then posterior globe involvement.

There are several recognized risk factors for postfiltration endophthalmitis. These are listed in Table 14-7. Bacterial conjunctivitis left untreated might spread transconjunctivally. Thin, cystic blebs that are particularly common following full-thickness procedures, especially trephination,[7,8,10,14] are more likely to become infected than thicker-walled blebs. Contact lens use in the presence of a filtering bleb might be hazardous.[20] Of obvious concern would be bleb trauma that would lead to a conjunctival hole and a Seidel positive leak. This would allow direct intraocular spread of surface organisms.

Table 14-7. Risk Factors for Postfiltration Endophthalmitis
1. Bacterial conjunctivitis
2. Thin-walled blebs
3. Contact lens
4. Trauma

Subjective complaints might include ocular pain, foreign body sensation, blurred vision, and tearing (Table 14-8). A history of a red eye with a discharge might be recalled. Fever and malaise should alert the clinician to the possibility of an endogenous metastatic endophthalmitis with a primary site of infection other than the eye.

Table 14-8. Symptoms And Signs of Endophthalmitis
1. Ocular pain
2. Foreign body sensation
3. Blurred vision
4. Tearing
5. Conjunctival injection
6. Chemosis
7. Bleb purulence/leak
8. Corneal edema
9. Hypopyon-uveitis
10. Vitreous debris
11. Hypotony

Examination might reveal conjunctival and ciliary injection, periorbital chemosis, bleb purulence (Fig. 14-19), corneal edema, uveitis-hypopyon (Fig. 14-20), and vitreal debris with loss of the red reflex. The IOP might be very low if a bleb leak is present (Fig. 14-21), or elevated when the sclerotomy is occluded with purulence and debris.

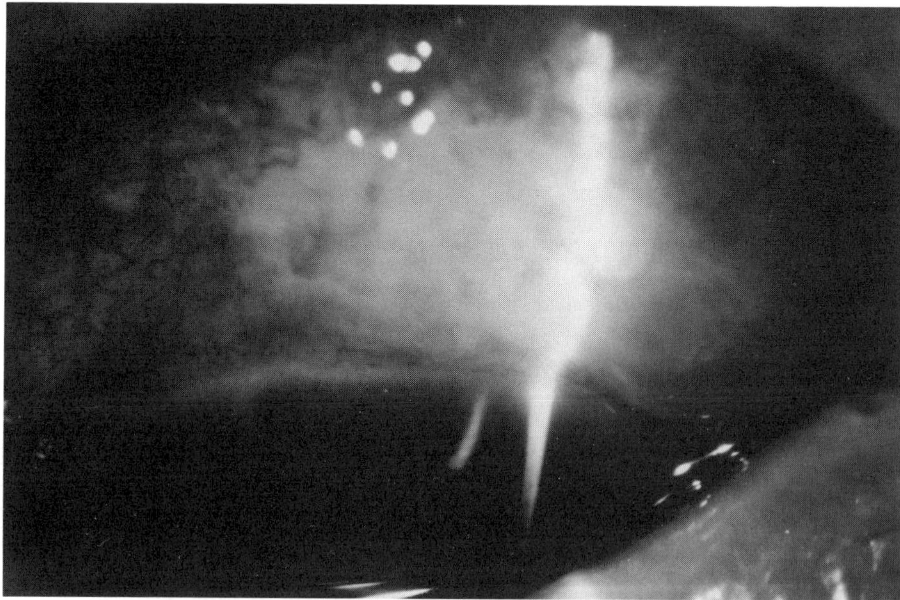

Figure 14-19. Infected filtering bleb.

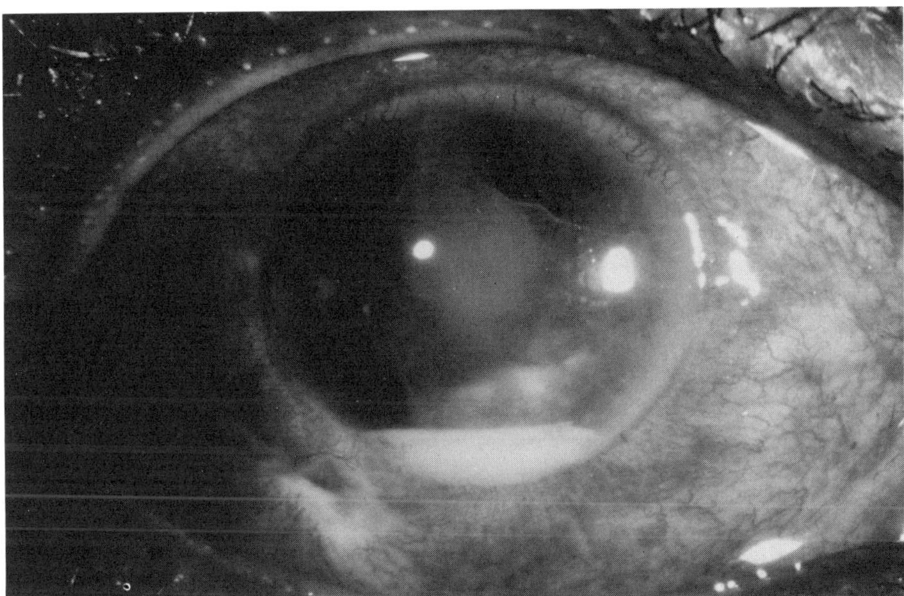

Figure 14-20. Hypopyon and fibrin clot in anterior chamber in an eye with late postfiltration surgery endophthalmitis.

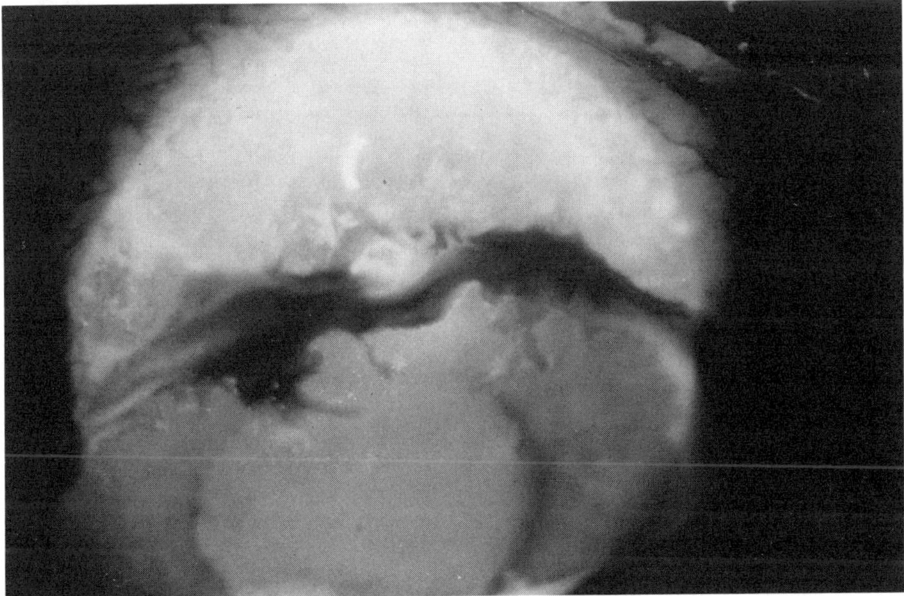

Figure 14-21. Seidel-positive leak in an infected filtering bleb.

Two forms of endophthalmitis have been identified based on the time of onset: early and late.[19] With early endophthalmitis the diagnosis is usually made within approximately three days of surgery. This resembles endophthalmitis associated with cataract extraction. With late onset infection, months to years typically lapse before the infection develops. Although pathogenesis might differ with transconjunctival bacterial migration in the latter and intraoperative contamination in the former, the workup and management are identical.

Diagnostic Workup

It is important to identify the organism responsible so that appropriate modifications can be made and specific antibiotics used. If an abscess has externalized with obvious drainage to the surface of the bleb, a conjunctival culture is usually helpful (see Table 14-9). However, the important sites for specimen collection are the anterior chamber and vitreous cavity.

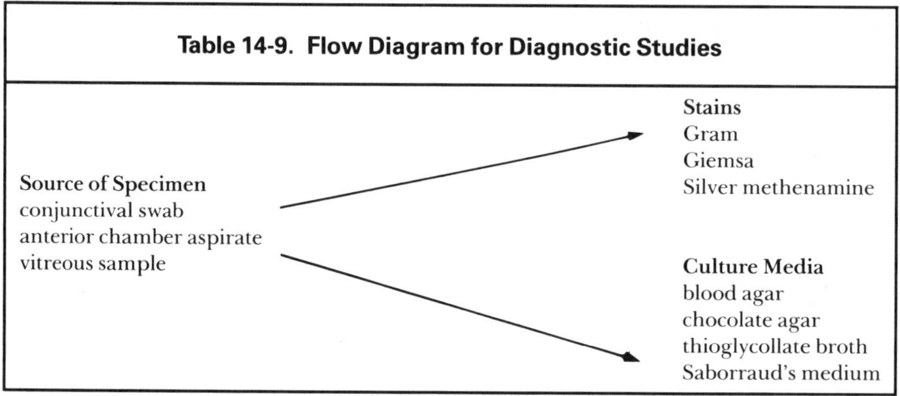

Table 14-9. Flow Diagram for Diagnostic Studies

Source of Specimen
conjunctival swab
anterior chamber aspirate
vitreous sample

→ **Stains**
Gram
Giemsa
Silver methenamine

→ **Culture Media**
blood agar
chocolate agar
thioglycollate broth
Saborraud's medium

When the vitreous is thought to be spared, as noted by slit lamp biomicroscopy and ophthalmoloscopy, then an anterior chamber tap might be sufficient without a vitreous tap. Usually, both the anterior chamber and vitreous cavity are sampled because positive cultures can be obtained from only one with the exclusion of the other.[23,24] If the media is hazy because of corneal edema or a cataract, B mode ultrasonography might be helpful in evaluating the retrolental area.[22] When the view is obscured, ultrasonography might identify vitreous infection with echoes signifying debris in the vitreous cavity (Fig. 14-22). It is also helpful to note the presence of a retinal detachment or choroidal detachment before embarking on a treatment plan.

In the performance of an anterior chamber aspiration, a 25 or 27 gauge sharp needle (5/8 inch) is directed peripherally through clear cornea starting near the limbus. A 1 to 2 mm tract is made through the cornea before intraocular entry to allow the incision to be self-sealing. Paracentesis of a 0.1-0.2 ml aliquot of aqueous into a 1ml tuberculin springe is sent for analysis. The anterior chamber should be reformed with balanced salt solution to prevent hypotony because it predisposes to ciliochoroidal detachment and suprachoroidal hemorrhage. Reformation should be done with a blunt 30 gauge cannula through the paracentesis track so that possible injury to the iris or lens can be avoided.

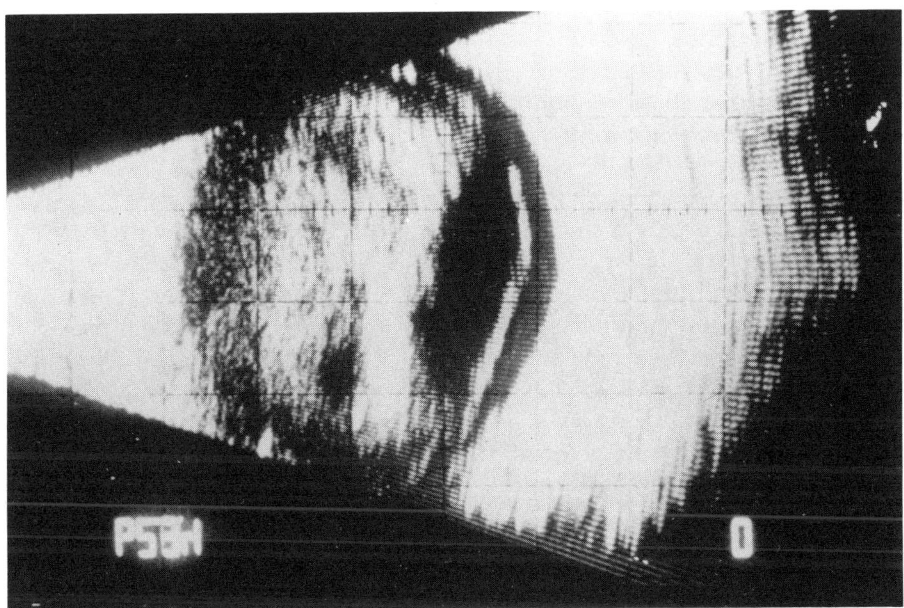

Figure 14-22. Ultrasound demonstrating vitreous extension of endophthalmitis.

The lens and an intact posterior capsule are relative barriers to bacteria, but are certainly not absolute in impeding the migration of organisms.[25] Therefore, one should not have a false sense of security in phakic eyes or where a posterior capsule has been left intact. A vitreous tap is strongly recommended should there be any suggestion of vitreal involvement. A pars plana approach should be utilized. The puncture site is made 4 mm from the limbus. After incising the conjunctiva and cautery application a partial-thickness scleral incision with a #67 Beaver blade precedes entry with either a MVR blade or a 20 gauge needle. Entry is made with the instrument tip pointed toward the optic nerve to avoid lens trauma or implant displacement. The vitreous sample is best collected by vitrectomy, but aspiration of liquid vitreous through a 20 gauge needle can be an alternative, although this latter technique places more tension on the vitreous gel and, therefore, promotes vitreoretinal traction. When direct observation of vitreous collection is impossible, the needle shaft can be clamped at 12 mm to ensure that while aiming toward the optic nerve the needle tip remains within the vitreous cavity. If a vitrectomy is planned for therapeutic reasons, an adequate sample for culture might be collected on a millipore filter (0.22 or 0.45 micron). In aphakic eyes a 22 gauge needle can be passed through the limbus and directed through the pupil or iridectomy into the vitreous cavity. An aspirate of 0.2 to 0.3 ml of liquid vitreous is obtained for analysis.

The specimen should be placed on glass slides to air dry for Gram, Giemsa, and silver methenamine stains. The latter is to look specifically for fungal elements. The slides might provide immediate information while waiting for the definitive culture results. Cultures should be made with several media that best support different pathogens: blood agar (general bacteria), chocolate agar (Hemophilus, Neisseria), thioglycollate broth (anaerobes), and Sabouraud's medium (fungi). Sensitivity to various antibiotics are assayed after the organism has been identified.

Although a sterile, noninfectious endophthalmitis might be erroneously diagnosed in up to 1/3 of the cases following cataract extraction,[24] it rarely will present a diagnostic dilemma in most cases of filtration surgery. There usually is no cortical debris or nuclear remnants inciting phacoanalyphylaxis nor an intraocular lens to confound the situation. When there has been a separate or combined operations for both cataract and glaucoma, however, a similar confusing situation might arise deciding whether an endophthalmitis is of a sterile or infectious variety. Infectious endophthalmitis is generally more rapidly progressive unless a low virulence organism, such as *Staphylococcus epidermidis* or *Propionibacterium*, is responsible.[26,27] A sterile inflammatory response will usually occur within the first two postoperative days, whereas an infection can occur at any time.

Treatment

Prophylaxis

Prophylaxis against infection has been recommended in three ways:

1. Preoperative topical antibiotics are given for 1 to 2 days to lower the conjunctival flora. This has been postulated to minimize the possibility of intraocular colonization in the immediate postoperative period.[28,29,30]
2. Intraoperative administration of antibiotics has been strongly recommended. It has been used in cataract extraction patients as an irrigating fluid with 8 mcg of gentamicin/ml passed through a millipore filter.[31] Subconjunctival injection of antibiotics upon completion of the surgery has been thought to appreciably reduce the postoperative incidence of endophthalmitis.[32,33,34] We prefer to use gentamicin 40 mg given in 1/2 cc. This is injected 180° away from the filtration site usually in the inferior fornix.
3. Postoperative topical antibiotics are routinely used for at least one week. However, it has been recommended that antibiotics be continued indefinitely with a once daily maintenance dose to avoid a subclinical conjunctivitis that might lead to intraocular infections.[30]

Special attention has been directed at very thin cystic blebs. No controlled study has established that prophylactic reduction of the bacterial conjunctival flora is beneficial or conversely that chronic use of an antibiotic selects a virulent organism that is resistant to the prophylactic antibiotic and predisposes toward infection. Perhaps alternating antibiotics at regular intervals would be helpful in getting broad suppression of bacteria.

Antibiotics

After a culture specimen has been obtained for suspected infectious endophthalmitis, intensive broad-spectrum antibiotic coverage is provided by three routes: topical, subconjunctival, and intravenous.[35-41] If significant vitreous involvement is suspected, an intravitreal bolus of antibiotic is also recommended as a fourth route. Specific recommendations are given in Table 14-10.

Table 14-10. Antibiotics for Endophthalmitis

Route	Drug	Dose	Frequency
Topical	Fortified Gentamicin	15mg/ml	qlh.
	Fortified Cefazolin	100mg/ml	qlh.
Subconjunctival	Gentamicin	80mg/ml	q½-ld.
	Cefazolin	300mg/ml 1/3ml	q½-ld.
Intravenous	Gentamicin	60-80mg	q6-8h.
	Cefazolin	1-2gm	q6-8h.
Intravitreal (0.lml)	Gentamicin	100mcg	q2d.
	(or Amikacin)	400mcg	q2d.
	Cefazolin	2.25mg	q2d.
	(or Vancomycin)	lmg	q2d.

The combination of a beta lactam antibiotic and aminoglycoside synergistically covers against a wide spectrum of bacteria including both the gram positive and gram negative rods that are the most likely organisms.[42] The topical antibiotics are given staggered so that drops are administered every 1/2-1 hour through at least the first 24 hours. It has been offered that amikacin should replace gentamicin as the first line aminoglycoside because a number of gentamicin-resistant organisms have been reported to cause endophthalmitis. Furthermore, amikacin is less toxic to the retina.[51]

Intravitreal injection of antibiotics has been increasingly strongly advocated to sterilize the vitreous cavity.[45-52] One possible detrimental effect might be macular infarction when vitrectomy and intravitreal injection of gentamicin are combined.[53] Because the vitreous gel is removed, the retina is exposed to a higher bolus of antibiotic and might be more toxic. To minimize the possible retinal toxicity of intravitreal antibiotics, the injection is placed anteriorly in the vitreal cavity, injected very slowly, and the dose reduced if a vitrectomy has been performed.

Some advocate the use of vancomycin and gentamicin as the initial drug combination because streptococcus is increasingly resistant to gentamicin and cefazolin.[51] This is especially important in light of the fact that streptococcus was the most common organism isolated in a large series of postfiltration endophthalmitis.[54] It has been suggested that cefataxine be the cephalosporin used since the blood-brain barrier (and presumably blood-eye barrier) is easily crossed unlike other drugs in its class.[55]

While using aminoglycosides systemically, renal function needs to be monitored with daily serum creatinine and BUN levels. Serum levels of the antibiotic are drawn for peak (one hour after dose) and trough (immediately before the next dose), twice weekly to help maximize the therapeutic effect and minimize toxicity. Once the organism is identified and antibiotic sensitivities are available, the antibiotic regimen should be adjusted as specified. After recovery from endophthalmitis, patients are instructed to seek medical attention immediately if a discharge or redness recurs. After an episode of endophthalmitis without previous chronic topical antibiotic prophylaxis, it might be decided that topical antibiotic therapy (e.g., erythromycin ointment) would be protective against a recurrence. Adjunctive therapy with a cycloplegic-mydriatic combination, such as atropine 1% and phenylephrine four times daily, helps in alleviating discomfort from ciliary spasm, breaking early posterior synechiae, providing a large pupil to better view the vitreous cavity, and strengthen the blood-aqueous barrier to better minimize the uveitis.

Steroids

The use of corticosteroids is a less clearly defined area, but one of great importance.[56,57] Although it reduces the hosts defenses against bacterium, steroids are also anti-inflammatory. The major benefits are to save the filtration bleb from scarring and to clear a cloudy vitreous mcre rapidly. The routes of administration are summarized in Table 14-11. Prompt administration within 24 hours after starting antibiotics helps limit inflammation that could lead to subconjunctival scarring. Of course, if there is progressive endophthalmitis, steroids should be withheld.

Table 14-11. Corticosteroids in Combination with Antibiotic Therapy for Endophthalmitis

Route	Drug	Dose	Frequency
Topical	Prednisoline	1%	q4h.
Subconjunctival	Dexamethasone	1ml of 4mg/ml	ql-2d.
Systemic	Prednisone	20mg	tid-qid po
Intravitreal	Dexamethasone	400mcg in 0.1ml	ql-2d.

Pros and Cons of Therapeutic Vitrectomy

The benefits of a therapeutic vitrectomy for endophthalmitis include: "debulking" of organisms, removal of toxins injurious to the retina and optic nerve, and limiting the potential of tractional retinal detachment. The disadvantages of vitrectomy include: iatrogenic retinal tear and detachment, vitreous hemorrhage, and increased risk of macular toxicity from intravitreal antibiotics. For early endophthalmitis with minimal vitreal involvement and a good red reflex or when dealing with a relatively indolent organism such as *S epidermidis* a core vitrectomy is not indicated. With a cloudy vitreous and a virulent organism, such as streptococcus, aggressive treatment with vitrectomy is warranted.

When the vitreous is infected, a vitrectomy can be quite useful.[58-63] If the organism is a virulent one, then intensive antibiotic therapy might prove insufficient. A vitrectomy would remove the vitreous (a good colonizing medium), debulk the bacterial mass, and allow better antibiotic circulation. A closed system—pars plana approach 4 mm from the limbus—is routinely used unless the patient is aphakic with no posterior capsule where a limbal incision is preferred. If the cornea is cloudy, then an open-sky limbal entry would be necessary. If a cataract obscures the view, a cataract extraction should be done. In an open-sky system, there is a significant risk for a glaucoma patient of developing a suprachoroidal hemorrhage.

Therefore, preplaced sutures are strongly recommended in that situation.[19] Should there be an intraocular lens present, its removal would not be necessary nor helpful in the recovery of the patient.[64]

Prognosis

The end result of an endophthalmitis is dependent on several factors: the virulence of the organism, the extent of infection compartmentalization when treatment is started, the rapidity of treatment initiation, and the sensitivity to the antibiotics chosen initially. Of course, the worst possibility is total loss of sight with a cosmetically unacceptable eye. Less extreme, but still unfortunate consequences would include loss of the filtration bleb and consequent, an elevation of IOP, corneal edema, cataract development, vitreo-retinal traction with retinal detachment, and loss of retinal function.

The type of organism is a strong determinant of outcome with organisms of low virulence, such as *Staphylococcus epidermidis* and *Propionibacterium*, having good prognoses with fairly conservative treatment with antibiotics alone. Interestingly, if there is a positive culture, those eyes generally fair worse than eyes in which a negative culture was obtained.[24,65] If the infection is fairly widespread at the time of diagnosis and the initial visual acuity is poor, then a fairly dismal outcome usually results. It appears that unless the eye is minimally involved with just the bleb area infected or a relatively nonvirulent organism involved, aggressive antibiotic therapy with corticosteroid adjunctive use and a vitrectomy should be promptly performed to help save the functional integrity of the eye.

References

1. Leopold IH, Apt L. Postoperative intraocular infections. Am J Ophthalmol 50:1225-1247, 1960.
2. McGrand JC. Post-operative intraocular infection. Trans Ophthalmol Soc UK 88:223-230, 1968.
3. Forster RK, Zachery IG, Cottingham AJ Jr., Norton EWD. Further observations on the diagnosis, cause, and treatment of endophthalmitis. Am J Ophthalmol 81:52-56, 1976.
4. Allen HF. Symposium: Postoperative endophthalmitis. Introduction: incidence and etiology. Ophthalmology 85:317-319, 1978.
5. Puliafito CA, Baker AS, Haaf J, Forster CS. Infectious endophthalmitis: review of thirty-six cases. Ophthalmology 89:921-928, 1982.
6. Berler DK. Endophthalmitis in 10,032 cataract operations. J Occup Ther Surg 1:159-162, 1982.
7. Abel R Jr., Binder PS, Bellows R. Postoperative bacterial endophthalmitis. Ann Ophthalmol 8:731-744, 1976.

8. Sugar HS, Zekman T. Late infection of filtering conjunctival scars. Am J Ophthalmol 46:155-170, 1958.
9. Hattenhauer JM, Lipsich MP Late endophthalmitis after filtering surgery. Am J Ophthalmol 72:1097-1101, 1971.
10. Kanski JJ. Treatment of late endophthalmitis associated with filtering blebs. Arch Ophthalmol 91:339-343, 1974.
11. Tabbara KF. Late infections following filtering procedure. Ann Ophthalmol 8:1228-1231, 1976.
12. Wilson P. Trabeculectomy: Long-term follow-up. BrJ Ophthalmol 61:535-538, 1977.
13. Jerndal T, Lundstrom M. 330 trabeculectomies—a follow-up study through 1/2-3 years. Acta Ophthalmol 55:52-62, 1977.
14. Freedman J, Gupta M, Bunke A. Endophthalmitis after trabeculectomy Arch Ophthalmol 96:1017-1018, 1978.
15. Mills KB. Trabeculectomy: a retrospective long-term follow-up of 444 cases. Br J Ophthalmol 65:790-795, 1981.
16. Paglen PG, Abbott RL, Webster RG Jr. Late onset bilateral endophthalmitis after trabeculectomy. J Occup Ther Surg 1(lA):33-34, 1982.
17. Shirato S, Kitazawa Y, Mishima S. A critical analysis of the trabeculectomy results by a prospective follow-up design. JpnJ Ophthalmol 26:468-480, 1982.
18. Pillai S, Limaye SR. Endophthalmitis following Scheie procedure. Glaucoma 6:96-98, 1984.
19. Katz LJ, Cantor LB, Spaeth GL. Complications of surgery in glaucoma. Early and late bacterial endophthalmitis following glaucoma filtering surgery. Ophthalmology 92:959-963, 1985.
20. Bellows AR, McCulley JP. Endophthalmitis in aphakic patients with unplanned filtering blebs wearing contact lenses. Ophthalmology 88:839-843, 1981.
21. Greenwald MJ, Wohl LG, Fell CM. A contemporary reappraisal. Surv Ophthalmol 31:81-101, 1986.
22. Chan IM, Jalkh AE, Trempe CL, Tolentino FI. Ultrasonographic findings in endophthalmitis. Ann Ophthalmol 16:778-784, 1984.
23. Forster RK, Abbott RL, Gelender H. Management of infectious endophthalmitis. Ophthalmology 87:313-318, 1980.
24. Bohigian GM, Olk, RJ. Factors associated with a poor visual result in endophthalmitis. Am J Ophthalmol 101:332-334, 1986.
25. Beyer TL, Vogler G, Sharma D, O'Donnell FE. Protective barrier effect of the posterior lens capsule in exogenous bacterial endophthalmitis. An experimental primate study. Invest Ophthal Vis Sci 25: 108-112, 1984.
26. O'Day DM, Jones DB, Patrinely J, et al. Staphylococcus epidermidis endophthalmitis: visual outcome following non- invasive therapy. Ophthalmology 89:354-360. 1982.
27. Meisler DM, Palestine AG, Vastine DW, et al. Chronic propionibacterium endophthalmitis after cataract extraction and intraocular lens implantation. Am J Ophthalmol 101:733-739, 1986.

28. Lobue TD, Deutsch TA, Stein RM. Moraxella nonliquefaciens endophthalmitis after trabeculectomy. Am J Ophthalmol 99:343-345, 1985.
29. Allen HF, Mangiaracine AF. Bacterial endophthalmitis after cataract extraction. II: Incidence in 36,000 consecutive operations with special reference to preoperative antibiotics. Trans Am Acad Ophthalmol 77:581-588, 1973.
30. Allen HF. Prevention of postoperative endophthalmitis. Ophthalmology 85:386-389, 1978.
31. Gills, JP. Prevention of endophthalmitis by intraocular solution filtration and antibiotics. J Am Intraocul Implant Soc 11:185-186, 1985.
32. Kolker AE, Freeman MI, Pettit TH. Prophylactic antibiotics and postoperative endophthalmitis. Am J Ophthalmol 63:434-439, 1967.
33. Christy NE, Hall P. A randomized, controlled comparison of anterior and posterior periocular injection of antibiotic in the prevention of postoperative endophthalmitis. Ophthalmol Surg 17(11):715-718, 1976.
34. Christy NE, Sommer A. Antibiotic prophylaxis of postoperative endophthalmitis. Annals of Ophthalmol 11:1261-1265, 1979.
35. Peyman GA, Paque JT, Meisels HJ, et al. Postoperative endophthalmitis: A comparison of methods of treatment and prophylaxis with gentamicin. Ophthalmol Surg 6:45-55, 1975.
36. Abel R Jr., Binder PS, Bellows R. Postoperative bacterial endophthalmitis III. Annals of Ophthalmol 8:1253-1265, 1976.
37. Diamond JG. Intraocular management of endophthalmitis: a systemic approach. Arch Ophthalmol 99:96-99, 1981.
38. Zaidman, GW, Mondino BJ. Postoperative pseudophakic bacterial endophthalmitis. Am J Ophthalmol 93: 218-233, 1982.
39. Rowsey JJ, Newsom DL, Sexton DJ, Harms WK. Endophthalmitis: current approaches. Ophthalmology 89:1055-1065, 1982.
40. Olson JC, Flynn HW Jr., Forster RK, Gelender H, Culbertson WW. Results in the treatment of postoperative endophthalmitis. Ophthalmology 90:692-697, 1983.
41. Baum J, Barza M. Endophthalmitis therapy, letter. Arch Ophthalmol 99:2054-2056, 1981.
42. Leopold, IH. Update on antibiotics in ocular infections. Am J Ophthalmol 100:134-140, 1985.
43. Insler MS, Cavanaugh MD, Wilson LA. Gentamicin-resistant pseudomonas endophthalmitis after penetrating keratoplasty. Br J Ophthalmol 69:189-191, 1985.
44. Lambert SR, Stern WH. Methicillin and gentamicin resistant staphylococcus epidermidis endophthalmitis after intraocular surgery. Am J Ophthalmol 99:725-726, 1985.
45. Peyman GA, May DR, Ericson, ES et al. Intraocular infection of gentamicin: toxic effects and clearance. Arch Ophthalmol 92:42-47, 1974.
46. Zachary IG, Forster RK. Experimental intravitreal gentamicin. Am J Ophthalmol 82:604-611, 1976.
47. Vastine DW, Peyman GA, Guth SB. Visual prognosis in bacterial endophthalmitis treated with intravitreal antibiotics. Ophthalmol Surg 10:76-83, 1979.

48. Fischer JP, Civiletto SE, Forster RK. Toxicity, efficacy, and clearance of intravitreally injected cefazolin. Arch Ophthalmol 100:650-652, 1980.
49. Baum J, Peyman GA, Barza M. Intravitreal administration of antibiotic in the treatment of bacterial endophthalmitis III. Surv Ophthalmol 26:204-206, 1982.
50. D'Amico DJ, Caspers-Velu G, Libert J, et al. Comparative toxicity of intravitreal aminoglycoside antibiotics. Am J Ophthalmol 100:264-275, 1985.
51. Tolano JH, D'Amico DJ, Kenyon KR. Intravitreal amikacin in the treatment of bacterial endophthalmitis. Arch Ophthalmol 104:1483-1485, 1986.
52. Pflugfelder SC, Hernandez E, Fliesler SJ, et al. Intravitreal vancomycin-retinal toxicity, clearance, and interaction with gentamicin. Arch Ophthalmol 105:831-837, 1987.
53. Conway BP, Campochiaro PA. Macular infarction after endophthalmitis treated with vitrectomy and intravitreal gentamicin. Arch Ophthalmol 104:367-371, 1986.
54. Mandelbaum S, Forster RK, Gelender H, Culbertson W. Late onset endophthalmitis associated with filtering blebs. Ophthalmology 92:964-972, 1985.
55. Laatikainen L, Tarkkanen A. Management of purulent postoperative endophthalmitis. Ophthalmologica 193:34-38, 1980.
56. Baum J, Rao G. Treatment of postcataract bacterial endophthalmitis with periocular and systemic antibiotic and corticosteroids. Trans Am Acad Ophthalmol Otolaryngol 81:151-162, 1976.
57. Baum J. The effect of corticosteroids in the treatment of experimental bacterial endophthalmitis. Am J Ophthalmol 80:513- 517, 1975.
58. Cottingham AJ Jr., Forster RK. Vitrectomy in endophthalmitis. Results of study using vitrectomy, intraocular antibiotics, or a combination of both. Arch Ophthalmol 94:2078-2081, 1976.
59. Peyman GA, Raichand M, Bennett TO. Management of endophthalmitis with pars plana vitrectomy. Br J Ophthalmol 64:472-475, 1980.
60. Eichenbaum DM, Jaffe NS, Clayman HM, Light DS. Pars plana vitrectomy as a primary treatment for acute bacterial endophthalmitis. Am J Ophthalmol 86:167-171, 1978.
61. Treister G, Glovinskiy Y. Vitrectomy in postcataract extraction endophthalmitis. J Occup Ther Surg 1:186-189, 1982.
62. Chen CJ. Management of infectious endophthalmitis by combined vitrectomy and intraocular injection. Ann Ophthalmol 15:968-979, 1983.
63. Olk RJ, Bohigian GM. The management of endophthalmitis: diagnostic and therapeutic guidelines including the use of vitrectomy. Ophthalmol Surg 18(4):262-267, 1987.
64. Driebe WT, Mandelbaum S, Forster RK, Schwartz LK, Culbertson WW. Pseudophakic endophthalmitis-diagnosis and management. Ophthalmology 93:442-448, 1986.
65. Forster, RK. Endophthalmitis-diagnostic cultures and visual results. Arch Ophthalmol 92:387-392, 1974.

Blockage of Internal Sclerostomy

L. Jay Katz, MD

Reasons for Filtration Failure

The failure of a filtration bleb can be divided into internal occlusions and external scarring.[1] When a filtering procedure results in the development of a bleb and IOP is lowered, it is disheartening to lose the beneficial effect of the surgery. In most cases, this is attributable to surface, subconjunctival scarring.[1] Histologically, a sheet of connective tissue covers the sclerostomy, perhaps emanating from the episclera.[2] In a limited number of situations, there is an internal obstruction of the sclerostomy seen gonioscopically. These eyes might be more easily treated to revive a failing bleb, because only a small area of obstruction is present. This is in contradistinction to the widespread surface scarring that usually requires another filtration operation. Failure to rapidly relieve the internal obstruction of the sclerostomy leads to flattening of the bleb and secondary external scarring.

Causes of Obstruction (Table 14-12)

Table 14-12. Causes of Internal Obstruction of a Filtration Fistula

Vitreous plugging
Ciliary processes rotating
Iris incarceration
Lens capsule fragment
Residual Descemet's membrane
Hemorrhage
Fibrin clot
Membrane (fibrovascular, epithelial downgrowth, endothelialization, etc.)

Internal occlusion of a sclerostomy can occur shortly after the surgery (within days to weeks) or much later (several months or longer). In an aphakic eye, vitreous gel can shift forward into the sclerostomy. Prevention is important in such situations. An anterior vitrectomy should be considered pre- and intraoperatively if vitreous is present in the anterior chamber. When the vitreous is behind the pupil but the anterior hyaloid face is broken, the vitreous gel can shift forward into the sclerostomy site.

Immediately prior to entering the anterior chamber and excising the internal block of a trabeculectomy, placement of a viscoelastic material through a paracentesis track keeps the vitreous behind the pupil while the globe is open and hypotonous.

Ciliary processes can rotate into the filtration tract, especially when the hole is small and posterior. A large internal block excision placed as far anteriorly as possible should avoid this complication. We strongly advise anterior sclerostomy sites, because the size of the internal block and whether trabecular meshwork is included in the excised block are unimportant in the success of the surgical outcome.[3,4] Excision and cautery of ciliary processes should be performed only when absolutely necessary, since they are highly vascular and prone to bleeding.

Iris extension into the sclerostomy can occur in several ways: following an inadequate peripheral iridectomy, anterior chamber reformation after a flat anterior chamber, and ocular compression (massage) for bleb resuscitation.[5] An iridectomy needs to be so broad that iris is not visible when looking through the sclerostomy site. When deepening an anterior chamber that has critically shallowed, injection of balanced salt solution, air, or sodium hyaluronate (Healon) through a paracentesis site should be continuous and slow while constantly under direct observation. Aggressive globe compression can promote iris obstruction of the sclerostomy, especially in the presence of a small peripheral iridectomy.

When a combined cataract extraction and filtration procedure is performed, large capsular tags can be carried into the sclerostomy by aqueous flow. Descemet's membrane, because it is quite thin and transparent, can be inadvertently left behind after the internal block excision. In order to not have these tissue remnants prove troublesome, one should specifically look for residual capsule pieces and Descemet's membrane fragments after completion of the sclerostomy and remove them.

Hemorrhage and fibrin clots are particularly undesirable because they are quite sticky and often lead to fibrous scarring if left unattended. There should be continual attention to hemostasis in the surgical field while operating. If a hyphema is present in a hypotonus eye, elevation of the head of the bed will keep the blood clot from sliding into and occluding the sclerostomy. Fibrin clots are usually seen in eyes with a marked alteration in the blood-aqueous barrier as, for example, eyes that have uveitis, immediately after a sector iridectomy, and diabetics, especially if there is iris neovascularization as with ischemic central retinal vein occlusions (CRVO). The fibrin clot usually responds dramatically to topical steroids with rapid shrinkage.

Various membranes can grow over the internal end of a filtration fistula. Fibrovascular membranes proliferate when iris neovascularization is present in diabetics and CRVO. Endothelialization with redundant Descemet's membrane occurs in eyes with iridocorneal endothelialization syndrome. Epithelial downgrowth and fibrous ingrowth are other recognized ways in which internal openings can be occluded after filtering surgery. A membrane of an often unknown source might cover the internal opening. It might or might not be pigmented. When unpigmented, it is difficult to see. These tend to occur later in the postoperative period.

Treatment

The revival of failing blebs has been attempted in several ways that work with varying success depending on the technique and the cause of the problem. From the external approach, Tenon capsule needle discission,[6] ocular compression,[7] transconjunctival argon laser photocoagulation of scleral flap

Table 14-13. Treatment of Internal Obstructions following Filtration Surgery
Argon laser
YAG laser
Internal surgical approach
External bleb revision

sutures or a surface clot,[8-9] and therapeutic ultrasound[10] have been found useful. For an internal occlusion there are also several options: argon laser photocoagulation,[11-14] Nd:YAG laser photocoagulation,[14-17] surgical blade or needle reopening of the sclerostomy,[2] and external revision of the fistula.

Argon Laser Therapy[11-14]

Several reports have detailed successful use of the argon laser to reestablish aqueous flow into the fistula in a small number of patients. The spot size ranged from 50 to 100 microns with energy of 1 to 2 watts, and a duration of 0.1 to 1 second. Up to several hundred spots were applied. It was thought that pigmented tissue and membranes respond best. Early failures and hypoactive filtering blebs were thought most likely to respond.

Yag Laser Photocoagulation[14-17]

In the group thought not to respond well to argon laser treatment, that is those with nonpigmented tissue obstructing outflow and late bleb failure, the Nd:YAG laser was on occasion effective in opening the internal sclerostomy. The power used ranged from 0.1 to 8.5 millijoules, 1 to 5 bursts, and up to 500 spots of application. Not only are translucent membranes cut, but also vitreous sheets can be transsected. Since there is no hemostasis with this laser, pretreatment has been recommended with argon laser for areas that appear vascular.

Internal Surgical Approach

Two surgical approaches have been described by Swan.[2] The first employed a goniotomy knife passed through the limbus across the anterior chamber into the surgical site while viewing through a gonio lens. The second technique made use of a spatula needle placed transcorneal immediately anterior the filtration site. An important point is that when these surgical aids were utilized in eyes with initially successful filtration operations, they were successful in lowering IOP in 75% of the cases. Whereas, if the initial filtering operations were unsuccessful, less than 20% of the incisions or needlings proved useful.

External Revision of the Bleb

If the internal occlusion cannot be visualized because of corneal opacification, edema, or other cause it might be necessary to revise the bleb. The original surgical site is uncovered and the sclerostomy site inspected and cleared of any material clogging it. This approach is best within one month of the initial surgery.

If it has been longer than two months following occlusion, it would be more prudent to prepare a new filtration site at another location because external scarring undoubtedly would be extensive.

References

1. Maumanee AE. External filtering operations for glaucoma: the mechanism of function and failure. Trans Am Ophthalmol Soc 58:319, 1960.
2. Swan KC. Reopening of non-functioning filters-simplified surgical techniques. Trans Am Acad Ophthalmol 79:342-348, 1975.
3. Spencer WM. Histologic evaluation of microsurgical techniques. Trans Am Acad Ophthalmol Otolaryngol 76:389, 1972.
4. Taylor HR. A histologic survey of trabeculectomy. Am J Ophthalmol 82:733, 1976.
5. Segrest DR, Ellis PO. Iris incarceration associated with digital ocular massage. Ophthalmol Surg 12:349-351, 1982.
6. Pederson JE, Smith SG. Surgical management of encapsulated filtering blebs. Ophthalmology 92:955, 1985.
7. Traverso CE, Greenidge KC, Spaeth GL, Wilson RP. Focal pressure: a new method to encourage filtration after trabeculectomy. Ophthalmol Surg 15:52, 1984.
8. Kurata F, Krupin T, Kolker AE. Reopening filtration fistulas with transconjunctival argon laser photocoagulation. Am J Ophthalmol 98:340-343, 1984.
9. Hoskins HD, Miliazzo C. Management of failing filtering blebs with the argon Laser. Ophthalmol Surg 15:731, 1984.
10. Yablonski M, Masonson HN, El-Sayyard F, et al. Use of therapeutic ultrasound to restore failed trabeculectomies. Am J Ophthalmol 103:492-496, 1987.
11. Ticho V, Zanberman H. Argon laser application to the angle structures in the glaucomas. Arch Ophthalmol 94:61-64, 1976.
12. Ticho V, Ivry M. Reopening of occluded filtering blebs by argon laser photocoagulation. Am J Ophthalmol 84:413-418, 1977.
13. VanBuskirk EM. Reopening filtration fistulas with the argon laser. Am J Ophthalmol 94:1-3, 1982.
14. Budenz DL, Brown SVL, Thomas JV, Blecher CD III, Simmons RJ. Laser therapy for internally failing glaucoma filtration surgery. Ophthalmic Laser Ther 1(3):169-176, 1986.

15. Praeger DL. The reopening of closed filtering blebs using the Nd:YAG laser. Ophthalmology 91:373-377, 1984.
16. Dailey RA, Samples JR, VanBuskirk EM. Reopening filtration fistulas with the Nd:YAG laser. Am J Ophthalmol 102:491-495, 1986.
17. Cohn HC, Aron-Rosa D. Reopening blocked trabeculectomy sites with the YAG laser. Am J Ophthalmol 95:293-294, 1984.

Complications and Management of Large Cystic Blebs

Mark B. Sherwood, MD

Large, thin-walled, cystic blebs (Fig. 14-23) may occur following filtration surgery, trauma, or inadvertently after cataract surgery. They present to the ophthalmologist for two main reasons. First, the large size of the bleb or its encroachment over the peripheral cornea can lead to defects in tear film spread or to visual difficulties. Second, the thinness of the bleb wall can predispose to perforation and an increased risk of endophthalmitis.

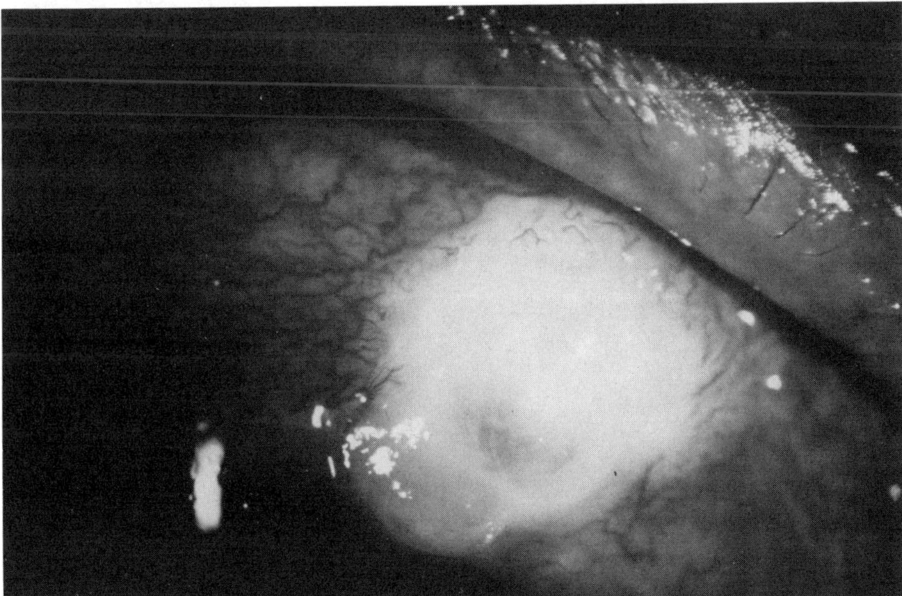

Figure 14-23. A. Large, thin-walled, cystic blebs.

The problems that can arise from these blebs range from minor symptomatic complaints, such as mild irritation of the eye, to sight-threatening complications, such as endophthalmitis. A list of possible symptoms and complications is given in Tables 14-14 and 14-15.

Table 14-14. Patient Symptoms from Large Cystic Blebs
Irritation and foreign body sensation in eye
Blinking difficulties
Difficulty with contact lens wear
Monocular diplopia
Apparent decreasing of visual field
Pain, redness, swelling (chemosis)—early endophthalmitis

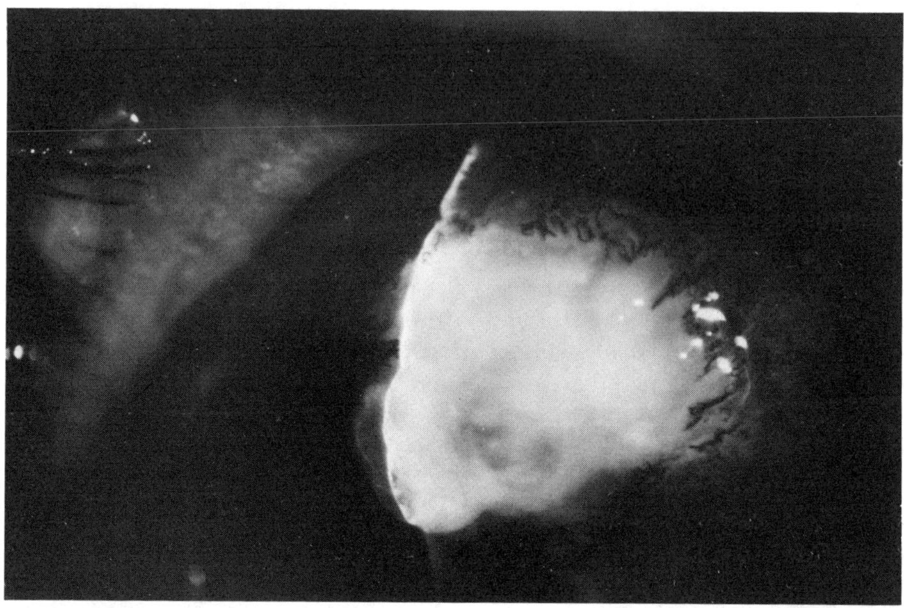

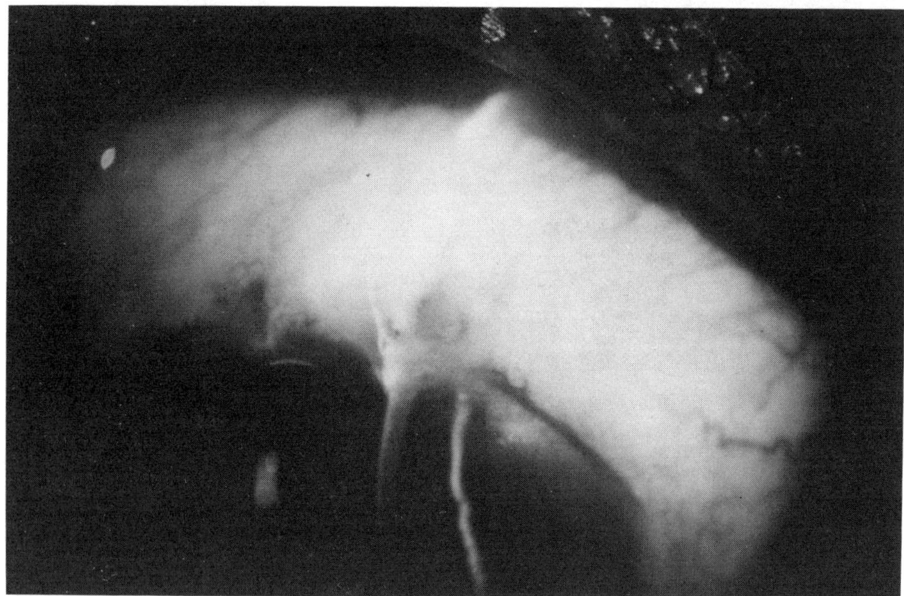

Figure 14-23. **B.** and **C.** Large, thin-walled, cystic blebs.

Superficial punctuate corneal erosions are common postoperatively adjacent to the bleb, particularly if the bleb is high. This is secondary to poor spreading of the tear film in these areas during blinking.

Dellen (Fig. 14-24) were noted following trabeculectomy in 9% of cases in one series,[1] again usually associated with large blebs. Use of frequent artificial

Table 14-15. Complications of Large Cystic Blebs
Superficial punctuate erosions adjacent to bleb
Dellen
Difficulty fitting contact lens
Leaking of bleb
Minute Seidel-positive spot
Gross leakage of aqueous
Hypotony
Macula edema
Endophthalmitis

tear drops (hydroxpropylmethylcellulose) and an ocular lubricant at bedtime is the recommended treatment. Reduction of topical steroid therapy has also been suggested. Most dellen clear without complication, but a minority (following about 2% of trabeculectomies) develop deep corneal ulceration; these resolve over several months, but leave a vascularized scar with localized stromal thinning.[2]

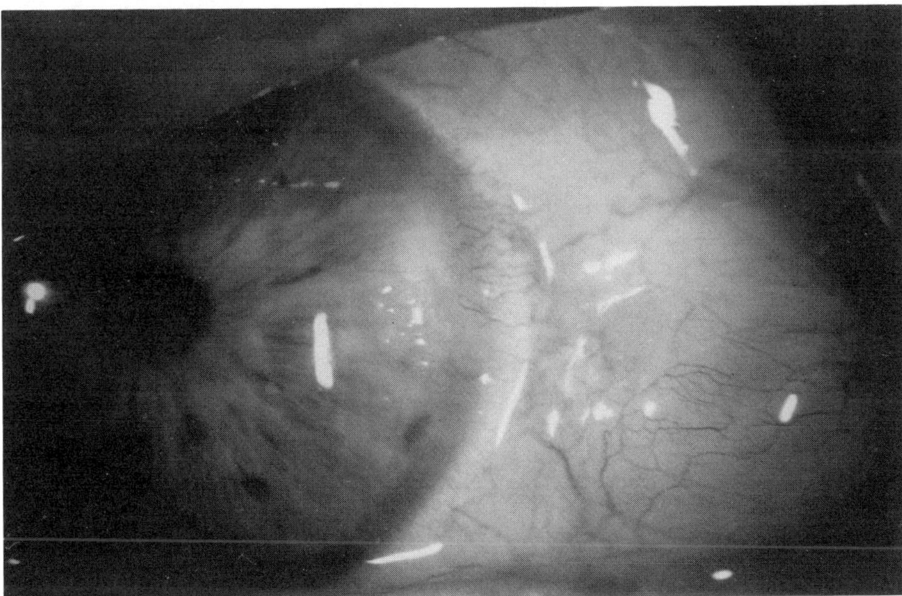

Figure 14-24. Dellen associated with a highly elevated temporal filtering bleb. **A.** Nonstained.

Late leaking from a thin bleb (Fig. 14-25) can lead to secondary hypotony with decreased visual acuity and sometimes associated macula edema. There might be a complaint of increased tearing. The leak can be confirmed by performing a Seidel test with a fluorescein strip. As there is a tract into the eye, the risk of bleb infection and endophthalmitis is increased.

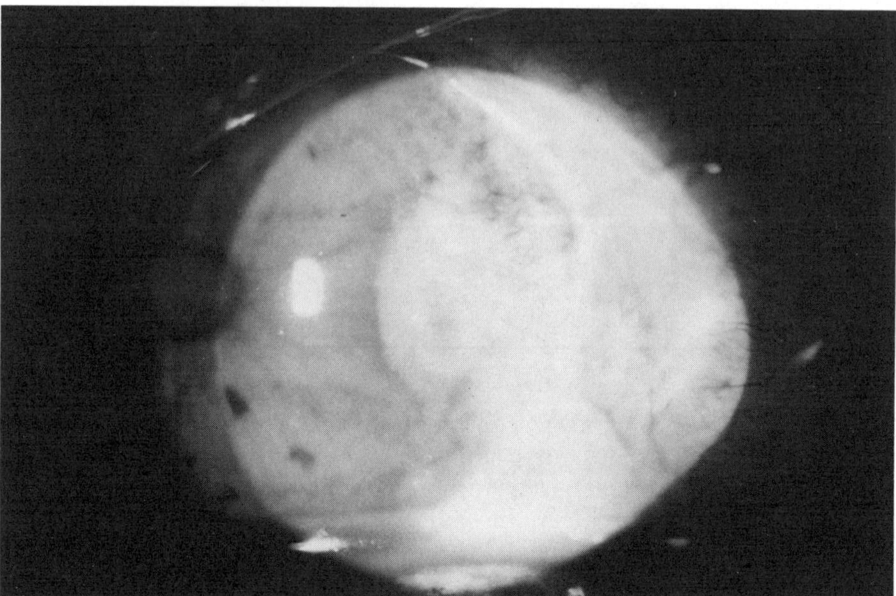

Figure 14-24. Dellen associated with a highly elevated temporal filtering bleb. **B.** With flourescein staining.

It is possible for any eye to develop an **endophthalmitis** following filtration surgery, but the incidence is far higher in thin-walled, cystic blebs. The complication tends to occur months or years after the initial trabeculectomy surgery.[2] Most eyes that develop endophthalmitis have a very poor final visual outcome despite intensive therapy at this stage. It is because of this small but definite potential for serious visual loss that prophylactic treatment of functional thin-walled, cystic blebs may be considered in some patients. Other patients have intolerable symptoms that necessitate intervention. A number of methods for the management of these blebs have been described and these are listed in Table 14-16.

Table 14-16. Methods of Treating Thin-walled Cystic Blebs
Argon laser therapy
Cryotherapy
Cauterization
Heat—diathermy
Chemical—Silver nitrate/trichloroacetic acid
Surgical repair

The two major factors to be considered when formulating a management plan are whether the bleb is leaking (Seidel-positive) and whether it is desired that bleb function be maintained.

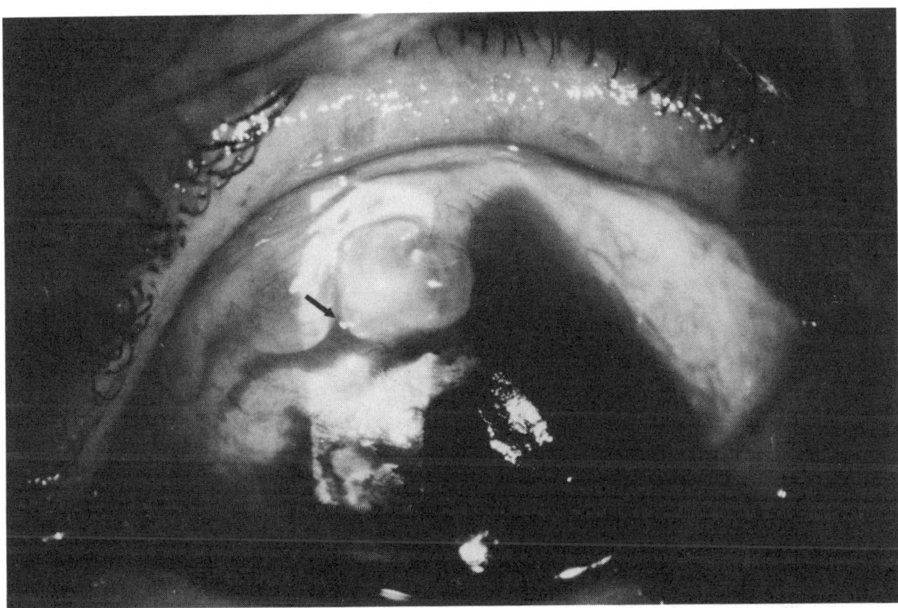

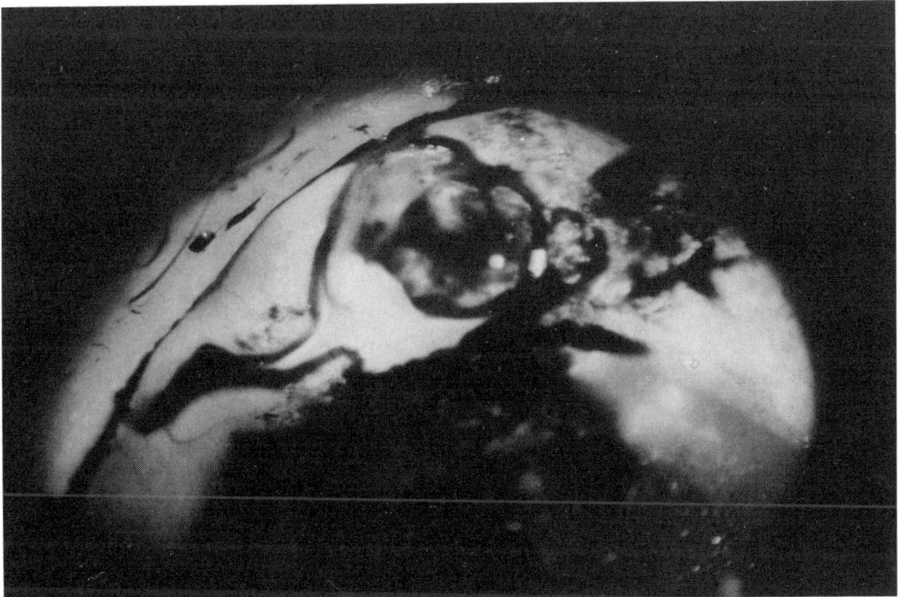

Figure 14-25. A. and **B.** Thin-walled cystic bleb with a minute Seidel-positive leak (*arrow*).

Medical Therapy for Overlarge Blebs

Laser Treatment

Argon laser therapy has been described[3] and is recommended for large cystic blebs that have at least a thin layer of underlying connective tissue rather than for those with a completely transparent wall. Flattening of the bleb is produced by the thermal effects of the laser, due to denaturation and contraction of proteins in the subepithelial collagen.

The procedure requires only topical anesthesia, following which the epithelium overlying the bleb is lightly abraided with a moistened cotton-tipped applicator. Sterile rose bengal strips are then employed to stain the surface of the bleb so that the energy of the laser beam will be absorbed by the superficial tissues. A setting of a 200- to 500-μ spot size, for 0.2 to 0.5 seconds, at 300 to 500 mW power is used and is adjusted to produce an end point of visible shrinkage of the bleb surface. About 100 burns are recommended per sitting. If there is charring or no further shrinkage of tissues in a particular region, treatment of that area should be discontinued. Small Seidel–positive leaks can occur after laser therapy, particularly in parts of the bleb where the overlying conjunctiva is extremely thin and transparent. Because no shrinkage is obtained in these very thin areas, the laser burns should not be delivered to these regions. Iatrogenic perforations tend to resolve spontaneously, but pressure-patching and CAIs may assist closure, should a Seidel-positive leak occur. No acute elevation of IOP or anterior chamber inflammatory reaction has been noted following laser therapy, and bleb function appears to be preserved.

Cryotherapy

Cryotherapy has also been used to shrink large cystic blebs.[4,5] It is particularly helpful for patients with unintentional filtering blebs following cataract surgery in whom total closure of the filtering site is desired. For glaucomatous patients with hypotony, where the aim of management is to relieve the subject's symptoms while maintaining adequate intraocular pressure control, the surgeon must reduce the amount of cryotherapy applied and carefully judge the area of bleb to be treated. More than one treatment session might be needed.

A retrobulbar block is required. The bleb surface is dried with a cotton-tipped stick, and coalescent freezes are applied to the bleb with the cryoprobe. The number of sites treated will depend on the size of the bleb and how much of the functional bleb is to be retained. Before starting the freeze, firm pressure is applied with the cryoprobe to bring the bleb surface tissues into apposition with the underlying sclera. Each application site may be treated with two or three, 30-second freezes at -50 to -80°C, in a freeze-thaw-freeze cycle. Topical cycloplegic and corticosteroid drops are prescribed postoperatively until the eye is quiet. A moderate uveitic reaction is common, and 20% of patients in one study[5] developed small peripheral anterior synechiae.

Cauterization

Shrinkage and thickening of cystic blebs has been reported following cauterization by heat[6] or diathermy[7] or chemically, using caustic agents such as silver nitrate or trichloroacetic acid.[8] This method, again, is mainly of use in the management of inadvertent blebs following cataract extraction. Treatment is associated with bleb cicatrization, and a loss of or decrease in filter function, which is difficult to titrate in the glaucomatous patient. Cautery to just the edges of the bleb has been described for glaucomatous eyes, which produces a smaller, but often thinner-walled, cystic bleb.

The use of the Birtcher hyfrecator, a small cautery unit, is reported in one study[7] for the management of symptomatic, thin-walled cystic blebs following cataract extraction. Under topical anesthesia alone, multiple light applications of minimum duration are applied to the bleb surface, which is kept dry with sterile cotton-tipped sticks. Perforation of the bleb with leakage of aqueous is common but does not lead to flattening of the anterior chamber.[7] The cautery can be repeated as necessary, the majority of patients requiring more than one treatment session to eradicate the bleb.

Cautery is not a totally benign procedure. Two cases of endophthalmitis related to tissue necrosis at the treatment site have been reported, although a less controlled cautery device than the hyfrecator was used in each case.[9]

Surgical Approach - Overhanging Blebs

Surgical excision of an overhanging bleb remains the mainstay of treatment for blebs in which function is to be maintained.

Large blebs that overhang the cornea lie on and in contact with the cornea rather than dissecting into its tissue planes. They can therefore be easily freed by blunt dissection with an iris spatula. Under local or general anesthesia the iris spatula is inserted beneath the lower border of the overhanging bleb, reflecting it up towards the limbus. The excess is excised parallel to the limbus, and the cut edges of conjunctiva are sutured to each other. The anterior chamber is not lost, because the overhanging part of the bleb is usually nonfunctional and because the scleral flap is not distributed. Intraocular pressure control was maintained using this technique in nearly all patients in one study.[10]

Thin Blebs That Leak

Medical Therapy

Many small leaks (see Fig. 14-25A and B) can be stopped by light to moderately firm patching of the eye with antibiotic cover for one or more days. Concommitant short-term use of aqueous suppressing agents such as a topical beta blocker and/or CAI is suggested. Topical steroids should not be given as they may slow healing. The patient is kept under close review. Care must be taken not to apply the patch too firmly or for too long, or bleb cicatization may be encouraged. In uniocular patients, where the leak is close to the limbus, a sterile, 15 mm bandage soft contact lens, or a collagen shield soaked in antibiotic, are acceptable alternatives to patching. Cyanoacrylate glue has been recommended by some, but in the author's experience has not proved very helpful. It can be difficult to apply the glue to a thin-walled leaking bleb and, as the globule of glue frequently assumes a collar-stud configuration, a larger conjunctival hole may be torn when the glue later falls out.

Surgical Repair

Rupture or persistent leaking of a bleb is more difficult to manage than overhanging of the cornea. If possible, repair should be avoided because decrease or failure of bleb function is quite common following this surgery.

If surgical intervention is required, the bleb may be reinforced by freeing and bringing down a conjunctival flap. This is sutured in place over the original bleb after abrading the corneal margin. Painting the surface of the bleb with 3.5% tincture of iodine has also been recommended.[11]

The alternative, which the author favors, is to excise the previous thin-walled bleb tissue, after mobilizing a conjunctival-Tenon's capsule flap from the surrounding host tissue. This latter is sutured to overly the peripheral cornea, in a similar fashion to the closure of a standard fornix-based filter procedure (Fig. 14-26). The anterior edge of the conjunctival flap should be pulled tightly over the peripheral cornea, partially indenting it, to provide a watertight (Seidel-negative) seal.

Replacing the previous thin-walled bleb surface with a thicker tissue covering, together with inflammation caused by the surgical procedure, frequently leads to decreased bleb function. Revision of the scleral flap, or fashioning of a new one, can be included at the time of bleb revision, if bleb function has previously been only marginal.

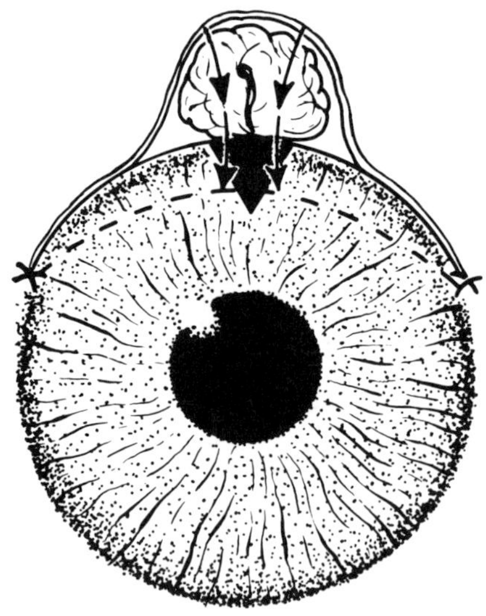

Figure 14-26. Surgical repair of a thin-walled leaking bleb. A conjunctiva-Tenon's capsule flap is mobilized from the surrounding tissue and is sutured to tightly overly the peripheral cornea. The original bleb wall can either be left in situ or excised.

References

1. Soong HK, Quigley HA. Dellen associated with filtering blebs. Arch Ophthalmol 101:385-387, 1983.

2. Hattenhauer JM, Lipsich MP. Late endophthalmitis after filtering surgery. Am J Ophthalmol 72:1097-1101, 1971.
3. Fink AJ, Boys-Smith JW, Brear R. Management of large filtering blebs with the argon laser. Am J Ophthalmol 101:695-699, 1986.
4. Douvas NG. Cystoid bleb cryotherapy. Am J Ophthalmol 74:69-71, 1972.
5. Cleasby GW, Fung WE, Webster RG. Cryosurgical closure of filtering blebs. Arch Ophthalmology 87:319-323, 1972.
6. Barkan H. Use of the Shahan thermophore in hypotony of the eyeball as a result of the Elliot trephining operation. Am J Ophthalmol 23:692-693, 1940.
7. Kirk HQ. Cauterization of filtering blebs following cataract extraction. Trans Am Acad Ophthalmol Otolaryngol 77:573-579, 1973.
8. Fitzgerald JR and McCarthy JL. Surgery of the filtering bleb. Arch Ophthalmol 68:453-467, 1962.
9. Yannuzzi LA. Discussion of cauterization of filtering blebs following cataract extraction. Trans Am Acad Ophthalmol Otolaryngol 77:579-580, 1973.
10. Scheie, HG, Guehl JJ. Surgical management of overhanging blebs after filtering procedures. Arch Ophthalmol 97:325-326, 1979.
11. Sugar HS. Complications, repair and reoperation of antiglaucoma filtering blebs. Am J Ophthalmol 63:825-833, 1967.

Tenon's Cysts (Encapsulated Filtering Blebs)

Mark B. Sherwood, MD

Tenon's "cysts," otherwise known as *encapsulated* (or encysted) *blebs*," develop in about 11 to 13% of patients following filtration surgery.[1,2,3] They are highly elevated, tense, localized blebs, and most commonly occur about three or four weeks after trabeculectomy. An example is shown in Fig. 14-27.

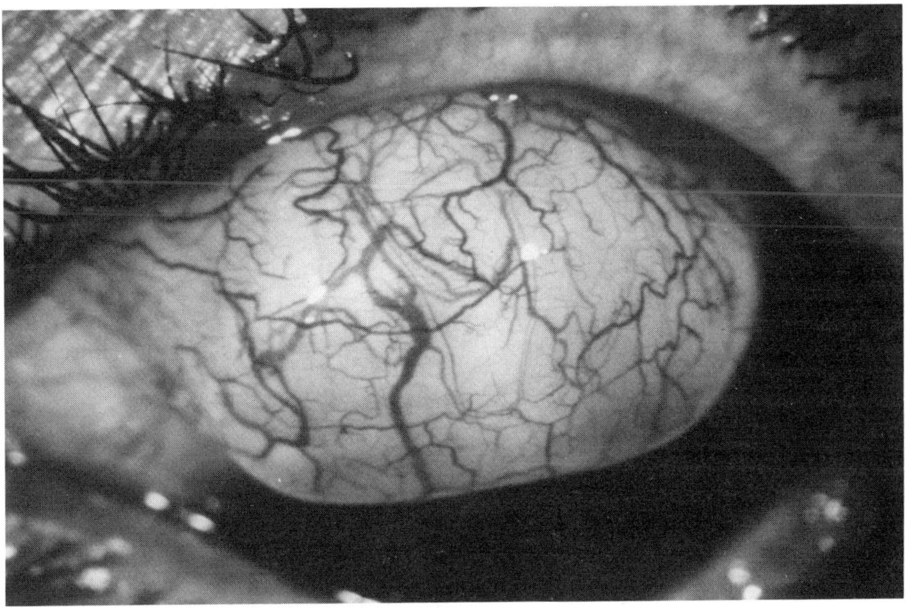

Figure 14-27. A Tenon's cyst or encapsulated bleb seen 3 weeks after filtration surgery. The bleb is highly elevated, localized, and injected.

The aqueous appears walled off beneath a thicken Tenon's capsule but the conjunctiva usually moves freely over the surface of the "cyst." Overlying microcystic intraconjunctival edema is generally not seen. There can be quite intense conjunctival injection locally. Histologically, the wall of the Tenon's cyst consists of an almost avascular sheet of fibrous connective tissue with some areas of active fibroblast proliferation and an acellular lining (Fig. 14-28).

Tenon's cysts present two main problems for the patient:

First, Tenon's cysts are associated with a rise in IOP after an initial period of pressure control following glaucoma surgery. The IOP might temporarily approach quite high levels, reaching a highest recorded peak of 40 mm Hg. or greater in 17% of patients in one study.[1] Patients with far advanced optic nerve glaucomatous damage are particularly vulnerable to further field loss from these pressure rises, and there is a danger of visual acuity decrease (central "snuff-out") especially in those with visual fields that split fixation.

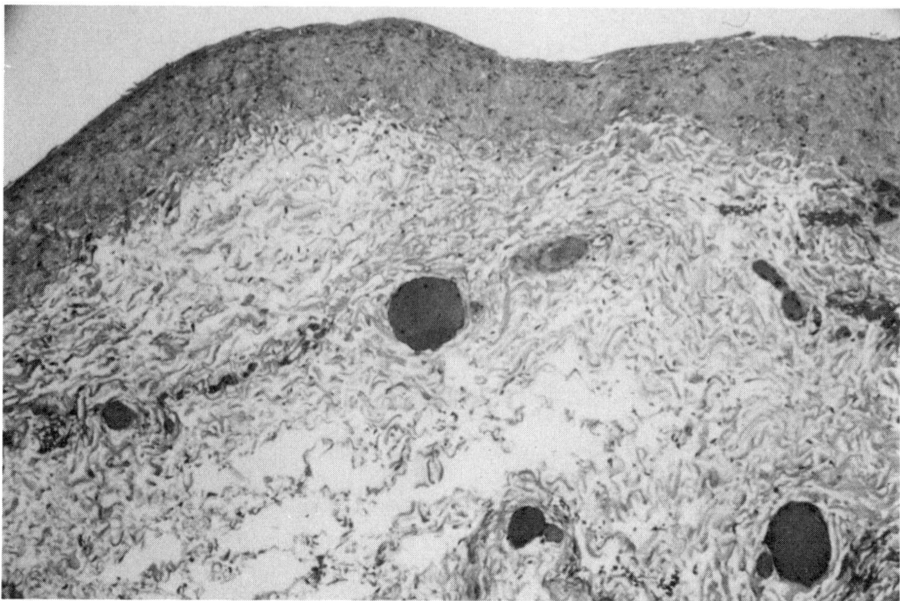

Figure 14-28. Histological section of a Tenon's cyst wall stained with hematoxylin and eosin. Note the dense, almost avascular sheets of fibrous connective tissue. (Magnification 25x.)

Second, Tenon's cyst blebs can be so elevated that they can interfere with upper eyelid movement. Dellen frequently form in the peripheral cornea at the base of the bleb because of poor spreading of the tear film, and this can lead to localized corneal stromal thinning. In addition, some patients are very upset by the unsightly appearance of the bulging of the lid, which can be obvious even with the eyelid closed.

The natural history is for gradual resolution of both the pressure rise and the extreme bleb elevation in most.[1,3] Following is a typical case.

Case Report

A 77-year-old woman with bilateral primary open angle glaucoma and high myopia underwent a superior, "Cairns-type" trabeculectomy, without tenonectomy, for progressive field loss in her right eye. Her left eye had only light perception vision. A limbal-based conjunctival flap was fashioned at surgery and closure was in two layers, using an 8-0 chromic collagen running suture.

Postoperatively, she had no hyphema, no Seidel-positive leak, and her anterior chamber remained well formed throughout. The patient was discharged on steroid, antibiotic, and dilating drops, each on a six hourly schedule.

Ten days postoperatively the IOP was 11 mm Hg. A diffuse bleb, with only moderate overlying conjunctival injection, was present. Seven days later the bleb still appeared satisfactory, although it was a little more localized, and the IOP had risen to 21 mm Hg. By four weeks following surgery, a high Tenon's cyst was apparent and the pressure was 36 mm Hg. The steroid drops, which had been reduced to twice daily at the previous visit, were stopped and topical dipivalyl epinephrine (Propine) commenced on a twice daily schedule. The patient was taught how to apply digital pressure to the eye and was asked to perform this massage four times a day. Because the patient had demonstrated intolerance to beta blockers and CAIs preoperatively, these were not prescribed.

After one week, although the bleb remained tense, the IOP had fallen to 22 mm Hg. By the following visit, the pressure was 13 mm Hg. The bleb remained localized but no longer tense. Microcystic conjunctival edema was noted superiorly at the margins of the bleb. The massage was stopped and after pressures between 10 and 11 mm Hg, were recorded at two further visits, the dipivalyl epinephrine drops were also discontinued. One year following surgery the patient had a low, somewhat localized, bleb and an IOP, on no medication, of 11 mm Hg. The Octopus visual field test was repeated at this time and showed no deterioration from the last presurgical field.

Risk Factors

The etiology of the complication is not fully established, but certain risk factors have been defined. These include prior surgery involving the conjunctiva[1,4] and Tenon's cyst formation in the other, previously operated eye.[1,5] There is a decreased incidence of Tenon's cyst formation in women, especially those under 50 years of age, and in patients undergoing surgery within two years of the diagnosis of glaucoma.[5] The type of surgery performed, either full-thickness or guarded, has not been proven to influence the rate of occurrence of Tenon's cysts, and a tenonectomy does not prevent it.[3,4] Pre- and postoperative medical regimens do not appear to be significant factors. It has been suggested that presurgical ALT is related to an increased incidence of cyst formation.[5,6]

Medical Management

Antiglaucoma medications can be reintroduced to reduce IOP. In the phakic eye, topical dipivalyl epinephrine (Propine) can be a good initial choice and appears particularly effective in the early postoperative period. Should this prove insufficient to control the pressure, agents that reduce aqueous production, such as topical beta blocker and/or an oral CAI can be added or substituted. Some recommend that these agents be used initially.[3] The use of frequent steroid drops to reduce inflammation and decrease fibroblast activity has been suggested.[4] It has not been proven, however, that these enhance the success rate of medical management.

Massage might be helpful[4,7] but before applying it, the internal sclerostomy site should be checked gonioscopically to ensure that there is no blockage. If vitreous or iris partially occlude the sclerostomy, they can be pushed through it by the massage treatment. If the filtration site is clear, the patient should be trained to apply digital pressure to the eye, through the lower eyelid, while looking upward (Fig. 14-29). We usually recommend compression for 5 to 10 seconds with the index finger, followed by removal of the pressure for 5 seconds and then its reapplication for a further 5 to 10 seconds. This can be repeated four times a day, or more frequently, as required. The massage

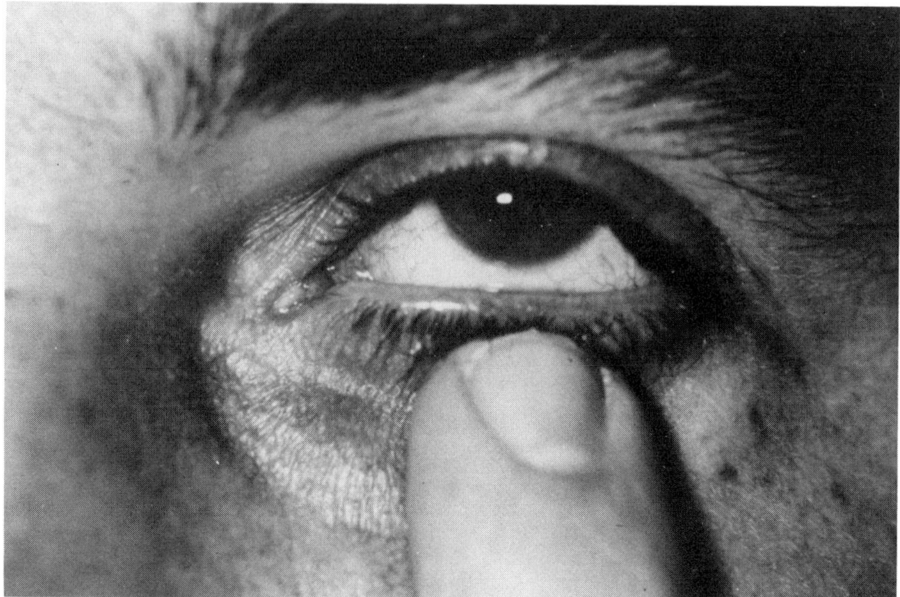

Figure 14-29. Ocular massage to improve bleb function. Digital pressure is applied to the eye through the lower eyelid.

should be supplemented at office visits by the surgeon compressing the bleb itself with an anesthetic-soaked cotton-tipped applicator while the patient is sitting at the slit lamp. The massage can be started early, as soon as there is a suspicion that the bleb is becoming localized, even if the IOP is still in the mid-teens.

Surgical Management

Two methods have been described for surgically treating Tenon's cysts.[2,4] The simpler approach consists of making a 2- to 4-mm slit in the side wall of the cyst using a narrow cutting instrument such as a Ziegler knife, an NVR blade, or even a 27 gauge needle. This can be performed under topical anesthesia. The procedure is facilitated by first injecting saline through a 30 gauge needle into the subconjunctival space alongside the bleb to separate the tissues. The knife traverses this elevated area, deep to the conjunctiva, and the small conjunctival entry hole can be placed at a point distant from the bleb site (Fig. 14-30). Antibiotic drops or ointment are applied and the eye patched for 24 to 48 hours. Leakage occurs through the conjunctival entry site for a few days but this stops by one week. Some surgeons routinely place a suture in the conjunctiva to close this leak.

The alternative technique involves complete excision of the Tenon's cyst (Fig. 14-31). The conjunctival and Tenon's capsule incisions from the previous trabeculectomy operation are reopened, or a new incision is made posterior to the upper border of the Tenon's cyst. The conjunctiva is detached from the underlying cyst wall with blunt scissors, and is reflected forward. The use of saline injection to separate the tissue planes is optional. Once the cyst is exposed it is dissected free from the sclera and removed using

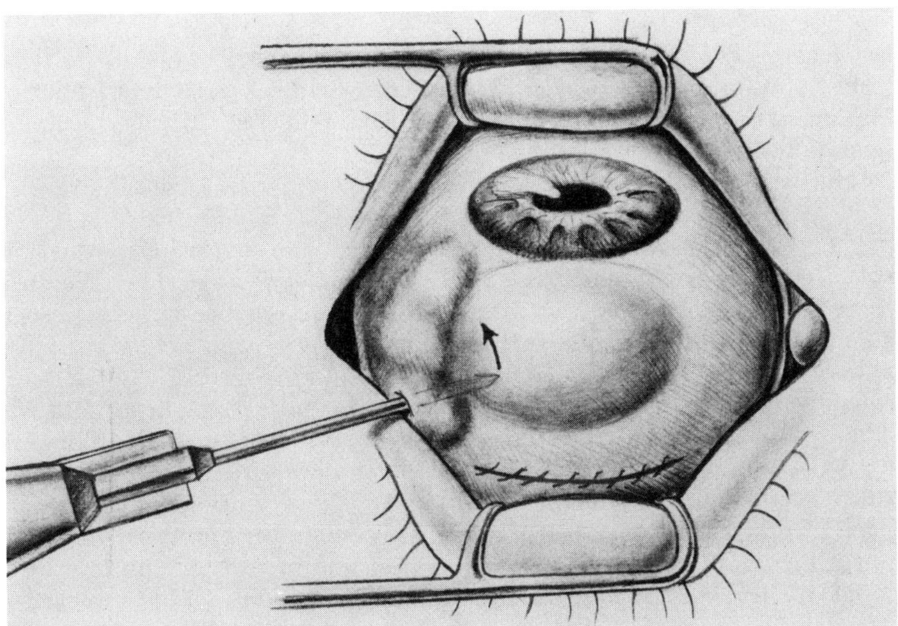

Figure 14-30. Needling of a Tenon's cyst. After the conjunctiva has been elevated by an injection of balanced salt solution, a needle or blade is passed subconjunctivally, from a peripheral site, and an incision made in the side wall of Tenon's cyst.

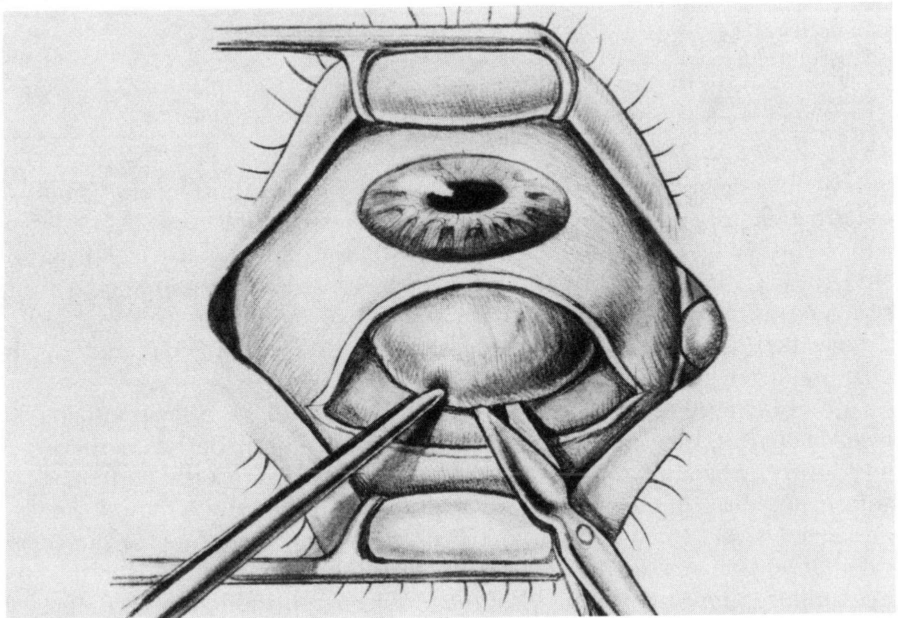

Figure 14-31. Surgical excision of a Tenon's cyst. The "cyst" is dissected clear of the scleral flap with Vannas scissors after being bluntly separated from the overlying conjunctiva.

non-toothed forceps and sharp Vannas scissors. Since the filtration site is now visible, aqueous should be seen leaking through from the sclerostomy. If aqueous leakage does not occur the filter site must be revised or a new sclerostomy made. The conjunctiva and Tenon's capsule are closed in a watertight fashion, preferably in two layers. The anterior chamber is filled with saline or Healon via the corneal paracentesis tract made at the original trabeculectomy operation, and a bleb is raised.

The decision whether to treat an eye with a Tenon's cyst medically or surgically will depend on a number of factors. These are listed in Table 14-17. In patients with far advanced cupping of the optic nerve or where fixation is split, the surgical option might be preferable at an early stage. This is because there is a relatively higher risk that the short-term pressure elevation associated with the cyst can cause further, clinically significant field loss. In the majority of cases, however, medical management will control the IOP at a reasonable level during the few weeks it takes for bleb function to improve. There was no significant difference in visual field loss between eyes that were treated medically, and control eyes that did not develop a Tenon's cyst in one study.[1] Returning bleb function is indicated by the appearance of microcystic edema in the conjunctiva surrounding the cyst and by reduction of IOP to normal levels. This takes on average about one month to achieve, with a range in our review of patients at the Wills Eye Hospital of 1 to 14 weeks.[1]

Table 14-17. Factors Influencing Decision for Medical or Surgical Treatment
1) Degree of optic nerve damage and visual field loss.
2) Height of the IOP spike.
3) Duration of the IOP rise.
4) Patient's attitude to the pressure rise and to a further surgical procedure.

The long-term prognosis for IOP control in eyes that develop Tenon's cysts in generally good. About 90% achieve pressures of 21 mm Hg, or less at a mean follow-up of a year and a half, whether they are managed medically or surgically.[1,2,3] It should be noted, however, that the blebs appear to function suboptimally, and a greater proportion of patients than usual (40 to 75%) will require continued supplemental medical therapy to maintain suitable pressures.[1,2,3]

It has been suggested that surgical intervention by retraumatizing an already operated area increases fibrosis and might compromise the success of any future procedures.[4] The needling procedure carries the added risk of subconjunctival hemorrhage and these irritant products could further enhance fibrosis. Recurrence of the Tenon's cyst, necessitating further surgical intervention, was seen in more than 30% of those needled and in 9% of the eyes undergoing cyst excision.[2] For these reasons, although most patients will do well with surgical revision, medical therapy is recommended. Perseverance and reassurance will be required in the face of patient doubts and disappointment that the "operation has failed." Explanation that the pressure rise is only temporary and that 90% of those treated medically will have good long-term IOP control, although with additional medical therapy in many cases, is important.

References

1. Sherwood MB, Spaeth GL, Simmons ST, el al. Cysts of Tenon's capsule following filtration surgery: medical management. Arch Ophthalmol 205:1517-1521, 1987.
2. Pederson JE, Smith SG. Surgical management of encapsulated filtering blebs. Ophthalmology 92:955-958, 1985.
3. Scott DR, Quigley HA. Non-surgical management of high domed blebs after filtering surgery. Ophthalmology 95:1169-1173, 1988.
4. Van Buskirk EM. Cysts of tenon's capsule following filtration surgery. Am J Ophthalmol 94:522-527, 1982.
5. Feldman RM, Gross RL, Spaeth GL, et al. Risk factors for the development of tenon's capsule cysts following trabeculectomy. Ophthalmology 96:336-341, 1989.
6. Richter CU, Shinglton BJ, Bellows AR, et al. The development of encapsulated filtering blebs. Ophthalmology 95:1163-1168, 1988.
7. Van Buskirk EM. Discussion of surgical management of encapsulated filtering blebs by Pederson JE, Smith SG. Ophthalmology 92:958, 1985.

Cataract Formation Following Filtration Surgery

L. Jay Katz, MD

Introduction

There is strong evidence that glaucoma surgery is cataractogenic.[1-18] In several series, a visually significant cataract developed following a filtration procedure. The incidence ranged from 2 to 53%, but in most larger series, approximately one-third of the eyes developed cataracts that dropped Snellen visual acuity at least two lines from the preoperative baseline. Since a cataract often leads to another operation, it is important to identify risk factors for the purpose of minimizing their effect, if possible, and to ably inform the patient of this potential complication before glaucoma surgery. The possible risk factors identified thus far include: pre-existing lens opacities, topical steroid use, uveitis, miotic use, direct lens trauma, and flat anterior chamber and hypotony (Table 14-18).

Table 14-18. Risk Factors for the Development of Cataracts following Filtration Surgery

1. Preexisting lens opacities
2. Steroid use
3. Uveitis
4. Miotic use
5. Lens trauma
6. Flat anterior chamber

Preexisting Cataract

Many of the patients undergoing surgery for glaucoma control are in the older age group where cataract prevalence is also high. Sugar noted that 8% of eyes in a control group (no surgery) had cataracts, whereas 30% had cataracts after glaucoma surgery.[11] He also reported cataract progression in almost one half of the eyes when unilateral surgery was performed while, in contrast, the lenses in the unoperated eyes did not opacify. It is often mentioned that significant cataracts are most likely to develop when there are preexisting lenticular opacities,[14,15,17] but D'Ermo reported that 16% of eyes with a clear lens developed a marked cataract after trabeculectomy.[1]

Topical Steroids

To control postoperative inflammation and scarring after filtering surgery topical corticosteroids are utilized. There has been convincing documentation that steroid eye drops can lead to posterior subcapsular cataracts, even in young eyes with previously clear lenses.[19-24] There appears to be a variable individual and perhaps racial susceptibility to steroid-induced cataracts.[25] Thus, a total dose relation effect is difficult to determine, although most report chronic use of topical steroids for several months to years before cataracts develop.

Uveitis

Intraocular inflammation promotes cataract development as seen with various uveitides. As with steroid-induced cataracts a posterior subcapsular opacity is the most common type of cataract. Postoperative iritis might be no different.

Reoperations, sector iridectomies, and underlying chronic uveitis are especially prone to have a significant anterior chamber reaction after surgery. An additional possible potentiator of lens change can be the formation of posterior synechiae that often develop with an iritis.[26]

Miotics

Parasympathomimetics, such as pilocarpine and carbachol, are recognized to cause lens opacification.[27] Markedly more cataractogenic are the anticholinesterases, such as echothiophate (phospholine iodide), whose use should be restricted to aphakes and pseudophakes. In the early postoperative period with coexisting inflammation and topical steroid use, miotic use might be synergistic in adversely affecting the lens clarity. In addition, miotics weaken the blood-aqueous barrier and would worsen an existing uveitis.

Direct Lens Insult

Any penetrating injury that disrupts the anterior lens capsule will characteristically lead to rapid lens opacification. During intraocular surgery in a phakic eye instruments can tear the lens capsule.[1] The most critical movements during filtration surgery would be the creation of the paracentesis track, excising the internal block or trabeculum, and the iridectomy. If entering through a pars plana approach to perform a vitrectomy or a vitreous aspiration for diagnostic or therapeutic reasons (e.g., endothalmitis and aqueous misdirection), the posterior capsule could be similarly traumatized.

Flat Anterior Chamber and Hypotony

Shallow or flat anterior chambers and hypotony have been implicated in hastening cataract formation,[7,9,10] although some dispute this.[28] Mills reported 61% of those eyes with a shallow anterior chamber and 46% with hypotony develop cataracts.[7] Lens-to-cornea apposition injures both the corneal endothelium and the lens epithelium. If they are not promptly separated, irreversible changes that result in corneal edema and cataract development can occur. It is yet unclear with lesser degrees of flat anterior chambers when reformation would be appropriate. Surgeons vary considerably in their approach with regard to timing of intervention and the type of intervention, whether it be merely anterior chamber reformation (using sodium hyaluronate, air, or saline) or combined with ciliochoroidal drainage through a sclerostomy.

With hypotony, ciliochoroidal detachment is usually coexistent. Alteration of aqueous dynamics and constituency that results with a choroidal detachment could adversely affect the lens metabolism and lead to opacification.

It is interesting to note that in the order of most likely to cause a cataract are the following: full-thickness filtration procedures, trabeculectomy, and peripheral iridectomy. It is that same identical order for likelihood of a flat anterior chamber.

Recommendations

There are several points worth emphasizing in dealing with cataract development after glaucoma surgery.

1. The patient should be advised that there exists approximately a 33% chance of significant visual decline, even with successful IOP control that would perhaps require another operation. Those with preexisting cataracts are most susceptible.
2. Topical steroids should be promptly discontinued when the external and intraocular inflammation has subsided. A tapering schedule should be followed.
3. Postoperative sterile inflammation needs to be addressed with topical steroids, cycloplegics to tighten the blood-aqueous barrier, and on occasion, oral steroids or nonsteroidal anti-inflammatory agents that inhibit prostaglandin synthesis.
4. Miotics, including pilocarpine, should not be used in the perioperative period. They should be stopped at least three days, preferably two weeks, before surgery, and not used for at least two months postoperatively.
5. To avoid iatrogenic lens trauma, the surgeon should always keep the instruments in direct view, especially when placed intraocularly. When making a paracentesis track, the tip of the needle or blade should never point toward the lens. The shaft of the instrument is depressed on the cornea while pushing in a horizontal plane. Firm fixation is achieved with a toothed forceps in the other hand. Direction of entry in this way is well controlled, with little chance of lens injury.
6. Steps helpful in preventing a flat anterior chamber include: a guarded rather than a full-thickness operation, viscoelastic placement into the anterior chamber for its two-day space occupying property, and liberal topical cycloplegic use to tighten the lens-iris diaphragm. The issue of anterior chamber reformation is a complex one, but clearly it is mandatory in the setting of lens-cornea apposition (grade 3). It should be promptly performed in patients with grade 3 flat anterior chambers because the duration of the flat chamber is critical. When there is a flat

anterior chamber without lens touch, then the timing of intervention is more controversial. One week would be the maximum waiting period for most situations before reforming the anterior chamber.

References

1. D'Ermo F, Bonaomi L, Doro D. A critical analysis of the long- term results of trabeculectomy. Am J Ophthalmol 88:829-835, 1979.
2. Greve EL, Dake CL, Klaver JHJ, Mutsacrts EMG. 10 year prospective follow-up of a glaucoma operation the double flap Scheie in primary open angle glaucoma. In: Greve EL, Leydhecker W, Railta C (eds): Second European Glaucoma Symposium. Helsinki, W. Junk Publisher, 1984, pp 237-247.
3. Jerndal T, Lundstrom M. 330 trabeculectomies-a long time study (3-5 years). ACTA Ophthalmol 58:947-956, 1980.
4. Keroub C, Hyams SW, Rath E. Study of cataract formation following trabeculectomy. Glaucoma 6:117-126, 1984.
5. Kolker AE. Visual prognosis in advanced glaucoma: a comparison of medical and surgical therapy for retention of vision in 101 eyes with advanced glaucoma. Trans Am Ophthalmol Soc 75:539-555, 1977.
6. Lawrence GA. Surgical treatment of patients with advanced glaucomatous field defects. Arch Ophthalmol 81:804-807, 1969.
7. Miles KB. Trabeculectomy: A retrospective long term follow-up of 444 cases. Br J Ophthalmol 65:790-795, 1981.
8. O'Connell EJ, Karseras AG. Intraocular surgery in advanced glaucoma. Br J Ophthalmol 60:124-131, 1976.
9. Shin DH. Trabeculectomy. Int Ophthalmol Clin 21(1):47-68, 1981.
10. Shirato S, Kitazawa Y, Mishima S. A critical analysis of the trabeculectomy results by a prospective follow-up design. Jpn J Ophthalmol 26:468-480, 1982.
11. Sugar HS. Postoperative cataract in successfully filtering glaucomatous eyes. Am J Ophthalmol 69:740-746, 1970.
12. Sugar HS. Cataract formation and refractive changes after surgery for angle-closure glaucoma. Am J Ophthalmol 69:747-749, 1970.
13. Sugar HS. Postoperative complications of adult glaucoma surgery. Eye Ear Nose Throat Monthly 54:29-38, 1975.
14. Warden NJ. Long term results of trabeculectomy. Trans Ophthalmol Soc NZ 29:89-90, 1977.
15. Watson P. Trabeculectomy—a modified ab externo technique. Ann Ophthalmol 2:199-205, 1970.
16. Watson PG, Barnett F. Effectiveness of trabeculectomy in glaucoma. Am J Ophthalmol 79:831-845, 1970.
17. Witmer R. Complications of trabeculectomy in recent advances in glaucoma. In: Ticho V, David R (eds): Excerpta Medica, New York, 1984, pp 313-316.
18. Zaidi AA. Trabeculectomy: a review and 4 Year follow-up. Br J Ophthalmol 64:436-439, 1980.

19. Becker B. Cataracts and topical corticosteroids. Am J Ophthalmol 58:872-873, 1964.
20. Burde RM, Becker B. Corticosteroid induced glaucoma and cataracts in contact lens wearers. JAMA 213:2075-2077, 1970.
21. Gasset AR, Bellows RT. Posterior subcapsular cataract after topical corticosteroid therapy. Ann Ophthalmol 6:1263-1265, 1974.
22. Spaeth GL, von Sallmann L. Corticosteroids and cataracts. Int Ophthalmol Clin 6:915-929, 1966.
23. Wood TO, Waltman SR, Kaufman HE. Steroid cataracts following penetrating keratoplasty. Am Ophthalmol 3:496-499, 1971.
24. Yablonski ME, Burde RM, Kokker AE, Becker B. Cataracts induced by topical dexamethasone in diabetics. Arch Ophthalmol 96:474-476, 1978.
25. Urban RC Jr., Cotlier E. Corticosteroid-induced cataracts. Surv Ophthalmol 31:102-110, 1986.
26. Phillips CI, Clark CV, Levy AM. Posterior synechiae after glaucoma operations: aggravation by shallow anterior chamber and pilocarpine. Br J Ophthalmol 71:428-432, 1987.
27. Levene RZ. Uniocular miotic therapy. Trans Am Acad Ophthalmol Otolaryngol 79:376, 1975.
28. Allen JC. Delayed anterior chamber formation after filtering operations. Am J Ophthalmol 62:640-643, 1966.

CHAPTER 15

Complications of Silicone Tube Drainage Devices

Mark B. Sherwood, MD

Setons have been described since the early 20th century[1] for use in cases of glaucoma refractory to standard filtration techniques. These include neovascular, juvenile, secondary, developmental, and aphakic glaucomas. Today's implants all employ a biologically inert (silicone or silastic) narrow bored tube to shunt aqueous from the anterior chamber to distant region of the eye, away from the main site of inflammatory reaction.

There are three principle "types" of seton in use (Fig. 15-1) although other devices have been described (White pump-shunt, Joseph valved implant, etc.). These are:

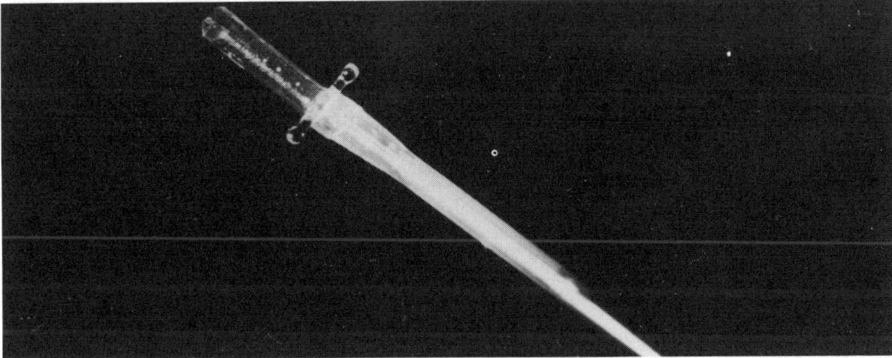

Figure 15-1. Commonly used setons. **A.** Original Krupin-Denver valved implant.

- The Krupin-Denver valve[2], which had a pressure sensitive one-way slit valve. Originally this had an unprotected distal tube orifice sutured to the sclera anterior to the equator of the eye. More recently, the long Krupin-Denver valve implant has been described; the distal end of this is covered by a #220 silastic explant. [2a]

- The Molteno Long Tube Implant[3], which employs a narrow tube to transport the aqueous to an area behind the equator of the eye. The tube is attached to either a single or double, 13 mm diameter circular methacrylic plate that provides the bed of a large area to which fibrous adhesion cannot occur.
- The Anterior Chamber Tube Shunt to an Encircling Band procedure described by Schocket.[4] This technique employs a 360° inverted retinal band to provide an encapsulated area at the equator of the eye, into

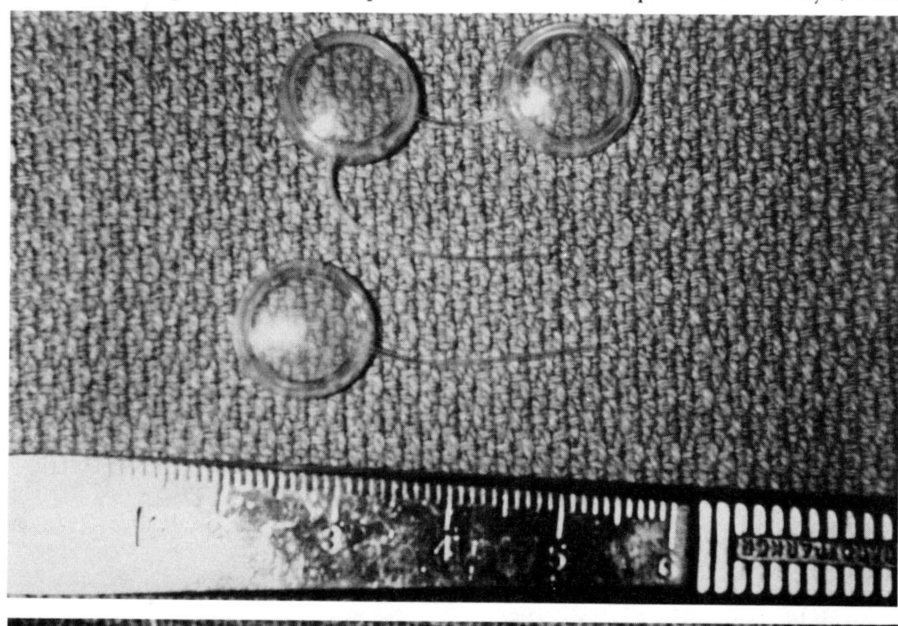

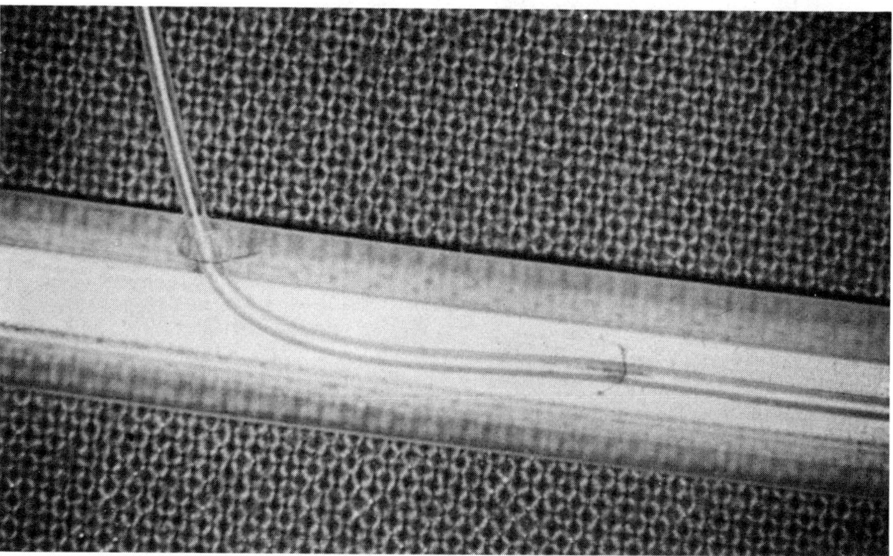

Figure 15-1. Commonly used setons. **B.** Molteno implant (single or double plate). **C.** Schocket implant (ACTSEB).

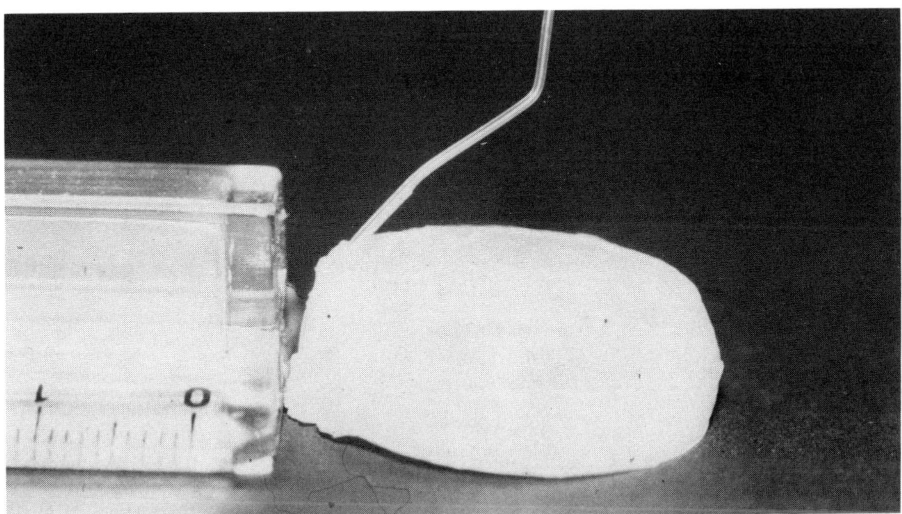

Figure 15-1. D. Joseph implant.

which aqueous can be shunted via a narrow tube. Diffusion into the retro-ocular space subsequently occurs from this encapsulated area.

Table 15-1 lists the success rates of a number of series in which setons were used. The complications of silicone tube surgery are summarized in Table 15-2.

Table 15-1. Success Rate of Seton Surgery in Published Series

Author	Type of Glaucoma	Success Rate (%)
Molteno Implant		
Molteno, et al.[5-8]	Neovascular	83
	Juvenile	95
	Uveitic	85
	Aphakic	94
Brown & Cairns[9]	Neovascular	75
	Non-neovascular	50
Minckler, et al.[10]	Mixed	66
Downes, et al.[11]	Mixed	58
Krupin-Denver Implant		
Krupin, et al.[12]	Neovascular	67
Sutton, et al.[13]	Neovascular	11
Forestier, et al.[14]	Mixed	93
Krupin, et al[2a] (long implant)	Neovascular	77
	Non-neovascular	82
ACTSEB – (Schocket procedure)		
Schocket, et al.[15]	Neovascular	96
	Non-neovascular	80
Sherwood, et al.[16]	Non-neovascular	82
Hitchings, et al.[17]	Mixed	92

Table 15-2. Complications of Seton Surgery

Early
- Hyphema
- Hypotony/Choroidal detachment
- Flat anterior chamber
- Endothelial touch by tube
- Pupillary block
- Blockage of the proximal orifice by iris, blood, or vitreous

Later
- Blockage of proximal orifice by iris or vitreous
- Endothelial touch by tube, with corneal decompensation
- Migration of tube out of the anterior chamber
- Tube exposure
- Blockage of distal tube orifice
- Insufficient aqueous absorption despite patent tube
- "Hypertensive phase" leading to possible further disc damage
- Increasing cataract in phakic patients

Less commonly
- Retinal detachment
- Delayed suprachoroidal hemorrhage
- Endophthalmitis
- Implant extrusion
- Phthisis

The early complications usually occur within the first few postoperative days while the ones listed in the later group can be seen several weeks or even many months or years after surgery. There is a degree of overlap, however, and problems such as corneal endothelial touch or proximal orifice occlusion can be seen either immediately postsurgery or many weeks later.[16]

There are five principle sites of complication. These are summarized in Table 15-3.

Table 15-3. Major Sites of Complication Following Seton Surgery

1) Anterior Segment Problems/Proximal End of Tube.
   a) Directly tube-related complications (occlusion of orifice, endothelial touch by tube)
   b) Indirectly tube-related (hyphema, flat anterior chamber, hypotony, choroidal detachment, pupillary block)
2) Along the course of the tube itself (exposure of tube, blockage from overtight suture)
3) Distal orifice of the tube (blockage secondary to fibrosis)
4) Insufficient aqueous absorption from "bleb" area despite a patent tube.
5) Other (distant) ocular problems (increased cataract risk, suprachoroidal hemorrhage, retinal detachment, endophthalmitis, etc.)

Anterior Segment Problems

Blockage of the proximal end of the tube in the anterior chamber of the eye occurs in 5% to 11% of cases in the various series.[15,16,18] There is loss of intraocular pressure control, and there can be a sudden sharp rise in pressure associated with pain and visual blurring. The orifice might be blocked by iris, vitreous, or blood clot. Blockage can be either related to poor initial positioning of the tube or can be secondary to shallowing of the anterior chamber. The latter is frequently associated with choroidal detachment. When the anterior chamber shallows, vitreous and/or iris are displaced anteriorly and can come into contact with a previously well-positioned tube. Peripheral anterior synechia formation can occur near or even surrounding the proximal end of the tube following a flat anterior chamber (Fig. 15-2) and can lead to later blockage. Occlusion of the proximal orifice usually occurs within a few weeks or months of surgery but can be seen even years later.[16]

Management consists of clearing the tube obstruction either with the Nd:YAG laser or surgically. The Nd:YAG laser has a poor success rate for unblocking the orifice, because often it is difficult to directly focus the laser energy on occluding tissue that has been sucked inside the tube lumen. It is reasonable, however, that laser treatment should be attempted first, before operative intervention, as it is less invasive. The surgical approach employs an iris spatula or thin cannula to sweep the occluding tissues away from the orifice. This maneuver can be performed via a small peripheral corneal tract, so that the conjunctiva is not disturbed. If the anterior chamber is flat, it can be reformed first with a viscoelastic using this same tract. Sometimes, if the tube tip is completely surrounded by PAS or if the orifice otherwise cannot be unblocked, the tube might need to be completely removed from the chamber and reinserted in a new position. This can be achieved by re-exposing the original trabeculectomy flap site and making a new stab incision either under this flap or beneath a newly fashioned one in a different quadrant. The distal part of the tube and gutter generally do not need to be disturbed. The patency of the tubing should be confirmed by injection of saline through the accessed proximal orifice.

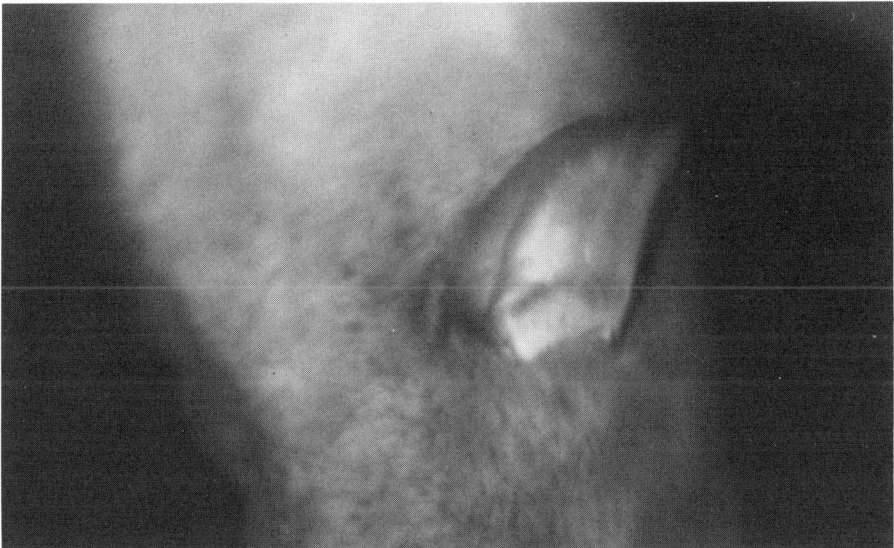

Figure 15-2. Iris surrounding proximal end of tube following an episode of shallowing of the anterior chamber. The tube orifice is patent still.

Corneal decompensation affecting visual acuity is rare following endothelial touch, but local corneal changes are almost inevitable and are seen early.[16] The long-term effects of peripheral contact are uncertain; each patient should be individually evaluated to determine whether shortening or reinsertion of the tube at another site is warranted. Serial, specular endothelial counts might be of help in making this decision. If the tube is overlong and is in contact with the endothelium centrally, it should be shortened. Any decrease in visual acuity because of corneal edema, secondary to tube touch, requires revision of the proximal tubing so that there is no further endothelial contact.

Avoidance of Anterior Segment Problems

These methods are summarized in Table 15-4.

Table 15-4. Avoidance of Anterior Segment Problems

1) Careful direction of stab incision into anterior chamber
2) Cutting tube tip with an anterior obliquity
3) Prevention of early flat chamber by:
– Use of a valved seton
– Use of a 23 or 25 gauge needle for the stab incision
– Filling the tubing and anterior chamber with viscoelastic
– Two-stage procedure or temporary suture placement around tubing
(– Tube insertion via a cyclodialysis tract)
4) Cauterization of the stab incision tract in neovascular glaucoma patients

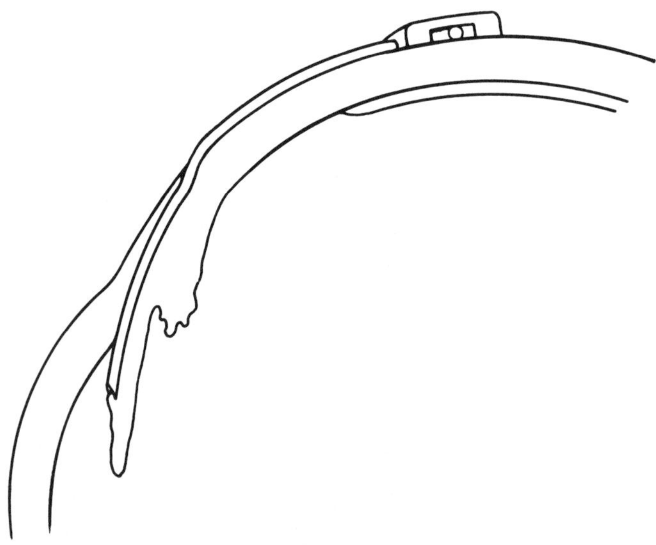

Figure 15-3. Tube directed too posteriorly. The tip is in contact with the iris, which increases the risk of later proximal orifice occlusion.

Correct alignment of the stab incision beneath the trabeculectomy flap is vital in positioning the tube in the mid-anterior chamber. If the tract is directed too far posteriorly, the tube will be in contact with the iris (Fig. 15-3) and if too anterior, with the corneal endothelium (Fig. 15-4). The best way to direct the needle for the stab incision is to place the point of the needle at, or slightly behind, the corneo-scleral junction and to advance the needle, parallel to the plane of the iris, into the anterior chamber.

An anterior core vitrectomy should be performed at the time of tube insertion in aphakic patients who have vitreous in the anterior chamber. It is also recommended for those in whom there is a later risk of vitreous coming into contact with the tube, should hypotony with choroidal effusion occur postoperatively. The presence of an anterior chamber intraocular lens in the eye is advantageous because it might help prevent forward displacement of iris and vitreous. The tube should be directed to pass in front of a lens foot process, in these pseudophakic eyes, with the orifice lying anterior to a peripheral portion of the optic (Fig. 15-5). This will prevent iris and generally vitreous contact with the proximal tube orifice.

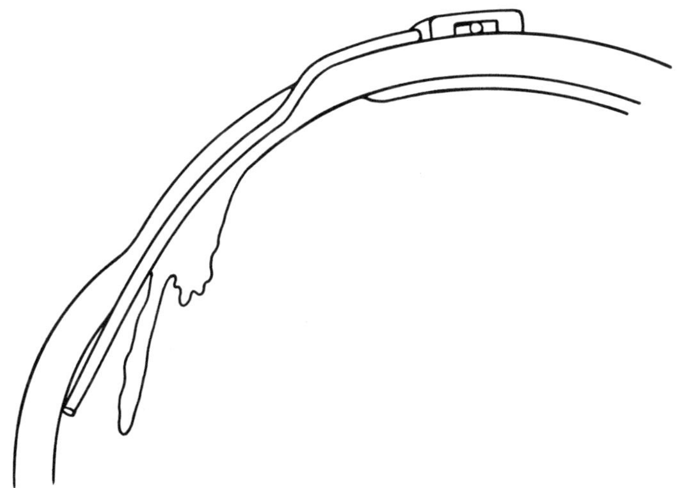

Figure 15-4. Tube directed too anteriorly. Contact between the tube and the endothelium leads to local corneal change and might lead to corneal decompensation.

Trimming the proximal tip of the tube obliquely, with the obliquity facing forward toward the cornea, has three advantages:

- The pointed end makes the insertion of the tube into the anterior chamber through the narrow stab incision easier.
- An opening of larger surface area is obtained and this is directed away from iris and vitreous, making occlusion less likely.

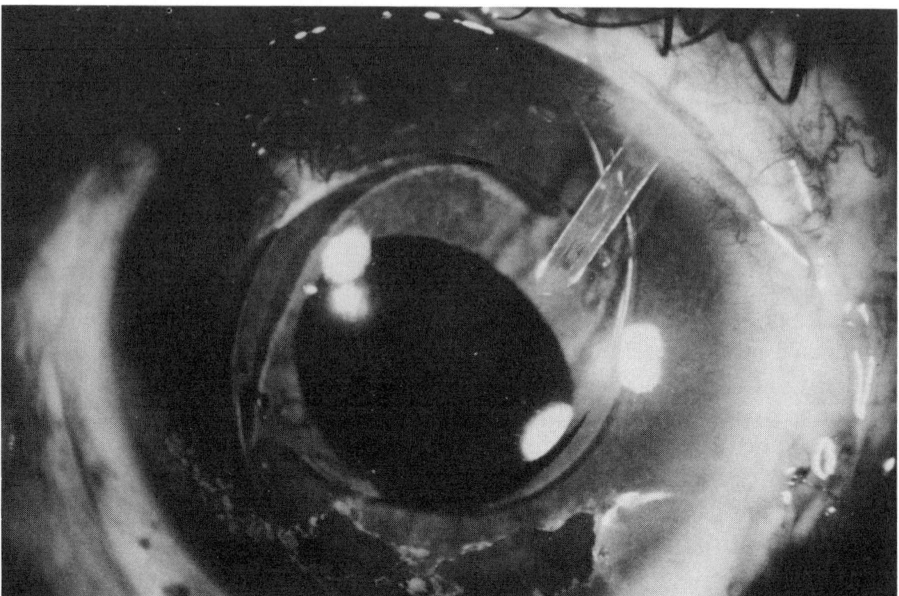

Figure 15-5. A. An anterior chamber IOL can be helpful in protecting the proximal tube orifice from occlusion by vitreous or iris.

- Should it become necessary, clearing iris or vitreous adhesions from the proximal orifice, by means of the laser, is easier. A knuckle of iris or vitreous is usually sucked into the tubing by the pressure difference between the anterior chamber and the drainage system. The laser can be applied directly to the base of the blocking tissue without the anterior wall of the tubing being interposed, if the orifice is cut obliquely.

A number of methods are described for the prevention of a flat chamber and hypotony in the early postoperative period. One or more of these can be incorporated at the time of the surgery.

A seton with a valve in it, such as a Krupin-Denver or Joseph implant,[2,19] can be used so that aqueous egress does not occur along the tube until a preset intraocular pressure is obtained.

Leakage of aqueous along the outside of the tubing is a major cause of flat anterior chamber if the tube is inserted into the anterior chamber beneath a partial-thickness scleral trabeculectomy flap. In these cases, even if the tube has a valve in it, hypotony can occur because of the formation of a filtering bleb with a lower resistance to the aqueous flow than the seton itself. To reduce flow around the tube, it is most important for the stab incision into the anterior chamber to be the same size as, or preferably slightly smaller, than the external diameter of the tube. This will provide a tight fit and can be achieved by using a 23 or 25 gauge round needle. A tight fit makes the actual insertion of the tube into the chamber technically more difficult, and an instrument to compress the tubing, such as a Shepard or curved McPhersons microforceps (Fig. 15-6), or a stiffening introducer, such as 30-gauge blunt infusion cannula (Fig. 15-7), might be required to aid insertion.

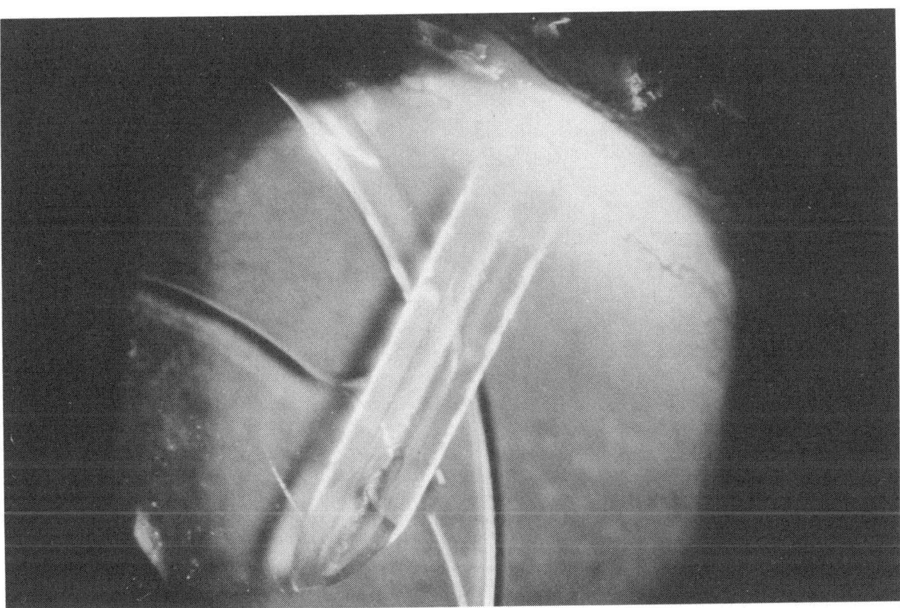

Figure 15-5. B. The tube is inserted to lie anterior to a peripheral portion of the optic. Notice the forward bevel of the tube orifice.

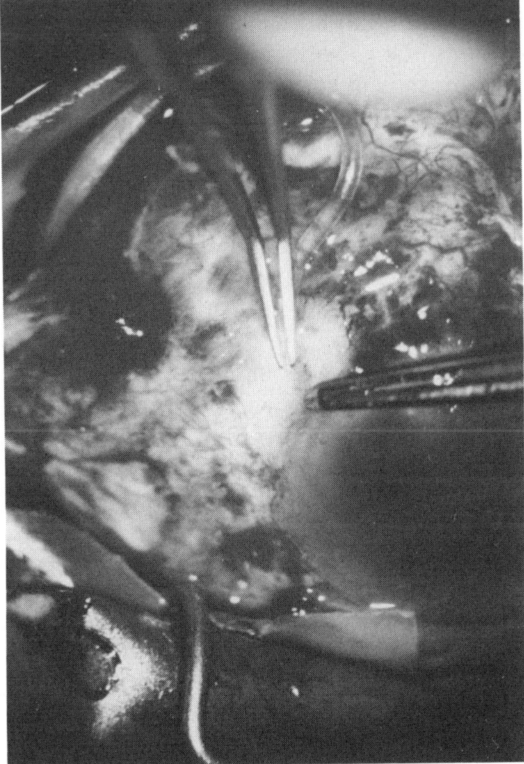

Figure 15-6. Tube insertion aided by compression using a curved McPherson forceps.

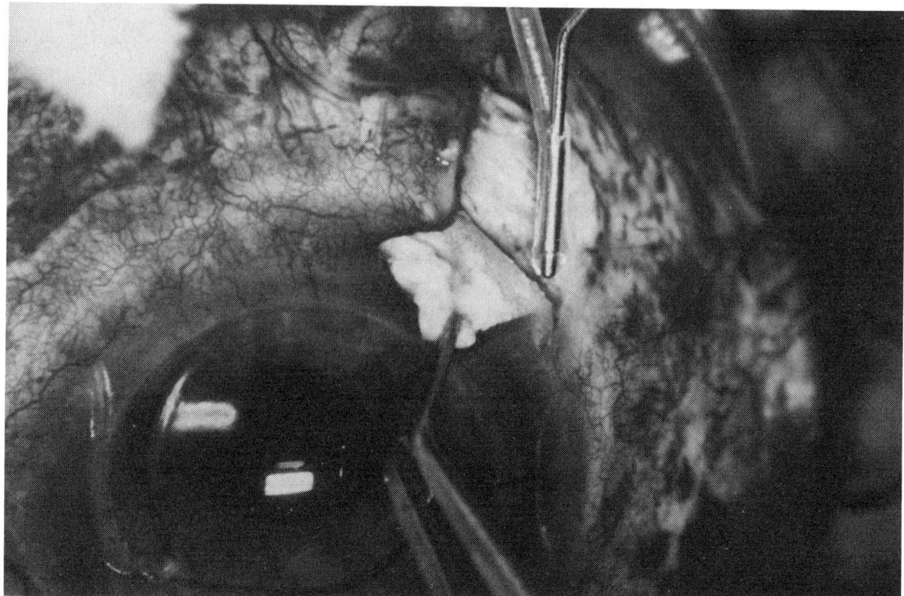

Figure 15-7. Tube insertion using a 30 gauge blunt cannula as a stiffening introducer.

Filling both the anterior chamber and the tubing with a viscoelastic can be combined with the use of the small entrance wound to further reduce the incidence of early hypotony and flat anterior chamber. The viscoelastic temporarily increases resistance to flow along the tube during the initial few days, when anterior chamber flattening is most likely to occur. Viscoelastic also has the advantage, particularly in eyes with neovascular glaucoma and prominent iris vessels, of decreasing the risk of hyphema because it isolates and stops bleeding points. Further, it aids insertion of the tube because of its lubricating and chamber-depth-retaining qualities.[4]

Molteno suggested a two-stage procedure for tube insertion.[20] In the first operation the acrylic plate is positioned on the sclera and the tube end tucked away beneath a rectus muscle. About two months later, the tubing is relocated and inserted into the anterior chamber. During the time between the two stages a fibrovascular capsule forms over the episcleral plate. Early hypotony is much reduced because the preformed bleb cavity curtails excessive aqueous bulk flow.

An alternative method to prevent early excessive aqueous drainage is to perform a one-stage procedure in which an absorbable suture such as 6-0 chromic collagen or polyglactin (Vicryl) is tied around the tube of the Molteno implant, near the episcleral plate, to temporarily occlude it. The suture is absorbed after several weeks and the tube then becomes patent. By this stage the bleb capsule is formed.[21] A further modification is to occlude the tubing with a 10-0 nylon suture in the suprascleral part of its course, posterior to the trabecular flap. This suture later can be divided with the Argon laser, using a Hoskins-style contact lens. The disadvantage of this method is that a donor scleral reinforcing patch cannot be used to cover the sutured part of the suprascleral tube and this might increase the risk of later tube exposure in patients with poor conjunctival tissues (see following section). The use of a prolene suture to occlude the proximal orifice of the tube, inside the anterior chamber, also has been proposed.[21] This again can be cut with an argon laser after a suitable time interval; the prolene fragments remain in the anterior chamber but are inert.

A narrow cyclodialysis tract can be employed to insert the tubing into the anterior chamber. This greatly reduces the incidence of flat anterior chambers and choroidal detachment when compared to the traditional trabeculectomy approach.[16] The disadvantage of the cyclodialysis tract approach for tube insertion is threefold:

- It is a more difficult procedure with risk of damage to the ciliary body or choroid and risk of peeling Descemet's membrane away from the corneal stroma if not performed correctly (see Chap. 17).
- There is an increased incidence of hyphema.[16] This is not a serious problem and the hyphema should clear spontaneously within a week or two.
- There is a much higher incidence of corneal endothelial touch by the tube, because the direction of the cyclodialysis tract naturally directs the tubing anteriorly. Use of a seton with an angulated proximal tube has been suggested to overcome this problem.[19]

In patients with neovascular glaucoma, hyphema can be a problem. Cauterization of the 25 or 23 gauge needle tract, by touching the inserting needle with a wet-field cautery, prevented hyphema in a consecutive series of 20 neovascular glaucoma eyes.[22] This is recommended for all patients with dilated iris or angle vessels.

Course of the Tube

Melting of the partial-thickness scleral trabeculectomy flap overlying the tubing (Fig. 15-8) is a frequent early finding, especially if the flap is sutured tightly over the tube. In itself this is no problem, but in some patients there is subsequent melting and perforation of the overlying conjunctiva, most commonly a few millimeters posterior to the limbus, leading to exposure of the tube (Fig. 15-9). The incidence varies markedly between different series, from 0% to 15%.[4,6,16,21] Prophylactic use of donor sclera to overlay the trabeculectomy flap and extrascleral tube (or inserting the proximal tubing into the anterior chamber via a cyclodialysis tract) should prevent tube exposure and is recommended for all cases. The further advantage of the donor scleral patch is that a partial-thickness trabeculectomy flap is no longer required for tube insertion. Instead, a full-thickness stab incision is made at the corneoscleral junction with a 23 or 25 gauge needle and the whole extrascleral length of the tube is covered with the donor scleral tissue (Fig. 15-10).

If tube exposure has occurred, management can include:

- Reinforcement of the exposed region by rotating a partial-thickness scleral flap from an adjacent area and then covering this with a

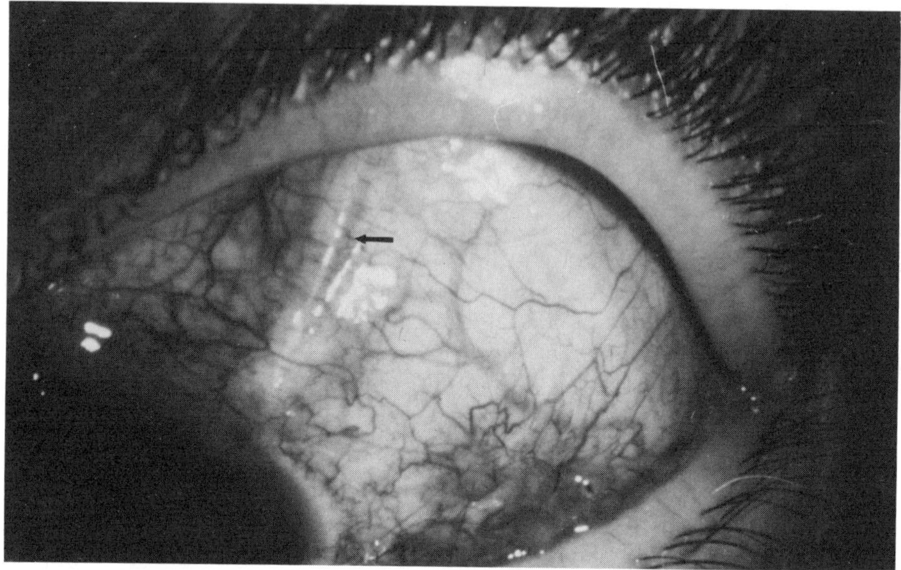

Figure 15-8. Silicone tube covered only by conjunctiva and tenon's capsule, having eroded through the trabeculectomy scleral flap.

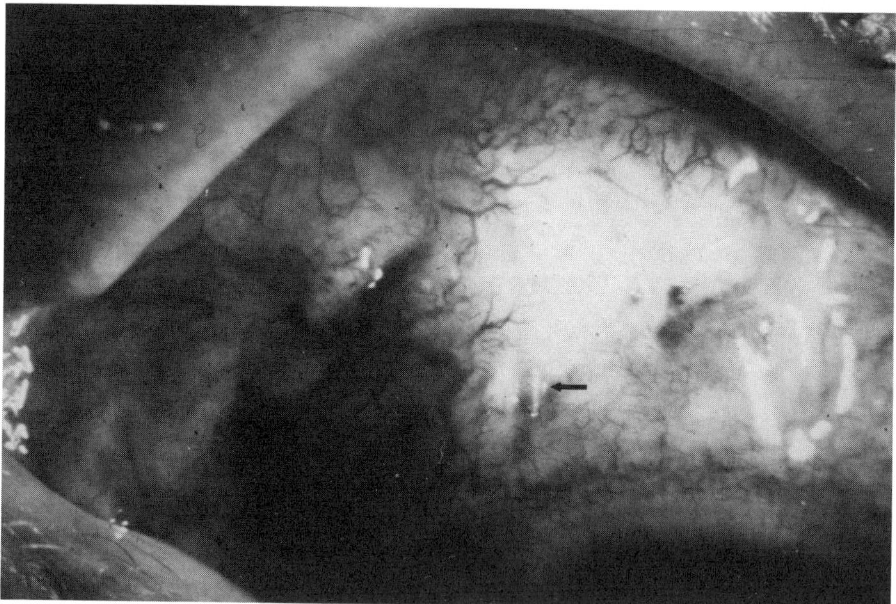

Figure 15-9. Exposed silicone tube having eroded through the overlying conjunctiva as well as the scleral flap (see arrow).

conjunctival flap mobilized from surrounding host tissues.[16] The partial-thickness scleral flap should not be sutured too tightly over the tube or further erosion might occur.

- Utilizing a patch of donor sclera to cover the tube instead of the host scleral tissue described earlier.[3,10] This is the simplest method and the one that is recommended as an initial revision procedure.

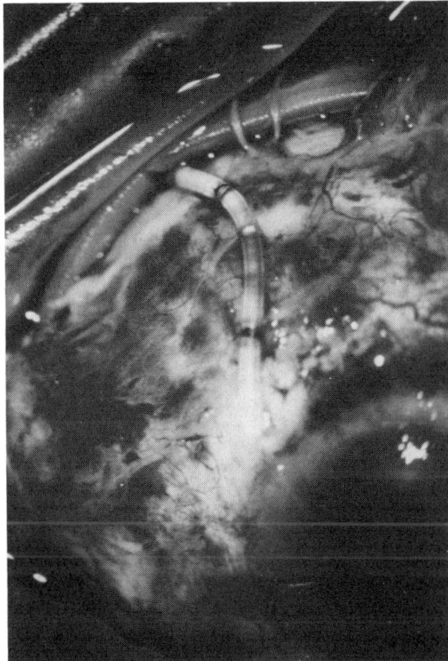

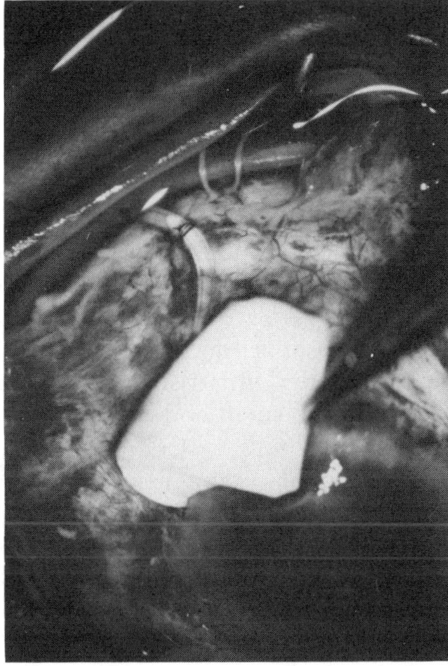

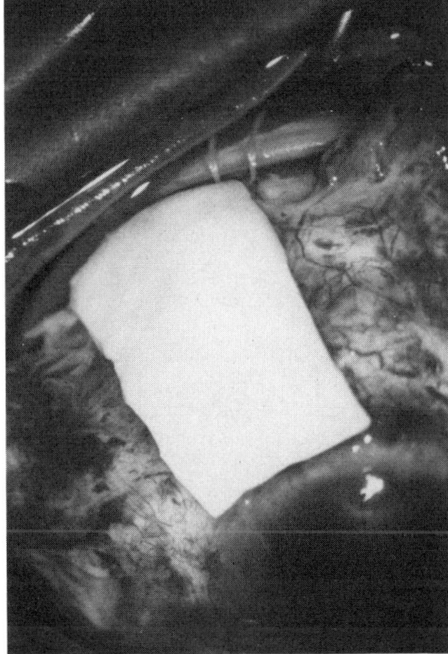

Figure 15-10. **A.** Tube inserted into the anterior chamber via a 23 gauge full-thickness stab incision. **B.** and **C.** Its entire extrascleral length is then covered with donor scleral tissue. The donor sclera implant is thinned, especially anteriorly, to prevent later corneal dellen formation.

- Total revision of the anterior portion of the drainage system by reinserting the tube in a new quadrant.[16] The prophylactic covering of the suprascleral tube with donor sclera tissue will further reduce the chance of recurrence of the tube exposure. This option is especially important in patients with conjunctival ischemia.

Blockage of the Distal Tube Orifice

In setons that do not have a guarded distal end,[2,23] fibrosis around the area of aqueous exit is a major cause of failure. Krupin now recommends the use of an inverted 220 silastic retinal band to cover the distal orifice of his device.[24] The idea described initially by Schocket of placing the tubing beneath a 360° encircling gutter greatly reduces the incidence of fibrous occlusion of the distal tube orifice, although it does not eliminate it completely (Fig. 15-11).[16,24] Lifting the distal end of the tubing away from the sclera and into contact with the under, grooved surface of the encircling band, by means of an extra suture, might reduce the risk of fibrous adhesion between the distal orifice and the underlying tissues (Fig. 15-12).

A series of small holes or slits can be made, either with an argon laser[22] or alternatively with the CU5 needle of a 10-0 nylon suture[25] (Fig. 15-13), in the part of the tubing that lies beneath the encircling element. Should distal orifice occlusion occur, these holes provide an alternate pathway for aqueous egress from the tube to the area under the band. It is recommended that these holes are made during the initial preparation of the Schocket implant, but they can be incorporated at revision surgery if occlusion of the distal orifice is found.

In the Molteno one-piece system, the circular acrylic plate provides a surface that resists fibrous tissue adherence. The tube opens directly onto the upper surface of the thin episcleral plate, which forms the floor of a bleb cavity. The area of the bleb cannot be reduced by fibrous scar formation to a size

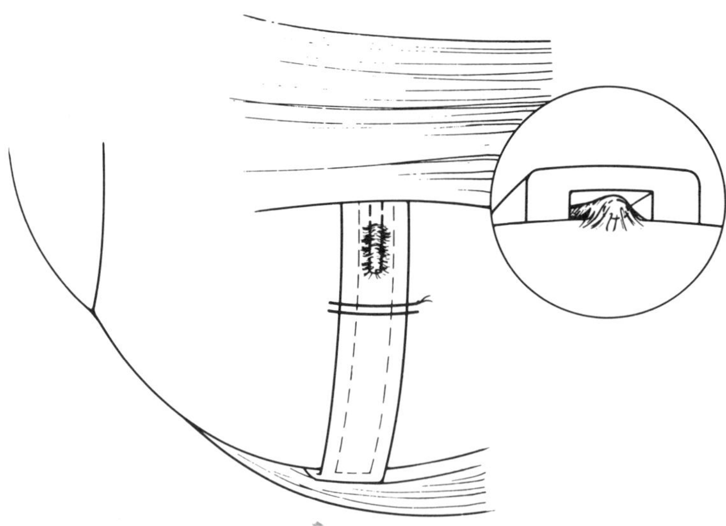

Figure 15-11. Although the incidence of distal orifice occlusion is much reduced by placing the tubing beneath an encircling band in the Schocket procedure, the complication is still seen.

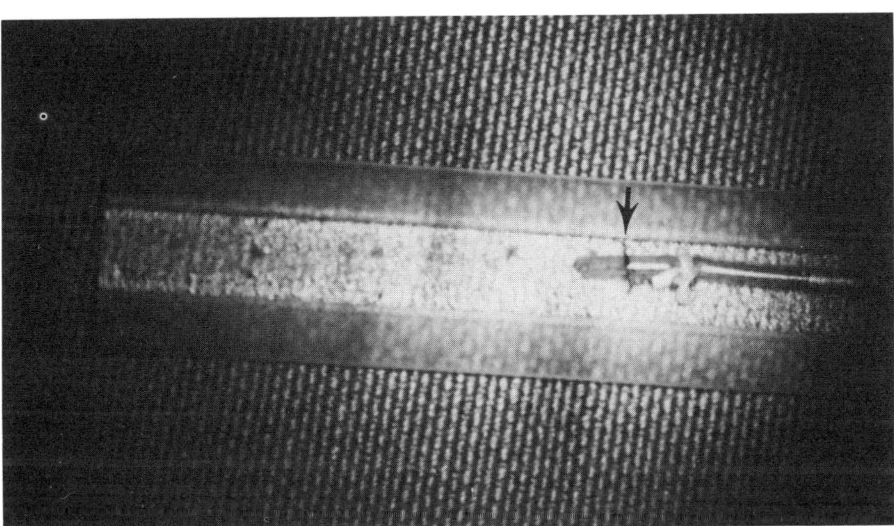

Figure 15-12. A 9-0 supramid or nylon suture is placed near the distal end of the tube to lift the distal orifice away from the underlying sclera (Schocket procedure).

any smaller than the surface area of the implant plate. The same idea of a one-piece system has been used in conjunction with a 360° encircling (Schocket-type) band.[19] Occlusion cannot theoretically be seen at the distal orifice in either of these two types of drainage device because there is no separate narrow-bored tubing to occlude. However, the author has treated one patient with congenital glaucoma who did develop blockage of a Molteno implant tube, at the site of attachment of the tube to the episcleral plate wall.

Insufficient Aqueous Absorption

Despite a fully patent tube delivering aqueous to the acrylic plate or beneath the encircling gutter (Fig. 15-14) in the Molteno and Schocket devices respectively, the intraocular pressure might still remain too high.

There are two important factors regulating the diffusion of aqueous away from the site of the plate or band:

- The thickness and density of the fibrous capsule overlying the plate or encircling band.
- The total surface area provided by the device.

To reduce thickening of the fibrous capsule overlying the episcleral plate Molteno recommends an antifibrotic regimen summarized in Table 15-5.

These drugs synergistically block the pathways of fibrosis. They are used for about 6 weeks following the second-stage surgery, particularly in younger patients.[6] Others disagreed that this regimen improved results and noted that 15% of patients could not tolerate the full course of the medications.[9] An alternative method for producing a more permeable fibrous capsule is to permanently heparinize the silicone implant using a heparin-quaternary ammonium compound-complex.[22] The increased permeability is histologically associated with a looser connective tissue structure.

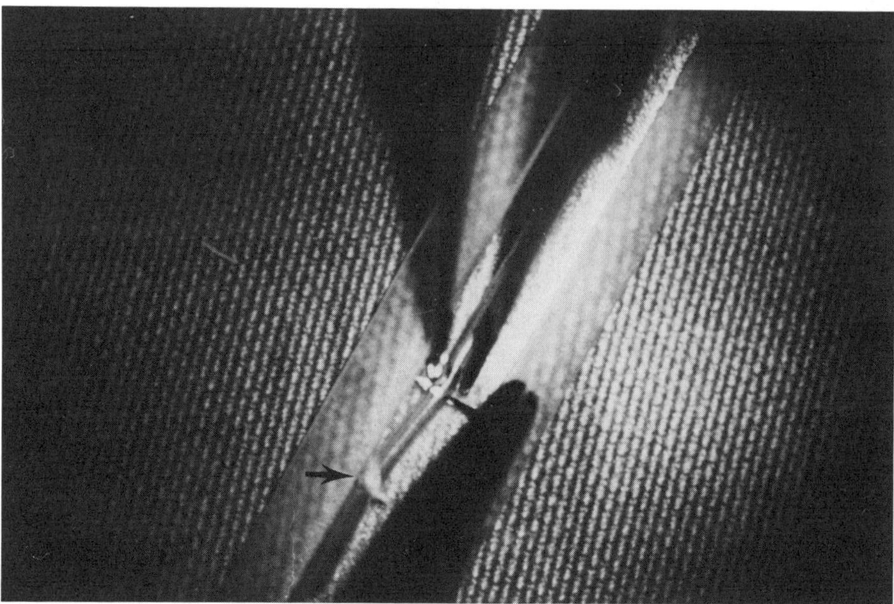

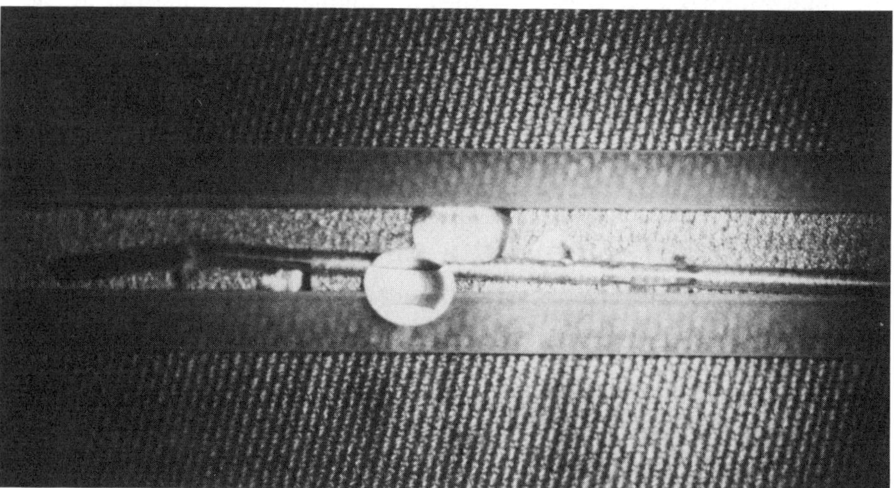

Figure 15-13. A. Slits made in the silicone tubing with a suture needle (CU5) act as an alternate pathway for aqueous egress from the tube, should the distal orifice become occluded. A dissolvable occluding suture has been deliberately placed in this case (see arrow) to prevent early excessive filtration and hypotony. **B.** Patency of the slits can be checked by injecting saline along the tube.

The easier of the two variables to clinically manipulate is the size of the implant. Molteno originally described a drainage device with a single 13 mm diameter methacrylic plate[26], which has a surface area of 135 mm^2. Subsequently, he developed a double- and even quadruple-plate system to increase the total surface area from which aqueous could be diffused. The four-plate

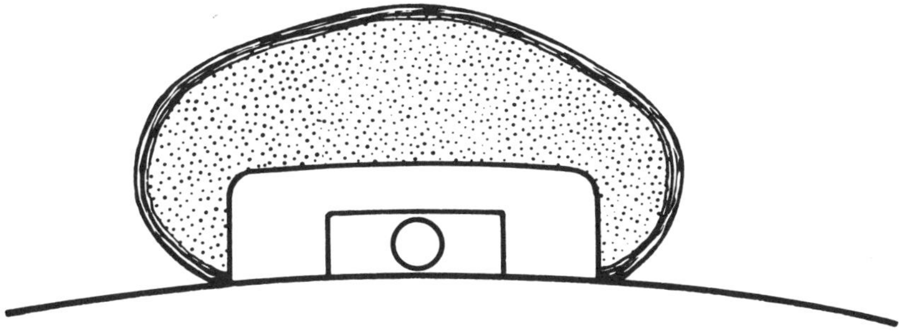

Figure 15-14. Elevated IOP can be seen, despite a fully patent tube, if there is excessive thickening of the fibrous capsule surrounding the episcleral plate or encircling band.

Table 15-5. Molteno Antifibrotic Regimen

Systemic		Topical	
Prednisone	10 mg tid	Dexamethasone	0.1% tid
Flufenamic acid	100 mg tid	Atropine	1% tid
Colchicine	0.3 mg tid	Epinephrine	2% tid

system tended to create excessive hypotony and is little used now. The two-plate implant is considered the best device when a large fibrotic response is expected.[27]

A 360°, inverted, no. 20 silicone encircling gutter was recommended by Schocket as the framework of an area around which a fibrous capsule would form. In the Joseph implant this has been enlarged to a 9 mm wide band, which has almost double the total surface area.[19] This modification was made following failure of IOP control in 7% of cases secondary to insufficient aqueous absorption, when using the original materials suggested by Schocket.[16] The greater surface area band is advantageous because some patients require only a 180° implant. Because access to only two quadrants is required, the operative technique is simpler in these cases. Should failure occur because of insufficient aqueous absorption, a further 180° of the band can be added in the remaining two quadrants, thus doubling the surface area.[17]

Other Ocular Problems

Progression of cataract was reported in 9 of 25 phakic eyes (36%) with neovascular glaucoma by Schocket.[15] Cataract extraction in these eyes led to reactivation of rubeosis iridis with hyphema in more than half the surgically treated cases. Other authors, studying mainly non-neovascular glaucoma patients, have not recorded such a high incidence of cataract progression following an aqueous shunt procedure.[10,16]

A traction retinal detachment was seen in one aphakic patient following adherence of vitreous strands to the proximal tube orifice.[16] This occurred secondary to serous choroidal detachment and a flat anterior chamber. Minckler and coworkers[10] reported retinal detachment in 6% of their patients following Molteno implant surgery, and a 6% incidence of vitreous hemorrhage. They also noted hemorrhagic choroidal detachment in 6% and phthisis in 4%.

Bacterial endophthalmitis is a rare complication but has been described.[10,11]

Artifical drainage tubes appear to be a major advance in the management of refractory forms of glaucoma poorly responsive to traditional filtration surgery. More and more surgeons have been using these implants in the last few years, but, as has been discussed here, they are not without significant potential complications. Attention to fine detail at surgery is very important in reducing the complication rate and close follow-up care is essential. Many of the problems are preventable or correctable but, in some early studies, greater than one-third of patients required some form of implant revision or other additional procedure.[10,16] Experience has led to modifications both in seton design and in the techniques of insertion, which it is hoped, will improve success rates and reduce complication rates in the future.

References

1. Zorab A. The reduction of tension in chronic glaucoma. Ophthalmoscope 10:258-261, 1912.
2. Krupin T, Podos SM, Becker B, et al. Valve implants in filtering surgery. Am J Ophthalmol 81:232-235, 1976.

2a. Krupin T, Ritch R, Camras CB, et al. A long Krupin-Denver valve implant attached to a 180° scleral explant for glaucoma surgery. Ophthalmol 95:1174-1180, 1988.

3. Molteno ACB, Straughan JL, Ancker E. Long tube implants in the management of glaucoma. SA Mediese Tydskrif 50:1062-1066, 1976.
4. Schocket SS, Lakhanpal V, Richards RD. Anterior chamber tube shunt to an encircling band in the treatment of neovascular glaucoma. Ophthalmol 89:1188-1194, 1982.
5. Ancker E, Molteno ACB. Molteno drainage implant for neovascular glaucoma. Trans Ophthalmol Soc UK 102:122-124, 1982.
6. Molteno ACB, Ancker E, van Biljon G. Surgical technique for advanced juvenile glaucoma. Arch Ophthalmol 102:51-57, 1984.
7. Molteno ACB. Uveitis with glaucoma treated by implants. SuidArikaanse Argief vir Oftalmologie 1:125-130, 1973.
8. Ancker E, Molteno ACB. Die chirurgische behandlung des chronischen aphakieglaukoms mit dem Moltenokunststoffimplantat. Klin Monatsbl Augenheilkd 177:365-370, 1980.

9. Brown RD, Cairnes JE. Experience with the Molteno long tube implant Trans Ophthalmol Soc UK 103:297-312, 1983.
10. Minckler DS, Baerveldt G, Heuer DK. Clinical experience with the single plate Molteno implant in complicated glaucomas. Ophthalmol 95:1181-1188, 1988.
11. Downes RN, Flanagan DW, Jordan K, et al. The Molteno implant in intractable glaucoma. Eye 2:250-259, 1988.
12. Krupin T, Kaufman P, Mandell AI, et al. Long-term results of valve implants in filtering surgery for eyes with neovascular glaucoma. Am J Ophthalmol 95:775-782, 1983.
13. Sutton GE, Popp JC, Records RE. Krupin-Denver valve and neovascular glaucoma. Trans Ophthalmol Soc UK 102:119-121, 1982.
14. Forestier F, Salvanet-Bouccara A. Valve de Krupin. Reflections sur la chirurgie du glaucome. Resultats personnels a propos de 20 valves de Krupin-Denver. J. Fr Ophthalmol 7:385-391, 1984.
15. Schocket SS, Nirankari S, Lakhanpal V, et al. Anterior chamber tube shunt to an encircling band in the treatment of neovascular glaucoma and other refractory glaucomas. A long term study. Ophthalmol 92:553-562, 1985.
16. Sherwood MB, Joseph NH, Hitchings RA. Surgery for refractory glaucoma. Results and complications with a modified Schocket technique. Arch Ophthalmol 105:562-569, 1987.
17. Hitchings RA, Joseph NH, Sherwood MB, et al. Use of one-piece valved tube and variable surface area explant for glaucoma drainage surgery. Ophthalmol 94:1079-1083, 1987.
18. Molteno ACB: The use of draining implants in resistant cases of glaucoma. Late results of 110 operations. Trans Ophthalmol Soc NZ 35:94-97, 1983.
19. Joseph NH, Sherwood MB, Trantas G, et al: A one-piece drainage system for glaucoma surgery. Trans Ophthalmol Soc UK 105:657-664, 1986.
20. Molteno ACB, Van Biljon G, Ancker E. Two stage insertion of glaucoma drainage implants. Trans Ophthalmol Soc NZ 31:17-26, 1979.
21. Traverso CE, Tomey KF, Al-Kaff A. The Molteno implant for the treatment of refractory glaucomas. Invest Ophthalmol Vis Sci (suppl) 28:271, 1987.
22. Schocket SS. Investigations of the reasons for success and failure in the anterior shunt-to-the-encircling-band procedure in the treatment of refractory glaucoma. Trans Am Ophthalmol Soc 84:743-798, 1986.
23. Honrubia FM, Gomez ML, Hernandez A, et al. Long-term results of silicone tube in filtering surgery for eyes with neovascular glaucoma. Am J Ophthalmol 97:501-504, 1984.
24. Krupin T: Surgical treatment of glaucoma with the Krupin-Denver valve. In Cairns JE (ed): Glaucoma. London: Grune and Stratton, 1986, pp 239-246.

25. Sherwood MB, Hitchings RA. The Schocket procedure. In Spaeth GL, Katz LJ, Parker KW: Current Therapy in Ophthalmic Surgery. Ontario, B.C. Decker, Inc., 1989, pp. 211-218.
26. Molteno ACB: New implant for drainage in glaucoma. Clinical trial. Br J Ophthalmol 53:606-615, 1969.
27. Molteno ACB. Use of Molteno implants to treat secondary glaucoma. In Cairns JE (ed): Glaucoma, London: Grune and Stratton, 1986, pp. 211-238.

CHAPTER 16

Complications of Surgical Iridectomy: Prevention and Management

Mark B. Sherwood, MD
Nina Tolat, MD
Ralph S. Sando, MD

The primary indication for iridectomy is elimination of pupillary block. The types of glaucoma for which an iridectomy is performed include acute angle closure, chronic angle-closure, secondary angle-closure or combined mechanism glaucoma. The Nd:YAG and argon lasers have replaced conventional surgery in recent years as the standard methods for making a peripheral iridectomy. A surgical iridectomy may still be required, however, in certain cases of inflammatory glaucoma in which a small laser iridectomy has repeatedly closed off; in patients in whom a patent iridectomy cannot be obtained with the laser because of media opacities or a very thick iris; and also in cases where an iris biopsy or an excision of a lesion is planned. Further, children who are too young to sit at a laser, some retarded patients, and those with head titubation may need general anesthesia and a surgical iridectomy (Table 16-1).

Table 16-1. Indications for Surgical Iridectomy

Repeated closure of laser iridectomy (inflammatory glaucoma etc)	
Unable to perform laser iridectomy due to hazy media	
Patient unable to sit at laser	– young children
	– retarded
	– head titubation.
Iris biopsy required	
In combination with other surgery (cataract extraction, PKP etc)	

It is often difficult to decide whether to perform an iridectomy or a filtering procedure in a patient with angle closure glaucoma.[1] In many patients, iridectomy combined with postoperative medical treatment is as successful as filtering surgery[2,3] and is associated with a lower incidence of complication; thus it is frequently the surgery of choice. If iridectomy is unlikely to provide adequate IOP control, however, initial filtration surgery is indicated to prevent the additional hazards and patient discomfort involved in performing two operations. Some authors recommend filtering surgery on the basis of the length of the acute attack[4], the tonographic facility of outflow[5,6], the amount of peripheral anterior synechiae[7,8], or the presence of visual field loss[9] (Table 16-2). Preoperative indentation gonioscopy with a Zeiss four-mirror goniolens is recommended in all cases to assess the amount of synechial angle closure.

Table 16-2. Choice of Operation – Factors Favoring Peripheral Iridectomy
1) Less than 180° peripheral anterior synechiae
2) Facility of outflow greater than 0.1
3) Healthy optic nerve with little or no visual field loss
4) Acute attack of short duration (less than 36-48 hours)

Prevention of Complications in the Surgical Technique

Most iridectomies can be performed with local anesthesia, either with a facial nerve block and topical anesthesia or with a retrobulbar block. The eye should be as quiet as possible, and a short course of hourly topical steroid, such as prednisolone acetate 1%, is helpful preoperatively if the eye is inflamed secondary to an acute glaucoma attack. The intraocular pressure ideally should be in mid-range. Very high pressures may predispose the eye to expulsive hemorrhage or malignant glaucoma, while low pressures make spontaneous prolapse of iris more difficult. Intravenous mannitol 20%, starting 45 minutes before surgery, is advocated if the intraocular pressure is above 30 mm Hg. A urinary catheter may be needed to prevent bladder overdistention if this infusion is given.

The surgical incision can be made either through clear cornea peripherally or alternatively at the limbus with a small conjunctival peritomy. For patients likely to require filtration surgery later, the clear corneal approach is preferable since the virgin state of the conjunctiva will be maintained. This approach is also favored if there are anteriorly placed peripheral anterior synechiae in the planned surgical quadrant. The limbal incision may allow easier prolapse of the iris and, in the rare event of a leak through the wound, will provide greater protection because of the conjunctival covering.

A common error is to make the incision too small or to cone the incision so that the deep part of the wound is shorter than the surface cut. Doing so can make both prolapse and reinsertion of the iris more difficult, especially in eyes with poor iris muscle tone following an acute glaucoma attack. An incision at least 2 mm wide at its base is recommended. The incision should be perpendicular rather than shelved, as this will further aid iris prolapse.

It is important to complete the final entry into the anterior chamber with one fairly rapid cut along the entire length of the incision. The pressure difference between the posterior and anterior chambers causes the iris to spontaneously prolapse. Care must be taken to avoid accidentally piercing the iris with the blade, since the pressure differential would then be lost. Once the chamber is entered aqueous will exit the eye and the iris will rise towards the blade. Delay should therefore be avoided at this stage. If the tip of the knife is inserted into the anterior chamber with the sharp edge uppermost, and the cut is made in an upward (external) direction, there is less risk of accidental injury to the iris.

Placement of an 8-0 polyglactin (Vicryl) suture when the wound is approximately two-thirds depth assists visualization when cutting the deep part of the incision and aids prolapse of the iris. The two loops of the suture are held by an assistant and are used to splay the edges of the incision apart. As soon as the iris prolapses following entry into the anterior chamber, release of the suture will trap a knuckle of iris in the incision. From there, it can be further exteriorized in a controlled fashion with forceps. The surgeon must not tug on the iris root when lifting the iris through the incision; a brisk hyphema will occur if the iris root is torn. Grasping the iris knuckle as anteriorly as possible and lifting it posteriorly will prevent traction on the iris root.

If, despite a well placed and sufficiently long incision, the iris will not spontaneously prolapse, extremely careful introduction of a fine-toothed forceps to grasp the iris and assist its externalization is suggested. This is done only as a last resort, since it significantly increases the risks of the surgery. Any posterior synechiae that tether the iris and prevent its passage through the incision need to be broken first with an iris spatula or blunt cannula. Viscoelastic materials can help maintain the anterior chamber during this maneuver but must be aspirated before the end of the procedure.

The cut piece of iris should be inspected to confirm that posterior pigment epithelium has been included in the iridectomy. This can be done by rubbing the excised tissue against the drapes or a gauze swab; a deposit of brown pigment should be seen.

The tip of a #21 irrigator is placed in the superficial part of the incision, and a gentle stream of balanced salt solution is used to flush away any remaining pigment epithelium and to help push the iris back into the anterior chamber. Gently stroking the peripheral cornea with a blunt instrument will also help return the iris to its proper position. The tip of the irrigator should not be inserted through the incision, and through the iridectomy, because this will introduce fluid into the posterior chamber, behind the iris, thus forcing the iris out of the eye rather than aiding in its reposition. Use of acetylcholine chloride (Miochol, Cooper Vision) may further assist in the repositioning of the iris if there are difficulties with reinsertion.

A previously prepared paracentesis tract will help in reforming the anterior chamber at the end of the procedure. The aim should be to leave the chamber slightly deeper than it was preoperatively. If recently formed peripheral anterior synechiae are present, these may sometimes be divided by a temporary, sudden, forceful overinflation of the anterior chamber with balanced salt solution, delivered via the paracentesis tract. An alternative is to introduce a bubble of air, which, if the eye is soft, can be maneuvered around the anterior chamber using a blunt instrument applied to the external surface of the cornea. These techniques can serve to separate the iris from the cornea and reopen the drainage angle.

At the end of the procedure, a check is made to ensure that the incision is watertight either by using a Weck cell swab or by performing a Seidel test with a fluorescein strip. Usually, one 10-0 nylon suture is sufficient to close the incision, but extra sutures should be placed if required. The knots are buried, especially if a corneal incision has been used.

Postsurgical Complications of Iridectomy

Many of the complications following a surgical peripheral iridectomy are the same as those following filtration surgery and are discussed in detail in Chapter 14.

Small hyphemas are common after iridectomy but usually resolve spontaneously. An anterior chamber washout procedure is very rarely required. If large dilated iris vessels are present, it may be prudent at the time of surgery to gently cauterize the exteriorized knuckle of iris before it is excised.

A shallow or flat anterior chamber following iridectomy is uncommon and is usually caused by a wound leak.[10,11] This can be prevented or repaired by adequate wound closure. Suprachoroidal effusion or hemorrhage, inadequate aqueous formation, or anterior displacement of the lens-iris diaphragm can also result in a shallow chamber. Ciliary block glaucoma (malignant glaucoma) is a rare but serious complication following surgical iridectomy. The flat anterior chamber in this case is associated with an elevated IOP. This complication is also discussed in more detail in Chapter 14.

Uncomplicated iridectomy may increase the risk of cataract formation, but this increase in risk is much less than the increased risk of cataract following filtration surgery.[12,13] The incidence of cataract formation being higher in eyes that have undergone iridectomy following an acute glaucoma attack than in fellow eyes that received prophylactic surgery[11,12] suggests that the acute attack itself is an important factor in lens opacification. Indeed, some authors report no increase in the incidence of cataract formation following prophylactic surgical iridectomy to the fellow eye,[10,11,14] although others disagree.[12,13]

Posterior synechiae can form, especially after operations on eyes inflamed following an acute angle closure attack. Mydriatics are not routinely required following peripheral iridectomy, but eyes at high risk for developing posterior synechiae should receive early and adequate dilation postoperatively, as well as frequent steroid drops. The IOP should be closely monitored.

Pupillary block persists when the iridectomy is trapped in the wound, when the pigment epithelium of the iris remains intact, or when posterior synechiae or fibrous ingrowth close the iridectomy. If an incomplete iridectomy is performed, the problem at the iridectomy site must be corrected, either surgically or with a laser, or a new iridectomy made at a different site. In many cases the preferred treatment is a new iridectomy.

Postoperatively the surgeon must carefully monitor IOP and inspect for any evidence of progressive synechial angle closure. If pressure control is inadequate despite maximum tolerated medical therapy, filtration surgery is indicated.

Table 16-3. Postsurgical Complications of Peripheral Iridectomy

1) Hyphema
2) Flat anterior chamber
3) Ciliary block (malignant) glaucoma
4) Possible increased risk of cataract
5) Posterior synechiae formation
6) Persistence of pupillary block due to occluded or incomplete iridectomy
7) Inadequate IOP control
8) Filtering bleb
9) Vitreous loss
10) Endophthalmitis

In summary, good surgical technique is of paramount importance in effectively and safely performing a peripheral iridectomy. The majority of intra- and postoperative complications can be prevented by careful adherence to the principles and precautions described above. Although it is much less commonly used now, a surgical iridectomy may still occasionally be required. The surgeon should be aware of the potential pitfalls that can accompany this apparently simple procedure and know how to handle them.

References

1. Galin MA, Obstbaum SA, Hung PT: Peripheral iridectomy. Ann Ophthalmol 9:833, 1977.
2. Murphy MB, Spaeth, GL: Iridectomy in primary angle-closure glaucoma. Arch Ophthalmol 91:114-122, 1974.
3. Forbes M, Becker B: Iridectomy in advanced angle-closure glaucoma. Am J Ophthalmol 57:57-62, 1964.
4. Epstein DL. Angle closure glaucoma. In Chandler and Grant's Glaucoma 3rd Ed. Philadelphia: Lea and Febiger, 1986, p.227.
5. Becker B, Thompson HE: Tonography and angle-closure glaucoma: Diagnosis and Therapy. Am J Ophthalmol 46:305-310, 1958.
6. Williams DJ, Gills JP Jr, Hall GA: Results of 233 peripheral iridectomies for narrow-angle glaucoma. Am J Ophthalmol 65:548-552, 1968.
7. Chandler PA, Simmons RJ. Anterior chamber deepening for gonioscopy at the time of surgery. Arch Ophthalmol 74:177-190, 1965.
8. Shaffer RN: Operating room gonioscopy in angle-closure glaucoma surgery. Arch Ophthalmol 59:532-535, 1958.

9. Gleber EC, Anderson DR: Surgical decisions in chronic angle- closure glaucoma. Arch Ophthalmol 94:1481-1484, 1976.
10. Douglas WHG, Strahan IM. Surgical safety of prophylactic peripheral iridectomy. Br J Ophthalmol 51:459-462, 1967.
11. Luke SK: Complications of peripheral iridectomy. Can J Ophthalmol 4:346-351, 1969.
12. Godel V, Regenbogen L: Cataractogenic factors in patients with primary angle-closure glaucoma after peripheral iridectomy. Am J Ophthalmol 83:180-184, 1977.
13. Sugar HS: Cataract formation and refractive changes after surgery for angle-closure glaucoma. Am J Ophthalmol 69:747-749, 1970.
14. Kirsch RE: Peripheral iridectomy for angle-closure glaucoma. Invest Ophthalmol 9:424, 1970.

CHAPTER 17

Complications of Cyclodialysis

James A. McAllister, FRCS

Introduction

In 1905, Heine described cyclodialysis as a useful surgical treatment in glaucoma.[1] He believed that disinsertion of the ciliary body from its scleral attachment allowed a communication to form between the anterior chamber and the suprachoroidal space. This allowed a new area for aqueous absorption and, therefore, effectively lowered IOP without external filtration. The mechanism of why cyclodialysis can lower IOP is still not fully understood. In 1922, Elschnig[2] felt the procedure suppressed aqueous production by producing ciliary body atrophy, which he demonstrated histologically.

Today, most people believe that absorption via the new communication into the suprachoroidal space is a likely mechanism, though it might be that detachment of the ciliary body itself, at least temporarily, reduces aqueous production. Whichever mechanism is responsible, Spaeth[3] suggests that a visible cyclodialysis cleft is probably essential for successful lowering of IOP.

The use of cyclodialysis has largely disappeared as a standard glaucoma surgical technique. Despite a low incidence of serious complications[4], its success rate is limited and because of changes in surgery, particularly cataract surgery and the success of modern trabeculectomy, cyclodialysis is rarely performed. Cyclodialysis clefts and suprachoroidal absorption can form part of the wanted or unwanted reason for pressure lowering in other procedures and certainly can result from trauma.

Indications

Historically, cyclodialysis was used in many types of glaucomas prior to the development of modern fistulizing surgery. It is now used occasionally in the management of aphakic glaucomas. It also has been used in phakic eyes when filtering surgery has failed and as a combined procedure with intracapsular cataract extraction where glaucoma and cataract coexist.

In secondary glaucoma, where the division of peripheral anterior synechiae is required to dissect the cleft, cyclodialysis has not been shown to be helpful as the angle rarely stays open. The synechiae tend to reform rapidly.

Patient Selection

Patients can be considered for cyclodialysis if they have aphakic glaucoma in association with some degree of open angle (Table 17-1). Secondly, it can be considered where other forms of glaucoma surgery have failed in phakic or aphakic eyes. In this latter group, where progression to cyclodestructive procedures in eyes with already markedly limited visual function might be the next step, cyclodialysis might be a technique still worth considering.

Table 17-1. Original Indications for Cyclodialysis
1. Aphakic glaucoma.
2. Failed filtering surgery in phakic and aphakic eyes.
3. Where open angle glaucoma and cataract coexist, it can be performed as a combined procedure with intracapsular cataract extraction.

Cyclodialysis can be used in combination with intracapsular cataract extraction but, with the advent of extracapsular surgery, filtering procedures such as trabeculectomy are preferably performed either prior to ECCE or as a combined procedure, making this approach obsolete (Table 17-2).

Table 17-2. Contraindications to Cyclodialysis
1. Secondary angle closure.
2. Glaucoma in which there is active uveitis.
3. Patients unable to tolerate long-term parasympathomimetics.
4. In patients extracapsular cataract extraction and posterior chamber lens implant.

When intraocular lens implantation was developed, it was initially with iris supported or anterior chamber intraocular lenses following intracapsular cataract extraction. These forms of implant were generally felt to be contraindicated in the presence of glaucoma. As a result, there is no supported study of cyclodialysis in this group.

In the last decade, with the dramatic change toward ECCE normally in combination with posterior chamber intraocular lenses, large numbers of glaucoma patients are benefiting from the advantages of internal optical correction. Preservation of the anterior vitreous face behind the intact, or subsequently laser dissected posterior capsule, has led to the use of pseudophakic trabeculectomy, either in combination at the time of cataract extraction, or as a pre-extraction procedure with extracapsular extraction at a later date.

The complication of filtering surgery is discussed elsewhere in this book but its greater success has led to almost complete disuse of cyclodialysis as a surgical technique.[5]

Operative Technique

Preoperative

Normal glaucoma medications should be continued until the time of surgery. If any patient is on cycloplegics, they should be discontinued one week in advance to permit the action of cholinesterase inhibitors at the time of and immediately after the surgery.

- Any existing uveitis should be controlled when possible before surgery is contemplated.
- The patient should be known to be able to tolerate cholinesterase inhibitors.
- The patient should be warned of postoperative blurring of vision for at least the first week with the likelihood of some degree of hyphema.

Anesthesia

Local anesthesia with a retrobulbar and facial block or general anesthesia can be used.

Technique

Cyclodialysis is normally performed in the upper temporal quadrant where possible and a previous iridectomy site should be avoided (to reduce the risk of rupturing the vitreous face). The conjunctival incision is made approximately 5 to 6 mm posterior to the limbus. Cautery is applied to the superficial sclera and a two-thirds thickness scleral incision made 3 to 4 mm long, circumferentially. A preplaced suture, such as 8-0 polyglactin, is positioned, and the dissection through the deepest third of the sclera is cautiously performed avoiding penetration of the ciliary body with the tip of the knife and reducing the risk of hemorrhage. A paracentesis is made into the anterior chamber at this stage. The cyclodialysis spatula is introduced into the scleral incision and advanced radially forward, between sclera and uvea. This procedure should be gentle with the tip up against the sclera to avoid bleeding. A cleft is produced as far as the scleral spur and the adhesion between the ciliary body and the scleral spur is broken gently so that the tip can be seen entering the anterior chamber for a distance of 2 to 3 mm.

It is important to make sure that the cornea is not dissected as the spatula enters the anterior chamber. The handle of the spatula is rotated (Fig. 17-1) so that the anterior end of the blade sweeps the iris surface on each side of its point of entry, opening the angle and tearing the iris from its attachment to the sclera rather than damaging the iris root itself (again likely to produce more bleeding). The cyclodialysis separation is made for approximately one-quarter to one-fifth of the circumference of the limbus; after withdrawal of the spatula the anterior chamber should be filled with balanced salt solution

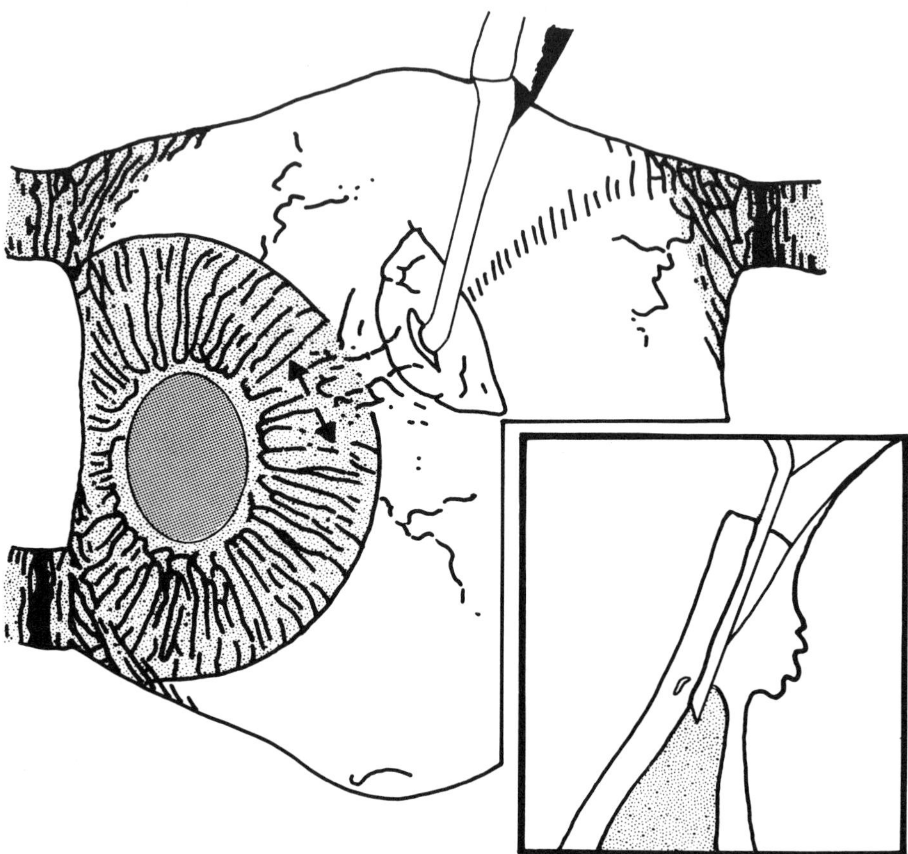

Figure 17-1. Cyclodialysis: beneath the conjunctival flap a small circumferential schleral incision is made into the supra choroidal space and a cyclodialysis spatula is passed anteriorly into the anterior chamber separating the ciliary body from the scleral spur. (Adapted from Shields, M.B.: A Study Guide for Glaucoma. Courtesy of Williams & Wilkins.)

using the paracentesis track. The scleral incision is closed with the preplaced 8-0 polyglactin sutures after the globe has been restored to a normal tension. Echothiophate is instilled at the end of the procedure; 0.125% in blue eyes and 0.25% in brown eyes. The use of viscoelastic left in the anterior chamber at the end of the procedure has not been shown to be helpful in reducing hemorrhage by tamponade.

This technique is a description of the fundamental method of making a cyclodialysis cleft by the external approach[6,7,8] but many modifications have been used, some including the use of setons.[9]

Postoperative Care

The patient is positioned on the side away from the cyclodialysis cleft to reduce the risk of a blood clot sealing the opening. Echothiophate is instilled every three hours for the first three days and twice daily for an indefinite period in an endeavor to maintain the cleft. Because of this long-term use of echothiophate (which itself might not be tolerated), phenylephrine 2.5% at night has been recommended to reduce the risk of iris cysts. An antibiotic steroid combination drop is instilled every three hours for the first three days and then four times a day until cessation of postoperative inflammation.

Assessment of the success of the procedure is usually possible by one month after surgery. A good prognosis exists where there is a visible cleft (Fig. 17-2) with no evidence of active inflammation and a continued normal IOP of around 15 mm Hg. Continued function normally requires the long-term use of echothiophate 0.125% twice a day.

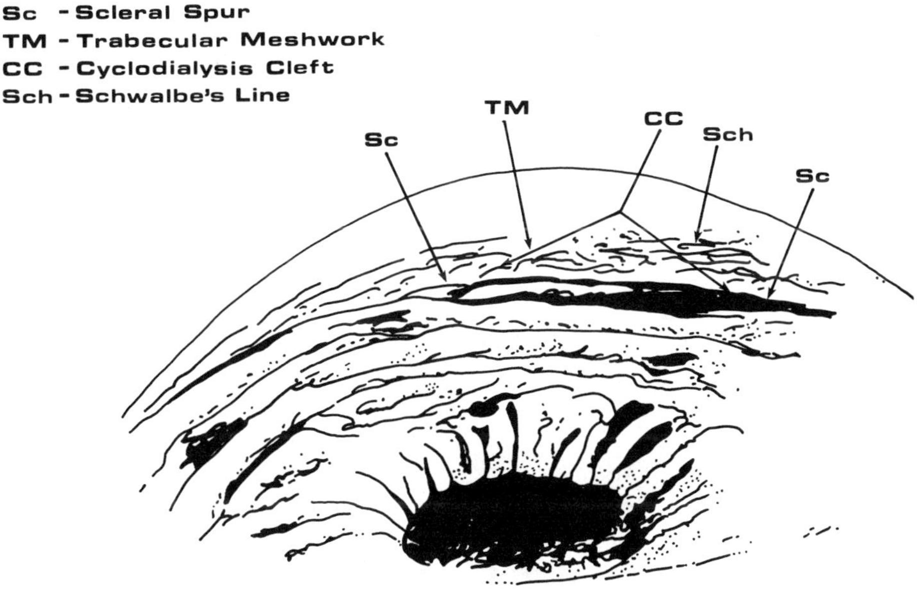

Sc - Scleral Spur
TM - Trabecular Meshwork
CC - Cyclodialysis Cleft
Sch - Schwalbe's Line

Figure 17-2. A gonioscopic feature of a cyclodialysis cleft which has been established. The cleft links the supra choroidal space with the anterior chamber of the eye. (Adapted from Becker-Shaffer: Diagnosis and Therapy of the Glaucomas, Fourth Edition. Courtesy of C.V. Mosby Co.)

A literature review of results suggests that with cyclodialysis alone, no more than a 50% success rate can be hoped for[3,4,10] and if anything, surprisingly, there is a higher success rate of around 75% in the combined procedure.[11-14] As the procedure has fallen into disuse, it would seem likely that the longer term results are poorer than suggested by the literature.

Significant variations in techniques include:

1. The combination of cyclodialysis has been performed with various implants that allow external filtration in addition to the effects of the dialysis itself. One of the classical examples is cycloretraction or iridocycloretraction described by Krasnov[6] in which two scleral strips are inserted along the cleft acting as an autogenous implant.
2. Cyclodialysis can form part of the method of function of trabeculectomy described by Watson[15] in which the internal sclerostomy extends further posteriorly to the scleral spur unroofing the anterior surface of the ciliary body. It is believed that this allows some aqueous absorption

into the suprachoroidal space as well as having the advantages of a filtering sclerostomy. The results and complications of this procedure are described in Chapters 13 and 14.

3. Q switched lasers, notably ruby and Nd:YAG, have been used to attempt to lower IOP in open angle glaucoma by dissecting (through a contact lens) into the anterior chamber angle. Trabeculopuncture (entering the trabecular meshwork),[16] goniopuncture (entering into Schlemms' canal and collection channels),[16] and cyclodialysis (creating a cyclodialysis cleft by laser),[17] have all been described and might be very similar. They have largely been unsuccessful.
4. Trabeculodialysis is a technique of modified goniotomy introduced to help in the management of secondary glaucoma from uveitis.[18] It is performed by introducing an irrigating goniotomy needle across the anterior chamber through a stab incision in the cornea at the opposite side of the eye. The needle is then passed across the anterior chamber normally into the inferior angle from above. Any synechiae are retracted and an incision is made posterior to Schwalbe's line with retraction of the trabeculum. This incision made over one quadrant of the eye can work partly by creating a cyclodialysis cleft from an internal approach. It has been shown to be safe and useful in the management of inflammatory glaucoma and in the particularly difficult problem of patients with juvenile chronic arthritis.[19] The procedure can be repeated and the complications are similar to cyclodialysis in that hyphema and exacerbation of intercurrent uveitis are not uncommon. Similarly, the success rate is around 50%.

Complications

Intraoperative Complications

Hemorrhage. The most common complication (Table 17-3) with this procedure is hemorrhage.[20] There can be slight hemorrhage during dissection of the sclera, but this is normally avoided with preparatory diathermy before incision. More massive bleeding can occur if the deeper scleral layer is cut too aggressively and the surface of the ciliary body is disturbed. This can be avoided as described in the technique by ensuring good visualization with a preplaced suture in the lip of the scleral incision. Gentle dissection is the key to performing the initial sclerostomy.

With the introduction of the cyclodialysis spatula, the ciliary body itself can again be torn; this can be avoided by keeping the spatula close to the sclera with the heel down against the outside surface and the end of the spatula close to the inner surface of the sclera as it slides into the anterior chamber.

During the same procedure, an anterior ciliary artery can be torn, but this should be avoidable by making the incision in midquadrant. Massive bleeding can occur occasionally when entering the anterior chamber, and the rapid introduction of an air bubble into the anterior chamber through an air cannula must be performed to tamponade the bleeding by maintaining IOP. A few minutes should be allowed before proceeding to complete the operation.

Table 17-3. Complications of Cyclodialysis

1. Intraocular bleeding.
2. Failure with worsening of vision.
3. Hypotony.
4. Stripping of Descemet's membrane.
5. Late development of cataract.
6. Rupture of lens capsule.
7. Persistent uveitis.

Despite the greatest of care, a small hyphema is almost routine in this procedure and is probably produced by tearing small iris vessels at the separation of the iris from the scleral spur.

Corneal damage. If the cyclodialysis spatula is not gently introduced into the anterior chamber and pushed too anteriorly, it can impinge on the cornea, separating Descemet's membrane, which can uncoil, or there can easily be direct damage to the corneal endothelium in a localized area. Less seriously, slight penetration of the stroma itself can occur. If this occurs, the spatula should be withdrawn and reintroduced more posteriorly.

Iris damage. The iris can be torn, producing an iridotomy or iridodialysis, if the anterior end of the spatula dips too posteriorly. Apart from bleeding from the iris, this can result in rupturing the vitreous face posteriorly in an aphakic eye or the lens capsule in a phakic eye.

Vitreous loss. The hyaloid face can be ruptured to produce vitreous loss in an aphakic eye. This normally can be avoided with careful observation of the anterior hyaloid face and by avoiding the site of a previous iridectomy, but if it does occur, it would require an anterior vitrectomy.

Damage to the crystalline lens. In the phakic eye, the lens capsule can be damaged, producing a local cataract or when more severe can result in general cataract formation developing subsequently.

Postoperative Complications

Early

Anterior Segment Hemorrhage. Normally, a small amount of hyphema is present but should resolve within the first few days postoperatively. A major anterior hemorrhage can be treated as any other traumatic hyphema with its possibly serious outcome.

Hypotony. One of the problems of cyclodialysis is that if it works, it might work too well. Postoperative hypotony can occur despite an apparent technically satisfactory procedure with a resultant serous choroidal effusion and the possibility of subsequent cystoid macular edema. Treatment of the choroidal detachment should be expectant unless the anterior chamber shallowing results in vitreo-corneal or lens-corneal contact or if it fails to resolve after several weeks. In this case, drainage of the choroidal detachment by posterior sclerotomy and reformation of the anterior chamber is required. Sometimes the choroidal effusion might be hemorrhagic and this should be treated similarly. It can be distinguished by transillumination or, of course, by the drainage of blood if sclerotomy is required and usually the patient is more likely to complain of pain.

Retinal Detachment. Retinal detachment is a rare complication that can occur in any intraocular procedure and requires treatment as appropriate. It is likely to result in failure of the cyclodialysis cleft.

Uveitis. Uveitis to some degree must always occur in the early postoperative period. The frequent use of topical steroids, usually in combination with antibiotics, is sufficient to control the inflammation. Echothiophate itself enhances vascular permeability, encouraging a fibrinous aqueous.

Complications of the Use of Cholinesterase Inhibitors. Sometimes, in the early postoperative period, the intense use of cholinesterase inhibitors will produce classical overactivity of the parasympathetic system.

Any of these symptoms, if severe, will necessitate discontinuation of the treatment which again jeopardizes success.

Late Complications

Failure with worsening of vision. The most common late complication is failure to control IOP, which occurs in around 50% of cases. The cleft can be seen to be healed or have associated synechial closure and result in consideration of further surgical or additional medical treatment.

Cataract. All intraocular procedures will increase the risk of cataract developing, although without direct contact of the lens surface, the frequency of producing cataract is difficult to quantify because many of these patients already have some degree of lens opacity and there are so many factors involved in the progression of lens opacities.

Hypotony. Prolonged hypotony can result in chronic cystoid macular edema or even phthisis.

In conclusion, the list of complications of cyclodialysis is significant and changes in surgical approach have rendered the procedure largely historical. Where all else has failed, there might be justification for its use.

References

1. Heine I. Die Cyclodialyse, ein Neue Glaukomoperation. Dtsch Med Wochenschr 31:834, 1905.
2. Elschnig A. Augenartzliche Operationslehre, Handbucke, Augenheilkunde, Spring, Berlin Vol.2, 1922.
3. Spaeth G.L. Ophthalmic Surgery, Principles and Practice, Philadelphia: Saunders, 1982, p. 322.
4. Sugar H.S. Experiences with some modifications of cyclodialysis for aphakic glaucoma. Ann Ophthalmol 9:1045-1052, 1977.
5. Chandler PA, Grant WM. Glaucoma 2nd Ed. Philadelphia: Lea & Febiger, 1979 p. 309.
6. Krasnov MM. Iridocyclo-Retraction. Br J Ophthalmol 55:389, 1971.
7. Aviner Z. Modified Krasnov's iridocyclo-retraction for aphakic glaucoma. Am Ophthalmol 7:859, 1975.
8. Ackerman J, Kanarek I, et al. A new approach to aphakic glaucoma a sub scleral filtering cyclodialysis. Glaucoma 1:176, 1979.
9. Gills JP. Cyclodialysis implants in humans. Am J Ophthalmol 61:841, 1966.
10. Paufique L, Sourdille PW. Arch Ophthalmol 79:551, 1969.
11. Sheilds MB, Simmons RJ. Combined cyclodialysis and cataract extraction. Trans Am Acad Ophthalmol Otolaryngol 81:286, 1976.
12. Simmons RJ, Thomas JV et al. Surgical indications and options in the management of co-existing glaucoma and cataract. Glaucoma 4(3) 92-98, 1982.
13. Galin M, Baras I, Sambursky J. Glaucoma and cataract—a study of cyclodialysis-lens extraction. Am J Ophthalmol 67:522, 1969.
14. McAllister JA, Spaeth GL. Intracapsular cataract extraction with cyclodialysis—a useful procedure. Klin Monatsbl Augenheild: p. 283-286, 1984.
15. Watson P. Trabeculectomy, a modified externo technique. Am Ophthalmol 2:199-203, 1970.
16. Van der Zypen E, Fankhauser F. The ultra structural features of laser trabeculopuncture and cyclodialysis. Ophthalmologica 179:189-200, 1979.
17. Krasnov MN. Q. switched laser goniopuncture. Arch Ophthalmol 92:37-41, 1974.
18. Hoskins HD, Hetherington J, Shaffer RN. Surgical management of the inflammatory glaucomas. Perspect Ophthalmol 1:173-181, 1977.
19. McAllister JA, Kanski, JJ. Trabeculodialysis for inflammatory glaucoma in children and young adults. Ophthalmol 92:(7), 1985.
20. Chandler PA, Grant WM. Glaucoma 2nd Ed. Philadelphia: Lea and Febiger, p. 307, 1979.

CHAPTER 18

Cyclocryotherapy

Joseph Caprioli, MD

Introduction

Cyclocryotherapy was introduced as an alternative treatment for intractable glaucoma by Bietti in 1950.[1] Since then, cyclocryotherapy largely replaced cyclodiathermy as the preferred technique of cycloablation for the treatment of advanced glaucoma. Early experimental studies demonstrated that structural and functional alterations produced by freezing the ciliary body caused substantial reductions of IOP. These studies provided support for the clinical use of cyclocryotherapy in open and closed angle glaucomas, glaucoma in aphakic eyes, neovascular glaucoma, glaucoma after penetrating keratoplasty, and congenital glaucoma. The relatively unpredictable results and high complication rates have generally caused cyclocryotherapy to be reserved for desperate cases of advanced glaucoma in aphakic eyes and for neovascular glaucoma. New techniques of filtering surgery, combined with the administration of antimetabolites such as 5-fluorouracil, offer an alternative for cases previously thought to be unoperable, and might further limit the use of cycloablation. This chapter will summarize the structural and functional effects of cyclocryotherapy on the eye and will review clinical techniques and results.

Anatomical and Physiological Alterations After Cyclocryotherapy

Temperatures

Early experimental studies of cyclocryotherapy were performed on rabbits and employed a variety of techniques. Cryosurgical probes were initially constructed of hollow metal cylinders that contained a mixture of dry ice and acetone or alcohol. These probes reached temperatures of approximately -80°C.[1,2] Later, liquid nitrogen probes provided probe temperatures which were variable from −20°C to −120°C.[3-7] Transscleral freezing sufficient to cause reproducible tissue disruption in the ciliary body required probe temperatures of −80°C or colder,[3] equivalent to ciliary body temperatures of approximately −7°C.[6] Much lower probe temperatures (−160°C) produced lower ciliary body temperatures (approximately −28°C) and caused extensive destruction and necrosis of the anterior segment.[6] A large temperature sink is provided by the high rate of ciliary blood flow. This requires very low probe temperatures to freeze the ciliary process, and limits the area of frozen tissue.[1,8] In enucleated monkey eyes, the lowest attainable ciliary body temperatures were 30° to 40°C lower than that in living monkey eyes for the same probe temperature.[8] This demonstrates the capacity of uveal blood flow to attenuate the steady state tissue temperature, at least in healthy monkey eyes. The temperature of the ciliary body reaches equilibrium 10 to 20 seconds after application of the cryoprobe to the sclera.[8] Freezing for periods greater than one minute does not expand the area of frozen ciliary tissue.[3]

Anatomical alterations

Histological examination of rabbit eyes immediately after transcleral ciliary freezing revealed marked edema, vasodilation, hemorrhage into the ciliary muscle and stroma, protein leakage into the anterior chamber, hyphema, and detachment of the ciliary epithelium with disintegration of the cells.[1-5] Similar anatomical changes were visible immediately after transcleral ciliary freezing in monkey eyes.

After resolution of the acute inflammatory response in the rabbit eyes, Bietti found atrophy of the ciliary body, resolution of the ciliary epithelial detachment with some disruption of its pigment, and mild irregularities to the thickness of the ciliary epithelium.[1] Rapid regeneration of the ciliary epithelium was noted in albino rabbits; the only visible alteration one week later was mild hyalinization of the subepithelial stromal vessels.[2,4,5] McLean and Lincoff noted no significant ciliary epithelial regeneration in pigmented rabbits,[3] and subsequent work showed that pigmented eyes demonstrated more tissue destruction after freezing than nonpigmented eyes.[5,7] Ciliary epithelial regeneration generally occurred in rabbits within two weeks after treatment. Permanent morphologic alterations included decreased stromal vascularity of the ciliary processes and some scattering of pigment throughout the ciliary body from disrupted pigmented epithelium.[1,2,5,7] Monkey eyes examined one to three months after treatment revealed flattening of the ciliary processes which were replaced with fibroblast-like cells, and absence of tight junctions between the nonpigmented epithelial cells. The trabecular meshwork suffered some endothelial damage that healed without sequelae, although the caliber of Schlemm's canal and the aqueous channels were decreased. Complete restoration of normal ciliary body morphology in monkeys uniformly occurred within 2 months after ciliary freezing in one study.[9] Electron microscopic examination of monkey eyes after cyclocryosurgery revealed proliferation of retinal pigment epithelial cells and glial cells from the region of the ora serrata, forming a mesh-like structure between the ciliary processes and the crystalline lens.[10] Proliferation and posterior migration of the equatorial lens epithelium was detected after cyclocryosurgery in rabbits and monkeys, though the lenses remained clear to gross examination.[4,8]

The structural alterations after cyclocryotherapy in human eyes has been studied by examining eyes enucleated at various times after treatment. The findings varied substantially. Quigley studied four enucleated human eyes after cyclocryotherapy.[8] Of these, two were removed immediately after treatment, the others four weeks and eleven weeks after treatment. Acute histologic findings included stromal edema, hemorrhage, and separation of the ciliary epithelium from the stroma. Eyes enucleated one to three months after treatment showed less of the ciliary processes. These were replaced by a mixed population of fibroblasts and pigmented cells that lacked tight junctions. No capillaries were present in the ciliary process stroma. Ferry studied 12 human eyes enucleated 12 days to 4 1/2 years after treatment.[11] Destruction and scarring of both layers of ciliary epithelium was present in all cases. The pigmented epithelium showed more evidence of damage than the nonpigmented epithelium. Chronic histologic changes also included scarring of the ciliary body muscle and the presence of a fibrous membrane overlying the ciliary body. Smith and coworkers observed variable morphologic changes 2 months to 2 1/2 years after cyclocryotherapy in three human eyes.[9] Structural abnormalities were completely absent in one eye; clinically, the same eye had a poor IOP response to treatment. Certain eyes, perhaps those of young healthy patients, might be capable of ciliary epithelial regeneration and might not realize a permanent reduction of IOP.

Physiological alterations

The physiological effects of cyclocryosurgery have not been well studied. Immediately after treatment, there is a rapid influx of plasmoid aqueous into the eye through the injured ciliary epithelium,[1,4,12] that contributes to an acute elevation of IOP immediately following treatment.[1,4,13] This hypertensive phase usually lasts between 2 and 6 hours and is followed by a hypotensive phase associated with visible anterior chamber inflammation. The inflammatory component usually resolves and the IOP stabilizes over the subsequent 2 to 4 weeks.

Alterations in aqueous humor dynamics after cyclocryotherapy have been studied with tonography in rabbits and monkeys. Small decreases in outflow facility have generally been measured.[2,3,7] Relatively larger decreases in aqueous production are held responsible for IOP reduction. Although potential changes in uveoscleral flow have not been studied, increased pressure-independent flow might be a factor, especially in eyes that become profoundly hypotonous.

Oxygen uptake studies in isolated rabbit iris-ciliary body preparations indicate a decrease of respiratory rate by 40% after cyclocryotherapy.[6] Blood flow to treated areas of rabbit ciliary body decreased by 50% compared to untreated controls.[14] In untreated areas, blood flow doubled compared to controls. This phenomenon was attributed to the shunting of blood from treated to untreated portions of the ciliary body. An alternative, perhaps more realistic explanation is that decreased IOP in the treated eyes might account for increased blood flow measured in the untreated areas because uveal blood flow is not autoregulated.

Rabbits pretreated with aspirin had lower levels of aqueous protein after cyclocryotherapy compared to control eyes. This suggested a role for prostaglandins in the cryosurgically induced inflammatory response.[12] However, permanent morphologic alterations induced by cyclocryosurgery in rabbits treated with aspirin did not differ from untreated eyes.[15]

Clinical Studies

A number of clinical reports document the use of cyclocryotherapy in uncontrolled glaucoma.[16,23] deRoetth reported the results of cyclocryotherapy in the treatment of advanced open angle glaucoma.[16] Six applications were made over the inferior half of the globe with a cryosurgical probe at −80°C; the superior half was treated if additional pressure reduction was required. Of the 141 eyes treated with one session of cryosurgery, 57% achieved a postoperative IOP less than 20 mm Hg. An additional 60 eyes required more than one treatment, of which 73% achieved a postoperative intraocular pressure less than 20 mm Hg.

Bellows and Grant studied cyclocryotherapy in 61 eyes with advanced uncontrolled open angle glaucoma. secondary glaucomas, neovascular glaucoma, childhood glaucomas (including congenital glaucoma), and angle closure glaucoma.[17] Overall, 59% of eyes had a reduction of intraocular pressure to less than 20 mm Hg. The group of patients with neovascular glaucoma had the worst IOP control and the highest frequency of complications. Later, Bellows and Grant reported long-term follow-up of cyclocryotherapy in 25 patients with aphakic open angle glaucoma.[18] Control was defined as a postoperative pressure less than 20 mm Hg and was achieved in 92% of all eyes.

Cyclocryotherapy has been considered by some to be the treatment of choice for neovascular glaucoma.[19,20] Despite control of IOP in patients with neovascular glaucoma with one or more treatments of cyclocryotherapy, the visual prognosis remains poor.[19,22] Krupin and coworkers analyzed the long-term results of cyclocryotherapy in 50 eyes of 46 patients with neovascular glaucoma.[21] A high incidence of loss of light perception (58%) and phthisis bulbi (34%) was reported. Significant alleviation of ocular pain was attributed to the procedure in the majority of patients. This might be related more to interruption of the sensory nerve supply rather than to adequate reduction of IOP.[23] The need for other forms of therapy in these eyes is widely recognized, because of the high incidence of serious complications including hypotony, phthisis bulbi, choroidal hemorrhage, hyphema, cataract, retinal detachment, and anterior segment ischemia. The morbidity following the procedure, however, might be more related to the devastating consequences of the disease itself rather than to the treatment per se.

Caprioli and coworkers reported the results of cyclocryotherapy in the treatment of advanced glaucoma in 96 eyes of 96 patients.[22] All patients had follow-up greater than 12 months (mean SEM = 29.0 ± 2.1 months). Three diagnostic groups were studied: aphakic open angle glaucoma, aphakic angle closure glaucoma, and neovascular glaucoma (phakic and aphakic). IOP was lowered to less than 21 mm Hg in 76% of eyes with aphakic open angle glaucoma, in 68% of eyes with angle closure glaucoma, and in 55% of eyes with neovascular glaucoma (see Table 18-1).

Table 18-1. Results of Cyclocryotherapy

Data	Aphakic Open Angle	Aphakic Angle-Closure	Neovascular	All
Follow-up(months)*	33.4 ± 1.8	28.4 ± 2.3	27.3 ± 1.9	29.0 ± 2.1
Preoperative IOP (mmHg)*	31.4 ± 2.0	31.4 ± 1.6	48.9 ± 3.1	41.2 ± 1.3
Final IOP (mmHg)*	18.6 ± 3.3	18.4 ± 1.4	19.4 ± 3.2	18.7 ± 1.2
Eyes with final IOP < 21 mmHg	13 (76%)	40 (68%)	11 (55%)	64 (67%)
Acuity change (lines)	−0.88 ± .54	−0.86 ± .37	−1.5 ± .29	−1.02 ± .26
Vision worse	7 (41%)	24 (41%)	14 (70%)	45 (47%)
Progression to NLP vision	3 (18%)	5 (8%)	6 (30%)	14 (15%)
Visual field worse*	4/14 (29%)	17/48 (35%)	10/14 (71%)	31/76 (41%)
Postoperative glaucoma medications*	1.20 ± .29	1.63 ± .17	0.76 ± .22	1.33 ± .13

IOP = intraocular pressure; NLP = no light perception.

* Values are expressed as mean SEM

(Modified from Caprioli J, Strang SL, Spaeth GL, Poryzees EH. Cyclocryotherapy in the treatment of glaucoma. Ophthalmol 92:947-954, 1985, published with permission, J.B. Lippincott Company).

Patients with neovascular glaucoma lost vision more frequently (70%) than patients with aphakic open angle glaucoma (41%) or patients with aphakic angle closure glaucoma (41%). The neovascular glaucoma group had the highest incidence of light perception loss and phthisis bulbi. In patients who had adequate visual field examinations (76 of 96 eyes), glaucomatous visual field loss was arrested in 71% of patients with open angle glaucoma, in 65% of patients with angle closure glaucoma, and in 29% of patients with neovascular glaucoma. There was a significant correlation between a postoperative IOP of less than 21 mm Hg and preservation of the visual field.

Clinical Technique

Cyclocryotherapy has been performed with a variety of techniques. The most reproducible and predictable results can be obtained when a standard method is used. One of the most useful methods is described here. Glaucoma medications are continued until the time of treatment, which can be performed without hospital admission. A topical corticosteroid is administered for three days preceeding treatment when possible. A retrobulbar injection of 4.0 cc of 0.75% bupivacaine provides prolonged anesthesia and significantly decreases postoperative discomfort. A cyclocryothermy unit that uses nitrous oxide gas provides a portable, convenient method of freezing (Kry-Med. Inc.), though any unit that provides a constant and reproducible probe temperature of −80°C is theoretically satisfactory. Transcleral freezing at this temperature achieves ciliary body temperatures of approximately −10°C within 10 to 15 seconds after application of the probe.

A probe diameter of 2.5 to 3.0 mm is used, though larger probes have been designed for retinal and ciliary cryosurgery.[24] The smaller probes allow optimal localization over the pars plicata. The probe is placed on the sclera directly over the pars plicata, usually leaving 2.0 to 2.5 mm between the limbus and the proximal edge of the probe, making sure firm contact is made. Each freeze is performed for 60 seconds. The correct placement of the probe is usually more anterior than is generally appreciated (see Fig. 18-1). In patients with unusually large or small eyes the exact location of the ciliary body might be in doubt. It is helpful in these cases to transilluminate the globe to visualize the pars plicata directly. In eyes previously treated with cyclocryotherapy, untreated areas of the ciliary body sometimes can be identified by this technique. The treated areas contain less pigment and will transilluminate, while untreated areas will be seen as a dark band.

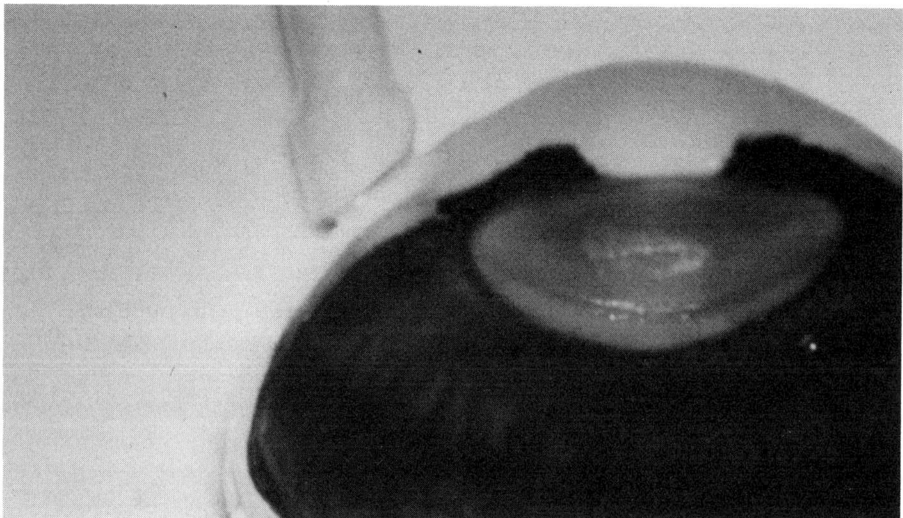

Figure 18-1. The correct placement of the cryosurgical probe in relationship to the pars plicata is demonstrated on an enucleated human eye.

Six equally spaced freezes are placed over 180° of the ciliary body. The initial treatment session is generally confined to the inferior half of the globe. If initial treatment fails to control IOP adequately, subsequent treatments are applied over the temporal 180° and finally over the superior 180°. Some clinicians prefer to leave a small portion of the ciliary body untreated in an effort to decrease the likelihood of postoperative phthisis bulbi.[18]

Patients are placed on topical atropine and corticosteroids. Previously used glaucoma medications are continued with the exception of miotics. IOP is monitored carefully during the first six hours after treatment, and significant elevations of pressure are treated with CAIs and/or osmotic agents. Topical atropine and corticosteroids are adjusted and tapered over the subsequent weeks depending on the degree of anterior segment inflammation. Glaucoma medications are adjusted as necessary to adequately control IOP; it is often possible to decrease or eliminate medications in the treated eye. It should be emphasized that great individual variability regarding the susceptability of the optic nerve to further damage requires careful visual field examination preoperatively and postoperatively whenever such testing is feasible. The visual field should be used as the critical outcome parameter whenever possible, rather than an arbitrarily set level of IOP.

Complications

Extensive anterior chamber reaction is a normal accompaniment of cyclocryotherapy in the immediate postoperative period. This can be associated with hyphema, especially in cases of neovascular glaucoma. Aqueous flare can persist for months or years because of chronic leakage of protein through disrupted tight junctions of the nonpigmented ciliary epithelium. Indeed, the presence of chronic aqueous flare might correlate with a permanent reduction of IOP. Cellular reaction in the anterior chamber usually resolves in several weeks. Acute cellular inflammation can be managed with topical cycloplegics and corticosteroids. In rabbits, the magnitude of the inflammatory response was found to be decreased by pretreatment with aspirin.[12] In humans, aspirin might increase the incidence of hemorrhage in cases of neovascular glaucoma and is not recommended. However, several days of pretreatment with topical corticosteroids might help blunt the inflammatory response, and should be administered when feasible.

Complications attributed to cyclocryotherapy by Bellows and Grant[17,18] were hyphema, choroidal detachment, retinal detachment, vitreous hemorrhage, chronic hypotony, unexplained loss of vision, transient elevation of IOP, intractable uveitis, macular edema, and corneal dellen. The overall complication rate was 27% in aphakic open angle glaucoma patients. Krupin and colleagues reported four cases of anterior segment ischemia after cyclocryotherapy for neovascular glaucoma in 50 eyes. In these eyes, 12 applications were made over the entire 360° circumference of the globe. Extensive cyclocryosurgery might further compromise a chronic ischemic ocular state and cause anterior segment necrosis. It therefore seems prudent to treat only a portion of the ciliary body at any given time. Retinal detachment,[17,25] ciliary body staphyloma,[26] and choroidal detachment with flattening of the anterior chamber[27] have also been reported after cyclocryotherapy for glaucoma.

Data from one study regarding serious postoperative complications and the need for additional cyclocryotherapy is summarized in Table 18-2.[22] Eyes which received initial 180° treatment required further treatment more frequently (52%) than eyes that received initial 360° treatment (24%). Hypotony was differentiated from phthisis bulbi (atrophy and shrinkage of the globe with loss of visual function) and was not considered a complication when it did not progress to phthisis. Postoperative phthisis bulbi occurred slightly more frequently in the 360° treatment group. Other complications included persistent inflammation, corneal decompensation, persistent pain requiring

Table 18-2. Results of 360° and 180° Initial Cyclocryotherapy and Complications

	Aphakic Open-Angle	Aphakic Angle-Closure	Neovascular	Total
INITIAL TREATMENT				
360°	9	29	12	50
Needed further CCT	2	7	3	12
Hypotony (without phthisis)	1	5	2	8
Complications				
Phthisis bulbi	2	2	2	6
Persistent inflammation	0	2	0	2
Corneal decompensation	0	3	0	3
Enucleation	1	2	0	3
Other	0	0	1 (CD)	1
Total	3	9	3	15
INITIAL TREATMENT				
180°	8	30	8	46
Needed further CCT	0	18	6	24
Hypotony (without phthisis)	2	4	1	7
Complications				
Phthisis bulbi	0	1	2	3
Persistent inflammation	0	2	0	2
Corneal decompensation	1	1	0	2
Enucleation	0	0	0	0
Other	0	2 (ME,PT)	0	2
Total	1	6	2	9
Total Complications (180° and 360° groups)	4 (24%)	15 (25°)	5 (24%)	24

CCT = cyclocryotherapy; CD = persistent choroidal detachment; ME = persistent macular edema; PT = ptosis

(Modified from Caprioli J, Strang SL, Spaeth GL, Poryzees EH. Cyclocryotherapy in the treatment of glaucoma. Ophthalmol 92:947-954, 1985 with permission).

enucleation, choroidal detachment, macular edema, and ptosis. Complications were more frequent in the group that received initial 360° treatment, (30%) then in the group that received initial 180° treatment (20%). Phthisis bulbi occurred most frequently in the neovascular glaucoma group. Hypotony without phthisis might be desirable in some patients with far advanced glaucoma who required very low pressures to arrest progressive visual field loss. Loss of light perception occurred in a substantial number of patients. This included 18% of the open angle aphakic eyes, 8% of the aphakic angle closure eyes, and 30% of the neovascular eyes.

Acute IOP elevation following treatment is of concern in patients with far advanced visual field loss. The marginal function of only a few surviving retinal ganglion cell axons might be compromised by an acute pressure increase. Cyclocryotherapy caused marked increases of IOP intraoperatively as well as postoperatively.[13] Intraoperatively, IOPs increase to between 60 and 80 mmHg during the freezing phase of cyclocryotherapy, then decrease to baseline values during the thaw phase (see Fig. 18-2). These IOP spikes can be avoided by cannulation of the anterior chamber and regulation of the IOP with a fluid filled reservoir connected to the cannula.[13] It is not known for certain what effect brief IOP spikes from cyclocryotherapy might have on an

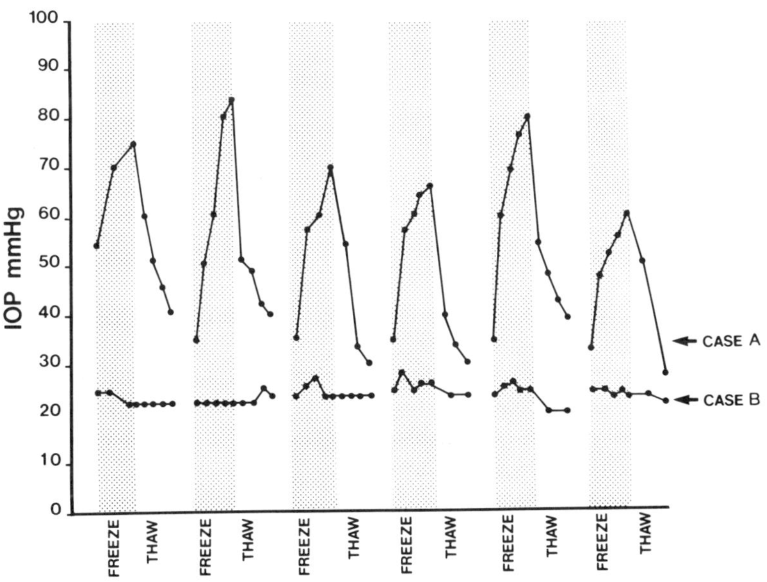

Figure 18-2. IOP during cyclocryotherapy. The shaded areas represent freeze cycles (60 seconds), and the adjacent unshaded areas represent thaw cycles (60 seconds). There was a period of approximately 30 seconds between the end of a thaw and the beginning of the next freeze. In case A a standard method of cyclocryotherapy was used and in case B manometric regulation of intraocular pressure was achieved. (Modified from Caprioli J, Sears M. Regulation of intraocular pressure during cyclocryotherapy for advanced glaucoma. Am J Ophthalmol 101:542-545, 1986. Published with permission.)

extensively damaged optic nerves. However, manometric regulation of IOP during the procedure might protect seriously compromised nerves from further damage, and might represent a safer method of treatment in these eyes.

New Cycloablative Techniques

In addition to cyclocryotherapy, transcleral cyclodestruction can be achieved with cyclodiathermy and cyclophotocoagulation with the ruby or Nd:YAG laser.[28,29] Cyclodiathermy for the treatment of glaucoma largely has been abandoned because of the overwhelming ocular inflammatory response and scleral necrosis that do not infrequently follow this procedure. Transcleral cyclophotocoagulation is discussed at length in Chapter 10.

Utilization of the transcleral route has the advantage of being less invasive than intraocular cyclophotocoagulation and is relatively easy. The most important disadvantage is the inability to visually monitor the tissue being treated and therefore recognize the treatment endpoint. A similar lack of standardization with cyclocryotherapy contributes to the rather poor predictability of the results.

Transpupillary cyclophotocoagulation[30] has been used to directly photocoagulate individual ciliary process with the assistance of a gonioscopic lens. Major disadvantages are the inability to treat the entire length of the ciliary process and difficult visualization even in eyes that are well dilated. With the advent of modern vitrectomy techniques and the ability to safely perform endolaser photocoagulation, endolaser cyclophotocoagulation for the treatment of glaucoma has been developed as an alternative technique.[31,33] The advantages offered by this method include enhanced visualization of the ciliary processes and a visible treatment reaction. Limiting factors are the need for a relatively clear cornea and a well dilated pupil. Because transpupillary visualization is frequently not optimal, the possibility of using an intraocular endoscope has been explored experimentally.[32,33] Important aspects regarding transpupillary and endoscopic endolaser cyclophotocoagulation require additional elaboration. Particularly important is knowledge of the optimal intensity and quantity of treatment needed to produce a desired clinical effect, and the definition of an appropriate treatment endpoint. Once this additional information has been acquired, the clinical utility of the newer techniques can be defined and compared to cyclocryotherapy for the treatment of advanced glaucoma.

Acknowledgment

The author wishes to thank Drs. Robert Bellows, Bruce Shields, and Kathleen Stoessel for reviewing this chapter.

References

1. Bietti G. Surgical intervention on the ciliary body. JAMA, 142:889-897, 1950.

2. Polack FM, de Roetth A Jr. Effect of freezing on the ciliary body (cyclocryotherapy). Invest Ophthalmol Vis Sci 3:164-170, 1964.
3. McLean JM, Lincoff HA, Cryosurgery of the ciliary body. Trans Am Ophthalmol Soc 62:385-407, 1964.
4. Conway J. Cryosurgery of the ciliary body. Proc Roy Soc Med 59:28-32, 1966.
5. Howard GM, deRoetth A Jr. Histopathologic changes following cryosurgery of the rabbit ciliary body. Am J Ophthalmol 64:700-707. 1967.
6. de Roetth A Jr. Ciliary body temperatures in cryosurgery. Arch Ophthalmol 85:204-210, 1971.
7. Edmonds C, de Roetth A Jr, Howard GM. Histopathologic changes following cryosurgery and diathermy of the rabbit ciliary body. Am J Ophthalmol 69:65-72, 1970.
8. Quigley HA. Histological and physiological studies of cyclocryotherapy in primate and human eyes. Am J Ophthalmol 82:722-732, 1976.
9. Smith RS, Boyle E, Rudt LA. Cyclocryotherapy. Arch Ophthalmol 95:284-288, 1977.
10. Yamishita H, Sears ML. Complications of cyclocryosurgery. Glaucoma 2:273-279, 1980.
11. Ferry AP. Histopathologic observations on human eyes following cyclocryotherapy for glaucoma. Trans Am Acad Ophthalmol Otolaryngol 83:90-113, 1977.
12. Chavis RM, Vygantas CM, Vygantas A. Experimental inhibition of prostaglandin-like inflammatory response after cryotherapy. Am J Ophthalmol 82:310-312, 1976.
13. Caprioli J, Sears M. Regulation of intraocular pressure during cyclocryotherapy for advanced glaucoma. Am J Ophthalmol 101:542-545, 1986.
14. Green K, Hull DS, Bowman K. Cyclocryotherapy and ocular blood flow. Glaucoma 1:141-144, 1979.
15. Haddad R, Grabner G, Braun F. Cyclocryokoagulation. Graefes Arch Ophthalmol 214:129-137, 1980.
16. deRoetth A Jr. Cryosurgery for the treatment of advanced chronic simple glaucoma. Am J Ophthalmol 66:1034-1041, 1968.
17. Bellows AR, Grant WM. Cyclocryotherapy in advanced inadequately controlled glaucoma. Am J Ophthalmol 75:679-684, 1973.
18. Bellows AR, Grant WM. Cyclocryotherapy of chronic open angle glaucoma in aphakic eyes. Am J Ophthalmol 85:615-621, 1978.
19. Feibel RM, Bigger JF. Rubeosis iridis and neovascular glaucoma. Am J Ophthalmol 74:862-867, 1972.
20. Boniuk M. Cryotherapy in neovascular glaucoma. Trans Am Acad Ophthalmol Otolaryngol 78:337-343, 1974.
21. Krupin T, Mitchell KB, Becker B. Cyclocryotherapy in neovascular glaucoma. Am J Ophthalmol 86:24-26, 1978.
22. Caprioli J, Strang SL, Spaeth GL, et al. Cyclocryotherapy in the treatment of advanced glaucoma. Ophthalmol 92:947-954, 1985.

23. Pinkerton RMH. The mechanism of symptomatic relief in cyclocryosurgery. Can J Ophthalmol 8:408-412, 1973.
24. Machemer R. Modified cryoprope for retinal detachment surgery and cyclocryotherapy. Am J Ophthalmol 83:123-124, 1977.
25. Burch PG, Morse PH. Retinal detachment following cyclocryothermy. Am J Ophthalmol 65:916-918. 1968.
26. Stewart RH, Garcia CA. Staphyloma following cyclocryotherapy. Ophthalmic Surg 5:28-29, 1974.
27. Kaiden JS, Serniuk RA, Bader BF. Choroidal detachment with flat anterior chamber after cyclocryotherapy. Ann Ophthalmol 1111-1113, 1979.
28. Beckman H, Kinoshita A, Rota AN, et al. Transscleral ruby laser irradiation of ciliary body in the treatment of intractable glaucoma. Trans Am Acad Ophthalmol Otolaryngol 76:423-436, 1972.
29. Fankhauser F, van der Zypen E, Kwasniewska S, et al. Transscleral cyclophotocoagulation using a Nd:Yag laser. Ophthalmic Surg 17:94-100, 1986.
30. Lee PF. Argon laser photocoagulation of the ciliary processes in cases of aphakic glaucoma. Arch Ophthalmol 97:2135-2138, 1979.
31. Shields MB, Chandler DB, Hickingbotham D, et al. Intraocular cyclophotocoagulation: histopathologic evaluation in primates. Arch Ophthalmol 103:1731-1735, 1985.
32. Shields MG. Cyclodestructive surgery for glaucoma: past, present and future. Trans Am Ophthalmol Soc 83:285-303, 1985.
33. Patel A, Thompson JT, Michels RG, et al. Endolaser treatment of the ciliary body for uncontrolled glaucoma. Ophthalmol 93:825-830, 1986.

CHAPTER 19

Congenital Glaucoma

L. Jay Katz, MD

History

During Hippocrates' time in the 4th Century B.C., physicians were aware of buphthalmic (Greek-ox eye) blindness, but it was not until 1869 that von Muralt recognized buphthalmos as a type of glaucoma.[1] As recently as 1939, a rather bleak prognosis was conceded despite treatment.[2] It became obvious that medical therapy was at most a temporizing solution until surgery. In 1893, deVincentiis attempted to incise the angle of glaucomatous eyes, but reported poor results.[3] The idea was successfully revived by Barkan in 1938 for congenital glaucoma, performing a goniotomy while visualizing the angle with a direct goniolens.[4] Goniotomy remains as the primary procedure for congenital glaucoma along with trabeculotomy ab externo, a procedure separately originated by Burian[5] and Smith[6] in the early 1960s.

Epidemiology and Pathogenesis

Congenital glaucoma can be divided into primary infantile or secondary associated with other ocular and systemic disorders.[7,8] Primary infantile glaucoma is quite rare, occurring in one out of 10,000 births.[8] Most are sporadic cases; however, familial transmission, usually by an autosomal gene, has been reported.[10-12] About three-quarters of the children have bilateral involvement.

There are several postulated mechanisms of IOP elevation.

Barkan thought that a membrane covered the angle which impeded aqueous outflow.[4] The membrane can be an embryonic remnant that would normally disappear with ocular maturation.[13] Histologic evidence has been lacking[14] because of preparation error or this may be the mechanism of glaucoma in only some of the cases.

Trabeculodysgenesis with anomalous development of the trabecular meshwork with an anterior iris insertion and thick iris processes (pectinate ligaments) has emerged as the prevailing theory for most cases of primary infantile congenital glaucoma.[14,15]

In the secondary congenital glaucomas, a variety of mechanisms exist. With Reiger's and Axenfeld's anomalies, an anterior chamber cleavage syndrome with iridocorneotrabeculodysgenesis exists. Elevated episcleral venous pressure retarding aqueous outflow, in some patients with Sturge-Weber syndrome, may result in "back pressure" glaucoma.[16]

Clinical Features

Signs

The classic triad of blepharospasm, epiphora, and photophobia can be attributed to corneal injury as a result of the elevated IOP.[17] With enlargement of the eye, breaks in Descemet's membrane (Haab's striae) can lead to symptomatic corneal edema.

Evaluation

In most situations a complete, meaningful examination must be performed under general anesthesia. Anesthesia can profoundly affect the IOP.[18-21] Halothane can rapidly lower the IOP to spurious values.[18,21] The agents that provide relatively "light" anesthesia have less effect on the IOP.[18-21] Ketamine has been strongly recommended for this property.[22,23] It is a potent analgesic effective within 10 minutes and lasting about 30 minutes. It does not lower IOP, but it elevates the IOP.[23]

A false IOP elevation noted with succinylcholine follows transient extraocular muscle contraction.[18] Therefore, the most accurate results occur with light anesthesia *before* succinylcholine administration and intubation. Special attention to the use of a long-acting anticholinesterase, such as phospholine iodide, is imperative when using succinylcholine. They inhibit cholinesterase, which inactivate succinylcholine. Therefore, prolonged apnea can ensue unless the anticholinesterase is discontinued at least two weeks prior to surgery. For abbreviated examinations chloral hydrate might prove adequate or in the very small infants feeding may prove enough of a distraction.[23]

Examination and evaluation of the adequacy of treatment is markedly different in the pediatric age group compared to adults. Visual function assessment as measured by Snellen visual acuity and perimetry is usually not possible. The parameters that have proven to be valuable in following progression include biometric axial length measurement by ultrasonography, optic disc photography, corneal diameter notation, and IOP determination by applanation tonometry.

Surgery

Goniotomy

The technique of goniotomy has been altered very little since Barkan's original description.[24-35] A modified, direct goniolens is placed on the cornea to visualize the structures (Fig. 19-1). A goniotomy knife with a sharp tip is passed through the limbus and across the anterior chamber toward the angle.

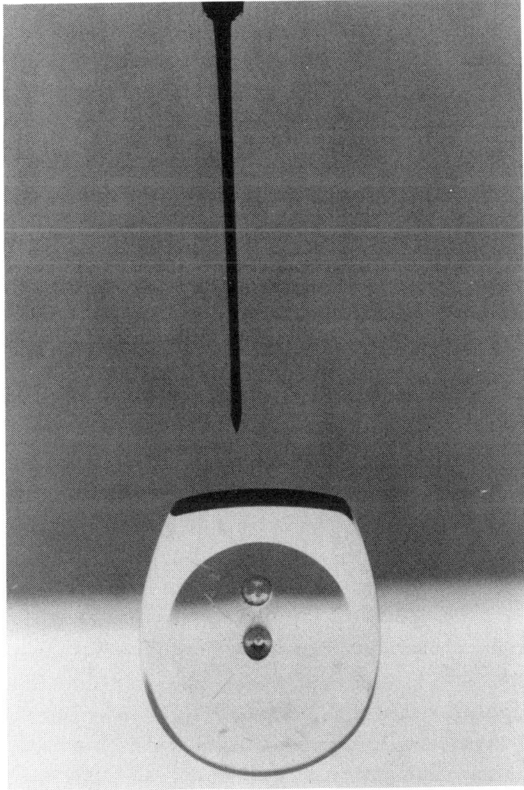

Figure 19-1. Goniotomy knife and direct goniotomy contact lens.

The tip is swept across the trabecular meshwork allowing the iris root to fall posteriorly (Fig. 19-2). Visual control of the blade direction is vital because tactile sensation is of no value[36] and the margin for error is small in an area that is about 400 microns in width. If resistance is felt with a grating sensation then the knife has been placed too deeply into sclera and can result in a hyphema.

With imprecision several intraoperative complications can be encountered (Table 19-1). These include iridodialysis, zonular rupture, (lens subluxation), traumatic cataract, cyclodialysis, Descemet's membrane detachment, and a shallow anterior chamber.[26, 27] A traumatic cataract occurs when the goniotomy blade tears the anterior lens capsule. When the goniotomy knife is used too far anteriorly, then a Descemet's membrane detachment with focal corneal edema can develop. Usually this would cover

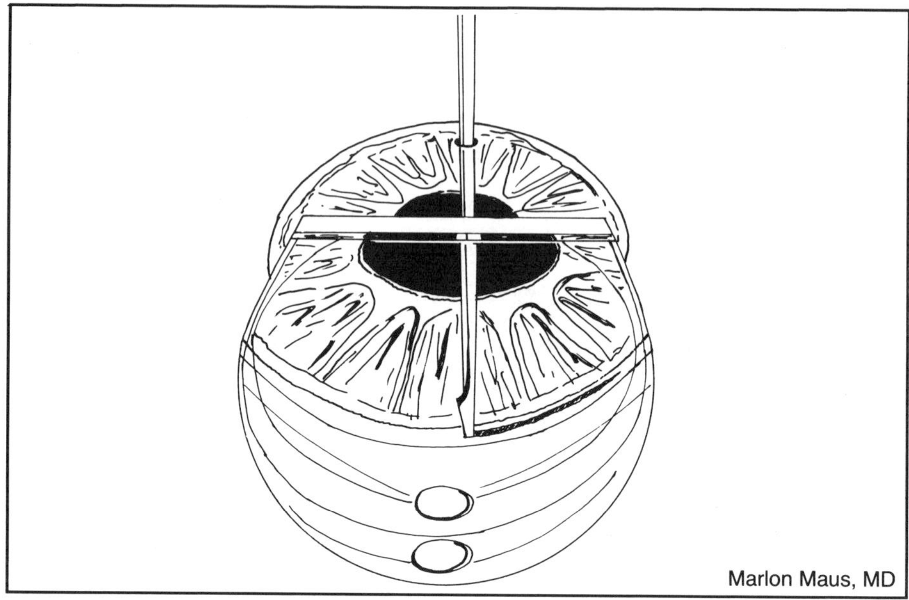

Figure 19-2. Goniotomy technique.

only a small area and spontaneously resolve. When the incision is placed too posteriorly then a hyphema, cyclodialysis, iridodialysis, or zonular rupture with lens subluxation can occur. Many are avoidable by keeping the surgical blade in view at all times. To minimize the chance of developing a flat anterior chamber and also to provide hemostasis, viscoelastics have been placed into the anterior chamber.[38]

Postoperatively, hyphemas are common and generally are absorbed quickly with no serious sequelae. However, total hyphemas have been reported requiring further surgery.[26] Peripheral anterior synechiae can adhere to the goniotomy site in the angle. Suggestions to avoid this problem include placing air or sodium hyaluronate (Healon) in the anterior chamber[38] and administration of a miotic, such as pilocarpine.[25] Late complications have been reported in 14% of the cases following goniotomy. These complications include elevated IOP pressure, retinal detachment, and corneal edema.[36] As with any intraoperative procedure, endophthalmitis can occur and detection can be challenging in an infant. Marked injection and photophobia can signal an infection and demands a return to the operating room for examination, and if needed, culture specimen from the anterior chamber and vitreous.

The risk of general anesthesia was underscored by Litinsky and coworkers where 1.8% (401 total cases) developed cardiopulmonary arrest requiring cardiopulmonary resuscitation measures.[37] It has been suggested that early age at onset and a corneal diameter greater than 14 mm adversely affect goniotomy outcome,[18,47,48] while others dispute this observation.[34]

The advantages of goniotomy are: the relative quickness, no conjunctival or scleral dissection, it is easily repeated, and a good success rate. The drawbacks include: the need for a clear cornea, a complete mastery of gonioscopy is essential, a poor response rate in certain cases, such as when there is aplasia of the pectinate ligament and after two previous goniotomes have failed, and several operations might be necessary for success.

Because these are significant potential complications, intraoperatively and postoperatively, goniotomy should be performed only by surgeons who perform this procedure on a fairly regular basis.

Table 19-1. Complications of Goniotomy

Intraoperative	Postoperative
Hyphema	Hyphema
Iridodialysis	Endophthalmitis
Zonular rupture/lens subluxation	PAS
Cataract	Retinal detachment
Descemet's membrane detachment	Corneal edema
Loss of anterior chamber	

Trabeculotomy

Trabeculotomy ab externo requires the dissection of a conjunctival flap and development of a 1/2 thickness limbal-based scleral flap.[40-46] Schlemm's canal is identified by a vertical "scratch-down" incision in a region straddling the blue zone (between clear cornea and scleral of the surgical limbus) (Fig. 19-3). In cases where Schlemm's canal is filled with blood, as when episcleral venous pressure is elevated, it is easily visible and blood reflux occurs when the canal is severed. Patience and keen observation, however, are required to note a more subtle slow aqueous leak when the canal has been opened.

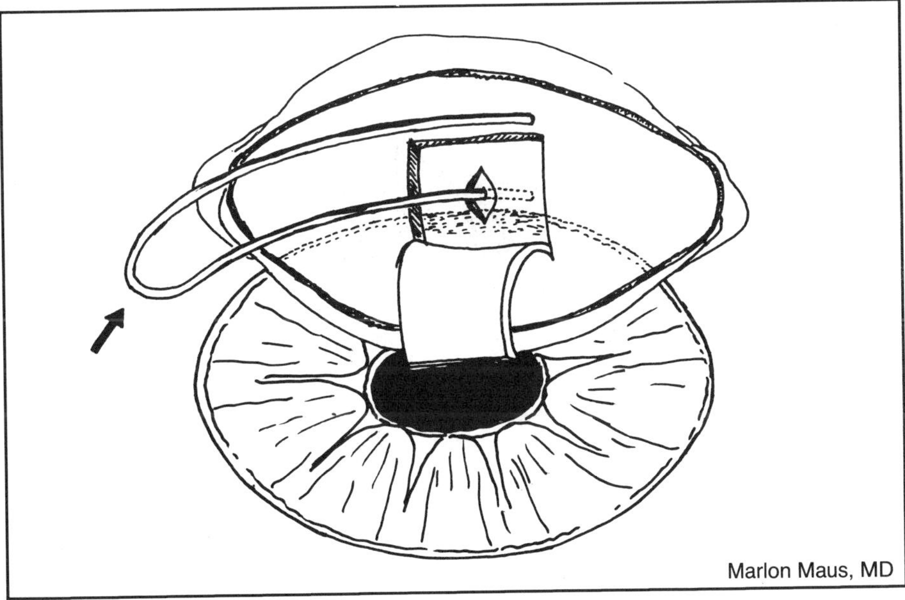

Figure 19-3. **A.** to **C.** Locating Schlemm's canal in preparation for trabeculectomy.

Insertion of a 5-0 nylon suture into the canal will ensure the proper orientation. If the suture "springs" back into position after flicking the external end, it is in the canal, but if it does not return to the original position the suture is not in the correct location, but more likely the suprachoroidal space or in the anterior chamber.

Introduction of a semicircular probe or trabeculotome (Fig. 19-4) into Schlemm's canal should follow the normal contour of the channel. Another

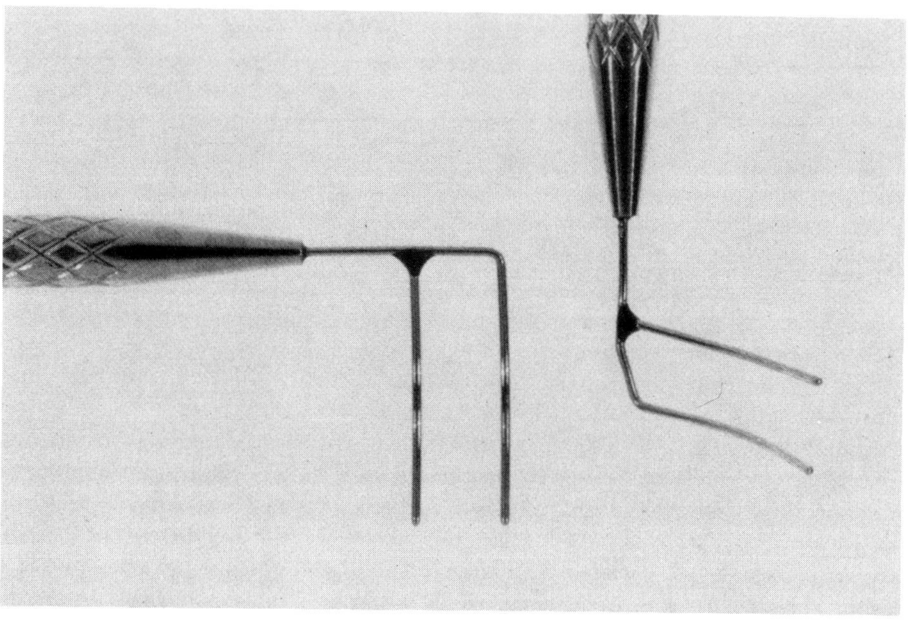

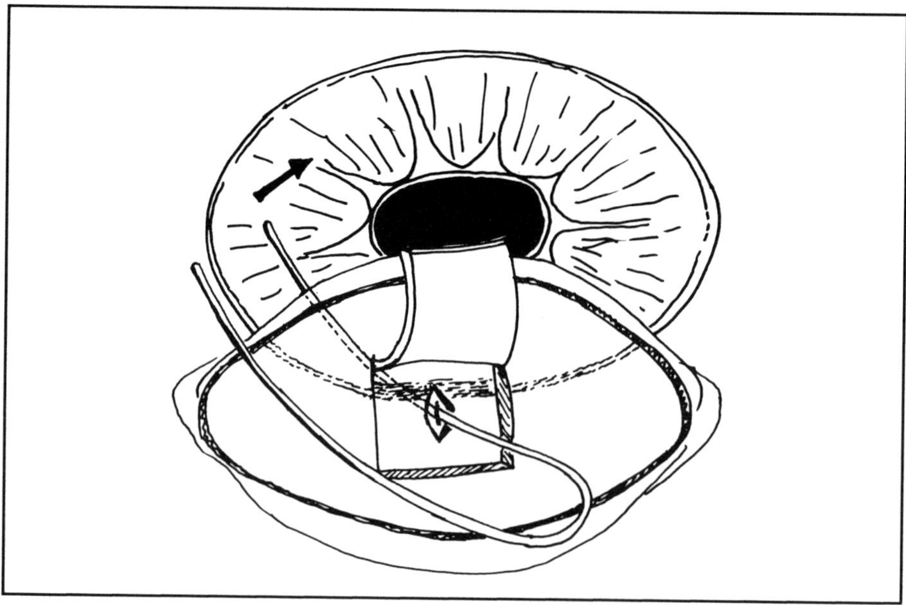

Figure 19-4. A. Trabeculotome for the left and right. **B.** Trabeculectomy technique.

"guide" probe is immediately above, attached to the same handle, which remains external and mirrors the position of the internal probe. With rotation of the trabeculotome the internal probe enters the anterior chamber and disrupts the juxtacanalicular tissue.

Intraoperative complications (Table 19-2) include: Descemet's membrane detachment if the trabeculotome probe enters the anterior chamber too far anteriorly instead of parallel to the iris plane, hyphema, iridodialysis, cyclodialysis, suprachoroidal hemorrhage if the suprachoroidal space is entered (Sturge-Weber patients are at high risk), and vitreous loss can occur if the surgeon assumes that the sclera will be of normal thickness. In buphthalmic eyes, the sclera is often thinned and the scleral flap should be made rather thin.

Table 19-2. Complications of Trabeculotomy

Intraoperative	Postoperative
Descemet's membrane detachment	Endophthalmitis
Hyphema	Flat anterior chamber
Iridodialysis	Cataract
Cyclodialysis	Inadvertent filtering bleb
Suprachoroidal hemorrhage	Corneal ulceration
Vitreous loss	

Postoperative problems can include a flat anterior chamber especially if subconjunctival filtration occurs; therefore, a tight closure of the scleral flap is recommended. In the early postoperative period, a filtration bleb will eventually disappear and healing with subconjunctival scarring occurs. However, there might be a persistent long-term filtration bleb that carries the risk of late postoperative endophthalmitis. Cataracts, early postoperative endophthalmitis, and corneal ulceration are other complications noted after trabeculotomy.[41]

The advantages afforded by trabeculotomy are: the surgical anatomy is familiar to most ophthalmologists, no gonioscopy skills are required, a cloudy cornea does not pose any difficulty, and if Schlemm's canal cannot be found (in 2% of the cases according to Harms and Dannheim[41]) conversion to trabeculectomy is quite easy. Disadvantages cited are: the disturbance of the conjunctiva leading to scarring, a negative influence on future filtration surgery should it be necessary, and it is a longer procedure than goniotomy. Comparative studies would indicate that end results with goniotomy and trabeculotomy are very similar.[47] More attempts might be necessary with goniotomy to control IOP adequately. On one surgical attempt one-third of the goniotomies and 83% of the trabeculotomies were successful.[44-48] The recurrence rate following goniotomy is 14% after six months,[34] 18% over a period of one year,[18] and 34% after 3 1/2 years.[30] The success rate of goniotomy in eyes with multiple congenital anomalies is quite low and is not recommended as the initial procedure.[22,35,48] These eyes would be best served by filtering surgery, such as a trabeculectomy or one of the alloplastic tube drains, or ciliodestructive procedures such as Nd:YAG laser transscleral cyclophotocoagulation and cyclocryotherapy. Although goniotomy is quicker and easier in "skilled" hands,[36] more potential complications are possible and more familiarity of the anatomy and skill is required than for trabeculotomy. Some experienced surgeons prefer goniotomy when corneal clarity permits,[36] but others perform a trabeculotomy[29,44] as the initial operation (Table 19-3).

Table 19-3. Relative Comparison of Goniotomy and Trabeculotomy for Congenital Glaucoma

Goniotomy	Trabeculectomy
quick no conjunctival dissection easily repeated	familiar surgical anatomy gonioscopy skills not required cloudy cornea not a hindrance easily converted to trabeculectomy

Visual Preservation

Reduction of vision because of deprivation amblyopia occurs in almost one-half the eyes, despite lowering of IOP by surgery. It must be remembered that the goal of surgery is to preserve sight, **not** to lower IOP. Successful control of the glaucoma is only part of the therapy required for these children. Since significant anisometropia and ametropia are common,[18,32,34] proper refraction and occlusion patching therapy are necessary. If the cornea is not clear, penetrating keratoplasty might be useful.

Only 37 to 58% of eyes have been reported to have better than 20/60 visual acuity.[18,40,49] Occlusion therapy and refraction was found useful in at least 50% of the cases of amblyopia.[23,49] In unilateral infantile glaucoma, patching is rarely helpful.[18] The incidence of strabismus has been reported as approximately 50%,[23] and about 20% of the children with congenital glaucoma in one series underwent strabismus surgery.[49]

References

1. Duke-Elder S.. System of ophthalmology, Vol III, Pt. 2, Congenital Deformities. St. Louis: CV Mosby, 1969, pp 548-565.
2. Anderson JR. Hydrophthalmia or congenital glaucoma. London: Cambridge University Press, 1939, pp 14-16.
3. deVincentiis C. Incisions dell angolo irideo nel glaucoma. Ann Ottalmol 22:540-542, 1893.
4. Barkan O. Technique of goniotomy. Arch Ophthalmol 19:217-221, 1938.
5. Burian HM. A case of Marfan's syndrome with bilateral glaucoma with a description of a new type of operation for developmental glaucoma. Am J Ophthalmol 50:1187-1192, 1960.
6. Smith R. A new technique for opening the canal of Schlemm. Br J Ophthalmol 56:833-843, 1963.
7. Hoskins HD, Hetherington J, Shaffer RN, Welling AM. Developmental glaucoma: diagnosis and classification. In Symposium on Glaucoma,

Transactions of the New Orleans Academy of Ophthalmology. St. Louis, CV Mosby, 1975, Ch 10, pp 194-197.

8. deLuise VP, Anderson DVL. Primary infantile glaucoma (congenital glaucoma). Surv Ophthalmol 28:1019, 1983.
9. Miller SJH. Genetic aspects of glaucoma. Trans Ophthalmol Soc UK 81:425-434, 1962.
10. Kwitko ML. Glaucoma in infants and children. New York: Appleton-Century-Crofts, 1973.
11. Moller PM. Goniotomy and congenital glaucoma. Acta Ophthalmol 55:436-442, 1977.
12. Morgan KS, Black B, Ellis FD, Helveston EM. Treatment of congenital glaucoma. Am J Ophthalmol 92:799-803, 1981.
13. Worst JGF. The pathogenesis of congenital glaucoma. Assen Netherlands Royal Van Gorcum: Springfield, IL.: Charles C Thomas, 1966.
14. Maumenee AE. The pathogenesis of congenital glaucoma: a new theory. Trans Am Ophthalmol Soc 56:507-570, 1958.
15. Sampaolesi R, Argento C. Scanning electron microscopy of the trabecular meshwork in normal and glaucomatous eyes. Invest Ophthalmol Vis Sci 16:302-314, 1977.
16. Phelps CD. The pathogenesis of glaucoma in Sturge-Weber syndrome. Trans Am Acad Ophthalmol Otolaryngol 85:276-286, 1978.
17. Becker B, Shaffer RN. Diagnosis and therapy of the glaucomas. St. Louis: CV Mosby, 1965.
18. Haas J. Principles and problems of therapy in congenital glaucoma. Invest Ophthalmol 7:140-146, 1968.
19. Dominguez A, Banos MS, Alvarez MG. Intraocular pressure measurement in infants under general anesthesia. Am J Ophthalmol 78:110-116, 1974.
20. Kornblueth W, Aladjemoff L, Magora F, Dor DB. Intraocular pressure in children measured under general anesthesia. Arch Ophthalmol 72:489-490, 1964.
21. Quigley HA. Childhood glaucoma: results with trabeculotomy and study of reversible cupping. Ophthalmology 89:219-225, 1982.
22. Quigley HA. Childhood glaucoma. Results with trabeculotomy and study of reversible cupping. Ophthalmology 89:219, 1982.
23. Rice NSC. Management of Infantile Glaucoma: Br J Ophthalmol 50:294-298. 1972.
24. Shaffer RN. New concepts in infantile glaucoma. Can J Ophthalmol 2:243, 1967.
25. Kwitko ML. The pediatric glaucoma. Glaucoma 5(3):261, 1983.
26. Costenbader FD, Kwitko ML. Congenital glaucoma: an analysis of seventy-seven consecutive eyes. J Ped Ophthalmol 4(2):9-15, 1967.
27. Worst JGF. The cause and treatment of congenital glaucoma. Trans Am Acad Ophthalmol Otolaryngol 68:677, 1964.
28. Lister, A. Technique of goniotomy. Br J Ophthalmol 49:594, 1965.

29. Worst JGF. Congenital glaucoma: remarks or the aspect of chamber angle otogenetic and pathogenetic background and mode of action of goniotomy. Invest Ophthalmol 7:127, 1968.
30. Moller PM. Goniotomy and congenital glaucoma. Acta Ophthalmologica 55:436, 1977.
31. Barkan O. A new operation for chronic glaucoma: restoration of physiological function by opening Schlemm's canal under direct magnified vision. Am J Ophthalmol 21:403-405, 1938.
32. Douglas DM. Reflection on Buphthalmos and Goniotomy. Trans Ophthalmol Soc UK 90:931, 1970.
33. Scheie HG. Goniotomy in treatment of congenital glaucoma. Arch Ophthalmol 42:266, 1949.
34. Broughton WL, Parks MM. An analysis of treatment of congenital glaucoma by goniotomy. Am J Ophthalmol 91:566-572, 1981.
35. Luntz, MM. Congenital, infantile, and juvenile glaucoma. Ophthalmol 86:793, 1979.
36. Shaffer RN, Hoskins HD. Goniotomy in the treatment of isolated trabeculodysgenesis (primary congenital [infantile] developmental glaucoma). Trans Ophthalmol Soc UK 103:581-585.
37. Litinsky SM, Shaffer RN, Hetherington J, Hoskins MD. Operative Complications of Goniotomy. Trans Am Acad Ophthalmol Otolaryngol 83:78-79, 1977.
38. Wilson RP, Lloyd J: The place of sodium hyaluronate in glaucoma surgery. Ophthalmol Surg. (17), 1:30-33, 1986.
39. Lister A. The prognosis in congenital glaucoma. Trans Ophthalmol Soc UK 85:5, 1966.
40. Morgan KS, Black B, Ellis FD, Helveston EM. Treatment of congenital glaucoma. Am J Ophthalmol 92:799-803, 1981.
41. Harms H, Dannheim R. Epicritical consideration of 300 cases of trabeculotomy "Ab Externa." Trans Ophthalmol Soc UK 89:491-499, 1969.
42. Rothkoff J, Blumenthal M, Biedner B. Trabeculotomy in late onset congenital glaucoma. Br J Ophthalmology 63:38, 1979.
43. Dannheim R. Trabeculotomy. Trans Am Acad Ophthalmol Otolaryngol 76:375, 1972.
44. McPherson SD Jr, McFarland D. External trabeculotomy for developmental glaucoma. Ophthalmology 87:302-305, 1980.
45. Allan L, Burian HM. Trabeculotomy ab externo. Am J Ophthalmol 53:19, 1962.
46. McPherson SD Jr. Results of external trabeculotomy. Am J Ophthalmol 76:918, 1973.
47. Anderson, DR. Trabeculotomy compared to goniotomy for glaucoma in children. Ophthalmology 90:805-806, 1983.
48. McPherson SD Jr, Berry DP: Goniotomy vs external trabeculotomy for developmental glaucoma. Am J Ophthalmol 95:427-431, 1983.
49. Biglan AW, Hiles DA. The visual results following infantile glaucoma surgery. J Ped Ophthalmol Strab 16:377, 1979.

CHAPTER 20

Cataract in the Glaucomatous Patient

Mark B. Sherwood, MD
Steven T. Simmons, MD

In the last 10 to 15 years there has been a revolution in the management of patients who have both cataract and glaucoma. The advances include:

- The change from ICCE to ECCE.
- The use of posterior chamber intraocular lenses.
- Combined cataract and trabeculectomy operations.
- The introduction of argon laser trabeculoplasty for the presurgical management of glaucoma.

Presently there are four major approaches to the surgical management of cataract in glaucomatous patients. These are listed in Table 20-1.

Table 20-1. Options for the surgical management of the glaucomatous patient with cataract
1. Cataract extraction with intraocular lens implantation alone
2. ALT, followed by cataract surgery a month or two later
3. Separate filtration surgery, followed by cataract extraction
4. Combined cataract and glaucoma surgery
a. Trabeculectomy
b. Guarded posterior lip sclerectomy
(c. Cyclodialysis)

In the patient with glaucoma, the major additional complication of cataract sugery is progression of optic nerve damage, resulting from insufficient IOP control. The loss of IOP control can be either brief, in the early postoperative phase, or there can be a long-term loss of pressure stability. Patients at high risk for further optic nerve damage must be identified; careful preoperative evaluation is therefore essential.

Preoperative Considerations

Factors important in formulating the most appropriate surgical approach are listed in Table 20-2.

Table 20-2. Preoperative factors in planning surgical approach

1. Degree of glaucomatous nerve damage and visual field deficit
2. Preoperative IOP
3. Preoperative antiglaucomatous medications
4. General health of patient
5. Etiology of glaucoma

The severity of glaucomatous optic neuropathy is the most important criterion. The greater the optic nerve damage, the more critical it is to avoid short-term pressure spikes in the initial postoperative period. Patients with split fixation or with small central islands of vision are particularly at risk of losing central vision following surgery.[1,2]

Long-term control of IOP is also vital in preventing progression of field loss. Many patients with glaucoma require an IOP in the mid- to low-normal range to maintain visual field stability. The results of further surgical intervention to lower an inadequately controlled IOP are not as favorable in the aphakic eye as in the phakic.[3,4] For this reason, the preoperative formulation of a surgical approach that will maximize the patient's chance of prolonged IOP control as well as his visual potential is critical.

The preoperative IOP greatly influences the choice of surgery. For patients in whom the IOP is well controlled on a minimal medical regimen, especially if they have only early or moderate field loss, ECCE with PC IOL implantation alone[5,6] or, if IOP control is more borderline, in combination with presurgical ALT[1], is appropriate. In about 20% of cases, the IOP control can be improved following cataract surgery alone, allowing a reduction in medication. More commonly, however, in about 30% additional medications are required.[6,7]

For those in whom the IOP is too high, despite medical therapy, a glaucoma procedure is required. This can be either ALT, if not previously performed, filtration surgery, or a combined procedure. In eyes where the principal problem is lack of IOP control and there is little cataract, ALT or filtration surgery alone can be considered. Visual acuity can be improved in some patients for whom miotics can be discontinued. Filtration surgery, however, might lead to worsening of the cataract and a need for later extraction.[8] If the main ocular problem, alternatively, is cataract with only moderate glaucomatous nerve damage, presurgical ALT, or a combined operation is indicated. The beneficial effect of laser trabeculoplasty is not lost with subsequent cataract surgery.[1,9] In patients with both dense cataract and advanced glaucoma the relative advantages of a single combined procedure versus separate filtration surgery followed by later cataract extraction is unclear. The surgeon's choice will be influenced by the knowledge that the success rate for glaucoma control following a combined procedure is not as high as with a separate filtration operation.[10] However, subsequent cataract extraction in eyes with a functional filtering bleb frequently diminishes bleb function and risks bleb failure, secondary to the inflammation produced.[7,11] In addition, there will be a delay in visual recuperation for several months because of the time interval between the filter and cataract operation.

For each patient, limitations in the ability to treat postsurgical IOP spikes must be weighed prior to selection of surgical approach. In the preoperative and postoperative periods, necessary alterations in ocular medical therapy can have a deleterious effect on IOP control. Miotics, especially anticholinesterase inhibitors, are usually discontinued preoperatively to allow better pupillary dilatation, to avoid intraoperative anesthetic complications, and to reduce postoperative ocular inflammation. In addition, miotics are often deferred in the initial postoperative period in an attempt to avoid posterior synechiae formation and breakdown of the blood-aqueous barrier. Following cataract surgery, epinephrine derivatives are relatively contraindicated because of the increased risk of cystoid macular edema.

The patient's general medical health can further decrease the physician's ability to administer antiglaucoma medications. For example, betablockers are relatively contraindicated in asthma, bradycardia, and in cardiovascular insufficiency. A history of nephrolithiasis or Addison's disease limits the use of CAIs. Osmotic agents should be avoided in patients with congestive heart failure or renal failure.

Whether secondary to ocular or general health problems, this reduction in the medical alternatives hinders the surgeon's ability to successfully treat a rise in IOP in the initial postoperative period. In one study, pressure spikes of 7 mm Hg, or more occurred in 62% of glaucomatous eyes undergoing ECCE and PC IOL implantation, either alone or in combination with preoperative ALT, as compared with 10% in nonglaucomatous eyes.[12] This number is reduced with combined procedures but is not totally eliminated.[13]

The etiology of the glaucoma can also limit the management options available. Patients with uveitic and other secondary forms of glaucoma respond poorly to ALT. Miotics also are relatively contraindicated in uveitic glaucoma because they cause alterations in the blood-aqueous barrier. As a result, separate filtration surgery or a combined procedure are usually necessary to minimize postsurgical IOP spikes and maximize long-term pressure control in these patients. In patients with narrow or closed angles it might be anatomically impossible to apply laser burns to the trabecular meshwork. Alternatively, patients with pseudoexfoliation glaucoma are known to respond particularly well to ALT.[14,15] As a result, laser therapy prior to cataract extraction might be especially beneficial in this latter group, but might not be a viable option in patients with a narrow angle glaucoma.

In conclusion, the preoperative assessment of the patient with a cataract and glaucoma is a most critical step (Fig. 20-1). By choosing the surgical procedure or procedures that will restore visual clarity and maximize IOP control most safely, the surgeon can often minimize later intraoperative and postoperative complications. This section highlighted only some of the major preoperative factors that must be considered. It is important that the surgeon tailor the procedure to suit each patient; for only by adjusting to individual differences can each patient be best served.

Intraoperative Considerations

Cataract surgery in glaucomatous patients is subject to the usual hazards of this type of procedure but certain complications occur more frequently in this group. The first and most common problem faced by the surgeon is difficulty in adequately dilating the pupil. This can be secondary to long-term miotic therapy or posterior synechiae. The two principal methods of obtaining sufficient surgical exposure for anterior capsulotomy and nuclear expression are:

- Sector (keyhole) iridectomy
- Multiple sphincterotomies

If posterior synichiae are present, they first must be divided using either an iris spatula or a blunt cannula. Prior injection of viscoelastic helps to maintain the anterior chamber during this procedure. Both sector iridectomy and sphincterotomies increase the incidence of hyphema. Postoperatively, sector iridectomies are associated with a higher incidence of pupillary-IOL capture. Although it rarely leads to clinical symptoms, this can largely be prevented by converting the sector iridectomy into a peripheral iridectomy after PC IOL insertion, using a single prolene suture placed near the pupillary margin. The disadvantage of closing the iridectomy is that future pupillary dilation is usually very poor, making fundal examination difficult. Closure of the iridectomy is therefore not recommended in diabetics or high myopes. Sphincterotomies increase the risk of synechial adhesion to the IOL, which can lead to later pupillary block. For this reason a surgical peripheral iridectomy is recommended whenever sphincterotomies are performed.

ECCE with PC IOL implantation is the cataract procedure of choice. ECCE, as opposed to ICCE, offers the benefit of a smaller incision, the ability to place a PC IOL, and the avoidance of later complications from vitreous in the anterior chamber. PC IOLs maximize the reduced visual field of the glaucoma patient. The insertion of a PC IOL at ECCE has been shown to have no deleterious effect on IOP control.[1]

Elevation of postoperative pressure can be caused by residual anterior chamber viscoelastic or by inflammation related to retained lens cortex. In patients with glaucoma it is particularly important to meticulously remove all viscoelastic and cortical material using an I&A device. It has been shown that irrigation of the anterior chamber alone will not adequately remove the viscoelastic.

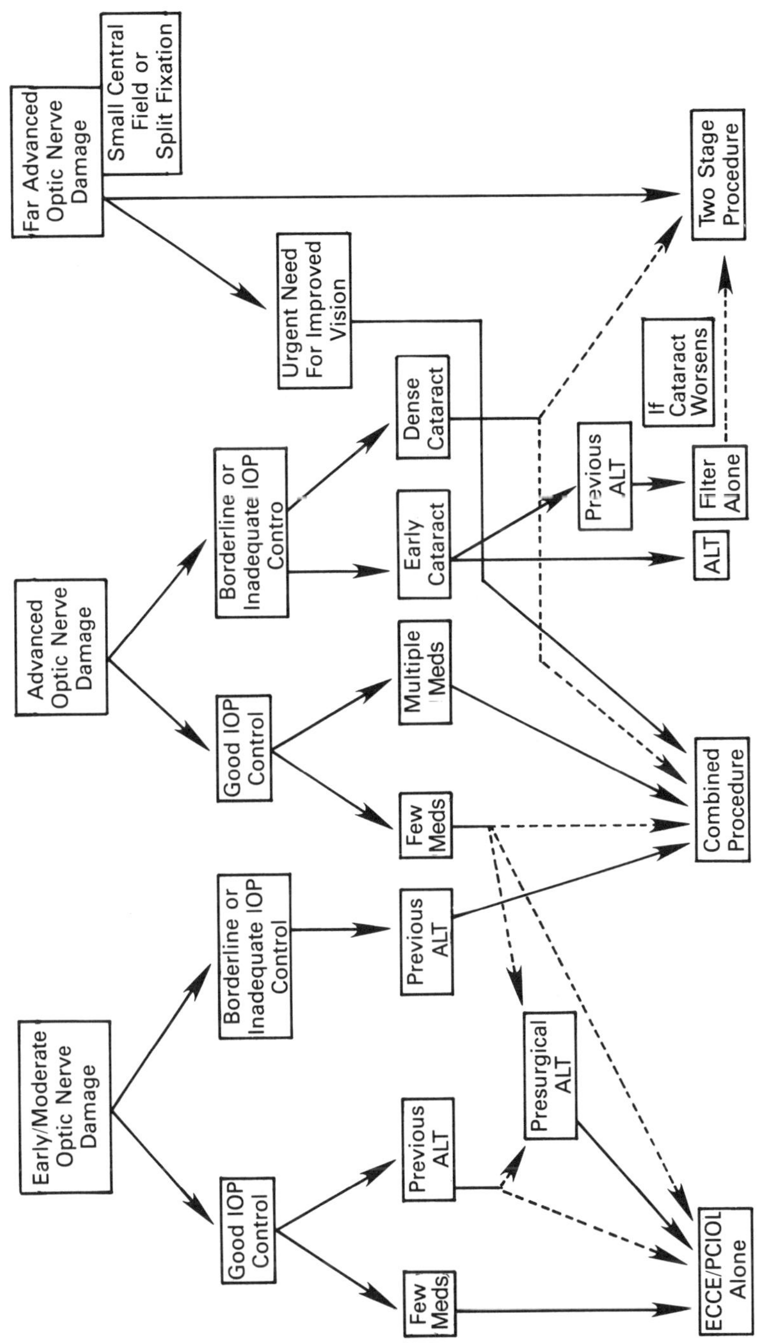

Fig. 20-1. Flow diagram of management options for patients with combined cataract and glaucoma.

In the event of inadvertent rupture of the posterior capsule and vitreous loss, a generous vitrectomy should be performed using an automated cutting instrument. This will usually prevent vitreous traction and possible later occlusion of the trabecular sclerectomy, should this be present. If sufficient posterior capsule remains, a posterior chamber intraocular lens can be inserted, with the loops placed in the ciliary sulcus. If there is insufficient residual posterior capsule, as a general rule no IOL should be inserted. Anterior chamber IOLs are relatively contraindicated in patients with glaucoma, especially if a filtration procedure has not been performed. In these latter patients a contact lens might provide the best alternative for visual rehabilitation. For those who have a filter, the surgeon needs to decide, for each individual case, the merits of anterior chamber IOL placement.

The location of the cataract incision and the placement of the sutures might influence the postoperative course. If cataract surgery alone is performed, the corneoscleral incision should be placed temporally, or a superior, clear-corneal approach used, to preserve a virgin area for future filtration surgery. If the incision is placed posteriorly, it is important that it be sufficiently shelved to avoid damage to the trabecular meshwork. Campbell and Grant[16] have demonstrated that the tying of cataract sutures, even without an incision, can profoundly affect outflow facility by causing compression of the trabecular meshwork and closure of Schlemm's canal. The use of a clear-corneal approach does not prevent this, because a similar distortion and decrease of outflow facility has been demonstrated with tying of corneal (penetrating keratoplasty) sutures.

For combined procedures, a guarded filter is preferred to the full-thickness type because of the increased potential hazard of over-filtration and flat anterior chamber in the pseudophakic eye; from contact between the PC IOL and the corneal endothelium. Cyclodialysis with cataract extraction used to be popular, particularly in combination with intracapsular cataract surgery[17,18], but is less commonly performed today because of its more unpredictable long-term results. Good results have been reported using a guarded posterior lip sclerectomy technique[5, 19] and with standard trabeculectomy flaps.[12,13,20] The guarded sclerectomy is quicker and easier to perform, requiring just a well-beveled cataract incision, from which a segment of the posterior lip tissue is excised using a scleral punch (Fig. 20-2). Care must be taken to ensure that the tip of a ciliary process is not accidentally caught in the jaws of the scleral punch when removing the corneoscleral tissue. Profuse bleeding will occur should this happen. Alternatively, a partial-thickness scleral flap can be dissected and the corneoscleral incision extended on either side of this (Fig. 20-3). The surgeon must choose either a fornix-based or a limbus-based conjunctival flap approach. No difference has been noted in long-term IOP control or functional bleb appearance between the two conjunctival flap approaches, although hyphema is more common in the limbus-based flap group. The advantages of the fornix-based flap are improved surgical exposure of the corneoscleral limbus and reduced operating time. It is important, however, to tightly secure the conjunctiva over the superior cornea at the end of the procedure, to avoid a conjunctival wound leak. The conjunctiva should

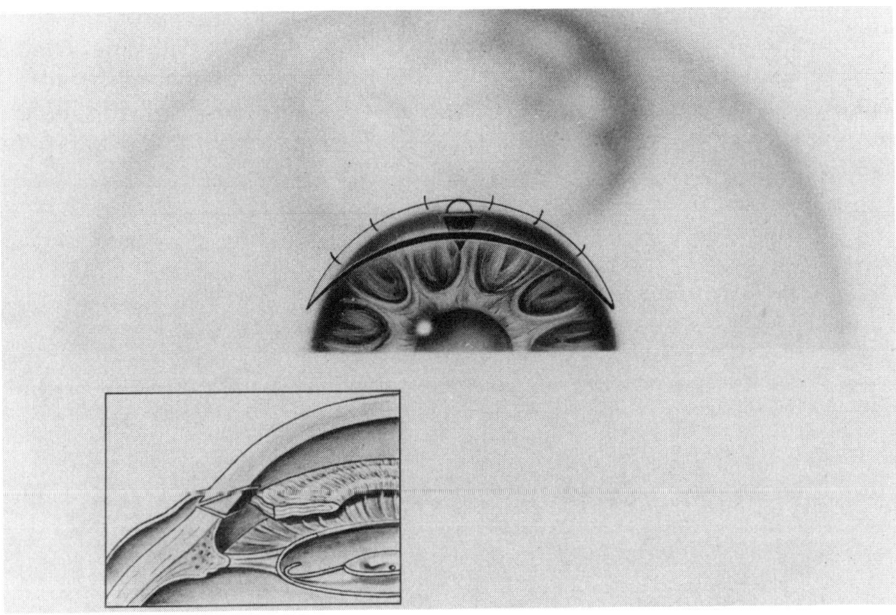

Fig. 20-2. Extracapsular cataract extraction, PC IOL implant combined with posterior lip sclerectomy. A wedge of tissue is excised from the posterior margin of the bevelled cataract incision (see inset) using a scleral punch. The amount of aqueous egress can be varied depending on the degree of overlap of anterior lip tissue and by the use of sutures that can be cut with a laser postoperatively to increase outflow. A fornix-based conjunctival flap is shown.

be placed on stretch and opposed firmly to the underlying cornea, slightly indenting it, using either interrupted or a running suture.

For patients with advanced glaucoma, some authors prefer the more laborious procedure of a clear-corneal cataract incision and separate trabeculectomy under a limbus-based flap (Fig. 20-4). This method has the advantage of reduced conjunctival manipulation and, should the filter later fail, provides other superior quadrant sites uncompromised by corneoscleral incision, for future guarded trabeculectomy. The scleral flap techniques can be further modified by use of releasable sutures (see Chap. 13). Releasable sutures can be particularly advantageous in combined procedures because they allow tight closure of the scleral flap initially, to reduce the risk of flat anterior chamber, and yet permit later increased aqueous flow in this group of patients who have a lower rate of long-term IOP control than those undergoing filtration surgery alone.

Postoperative Complications

In performing cataract surgery, the primary goal is to improve visual acuity. In the most recent studies on ECCE,[1,12,21] combined procedures,[5,12,13,22] and separate procedures,[6] the visual improvements were comparable, no procedure having a clear advantage. An unexplained slower visual recovery has been noted, however, in both the combined and separate procedures.[5,13] The incidence of posterior capsule opacification and cystoid macular edema has not been shown to be increased in this population or between the different procedures. Shields[6] has reported an increased incidence of vitreous loss and capsular rupture with separate procedures. This might be a result of the

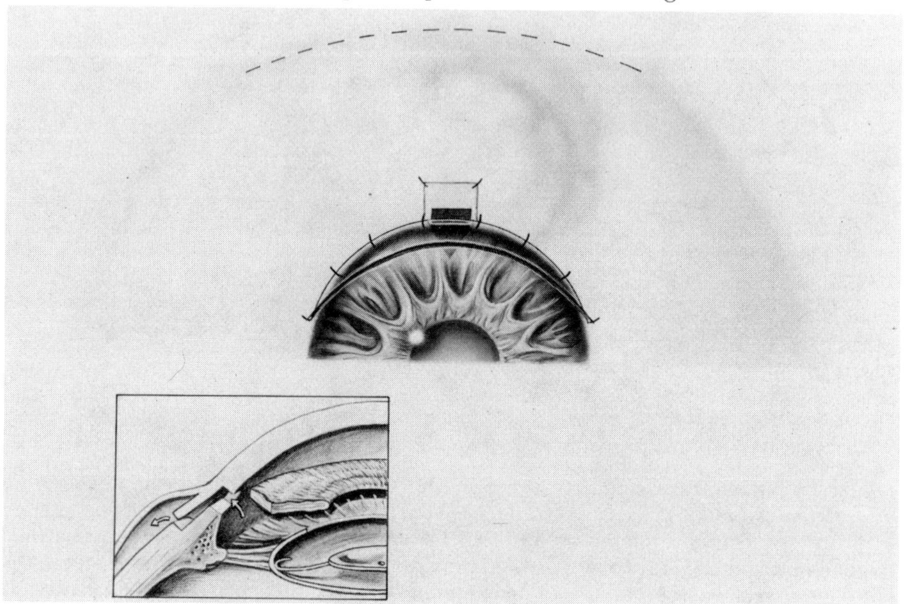

Fig. 20-3. Extracapsular cataract extraction, PC IOL implant combined with a guarded trabeculectomy. A fornix-based (solid line) *or* limbal-based (dotted line) conjunctival flap can be employed. The deep sclerectomy forms part of the cataract incision and is covered, in the usual way, by the partial-thickness scleral flap.

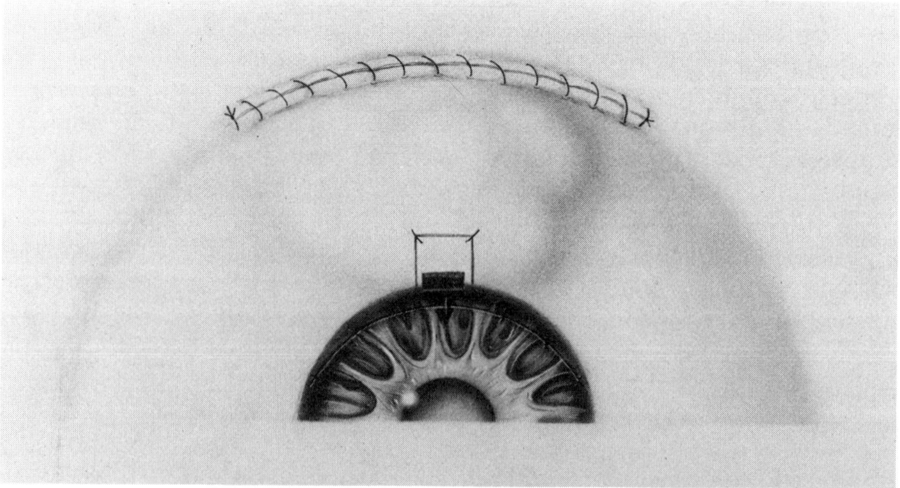

Fig. 20-4. Corneal section extracapsular cataract extraction, PC IOL implant, combined with a guarded trabeculectomy using a limbal-based conjunctival flap. This technique is essentially an entirely separate cataract and filtering procedure performed at the same anesthetic.

unfamiliar locations of the corneoscleral incision (inferotemporal and clear-cornea). An increased incidence of vitreous loss has also been reported in some secondary glaucomas, such as pseudoexfoliation because of zonular dialysis[23]; however, no such propensity has been demonstrated in primary open angle glaucoma.

Postoperative astigmatism can occur in all types of cataract surgery. Neither combined procedures nor separate procedures have been shown to increase the amount of astigmatism over that of cataract surgery alone. However, the ability to manipulate the astigmatism might be hampered because of the inability to release tight sutures under a functioning conjunctival filtering bleb. The use of the argon laser together with the Hoskins lens has greatly reduced this problem. With this lens, corneoscleral sutures can be released without damage to the overlying conjunctiva and without producing a bleb leak.

The most frequent postoperative complication in glaucoma patients is an elevation of IOP above baseline in the first week following an ECCE.[1] These pressure elevations are transient in most patients and are not prevented by preoperative ALT.

A combination of trabeculectomy and ECCE offers some protection against initial pressure elevations, but this protection is not absolute. One study found IOPs 7 mm or more above the preoperative baseline in a third of their patients undergoing a combined procedure and, in over 20%, a spike of 15 mm Hg, or greater was recorded.[13] These elevations usually responded rapidly to ocular massage and aqueous suppressants. The ability to quickly normalize the IOP with ocular massage is a major advantage of the combined procedure. It is important that patients with glaucoma be followed very closely in the initial postoperative period because of the high incidence of pressure fluctuation. This will enable the surgeon to initiate necessary therapy if the IOP rises and to minimize the threat of optic nerve damage.

Long-term IOP control is significantly improved following combined procedures.[5,12,13,22] This improved control is seen despite the fact that only 12 to 14% of blebs are elevated and appear functional after 12 months.[5,13] Many reasons can be hypothesized for the low success in obtaining functional-looking conjunctival filtering blebs. These include the increased inflammation caused by the combined procedure, the pseudophakic status, and the surgeon's hesitancy to produce over-filtration in the initial postoperative period. The type of conjunctival flap (limbus or fornix-based) does not significantly alter success rate.[13]

A common complication of combined procedures is hyphema, the incidence ranging between 30 and 50%. Hyphemas are, however, usually small and do not significantly affect the visual outcome. They also do not appear to be associated with an increased incidence of IOP elevation in the initial postoperative period. The increased chance of fibrin in the anterior chamber following combined procedures makes it important to dilate the pupil of these patients periodically, to avoid posterior synechiae formation.

Flat anterior chambers are surprisingly rare postoperatively in combined procedures.[5] However, when the anterior chamber does shallow in these cases, it is important to determine the cause of the shallowing and initiate the appropriate therapy (discussed in detail in Chapter 14). Reformation of the anterior chamber should be performed at an early stage to avoid any IOL-corneal endothelial touch, which would have a profound and rapid deleterious effect on corneal clarity.

The presence of an already functioning filter offers the greatest protection against an elevation of IOP initially following cataract extraction. Unfortunately, there are disadvantages to a two-stage approach. These include the delayed visual recuperation, the "unfamiliar" location of the cataract incision (inferotemporal or clear corneal) and the danger of postcataract surgery bleb failure. The delay in visual recovery is often greater than seven months because many surgeons recommend waiting approximately four to six months between procedures. Following cataract extraction, only 60 to 70% of the conjunctival filtering blebs will still be present one or two years later.[6] This is discouraging, yet much better than the percentage of functioning conjunctival filtering blebs present following combined procedures. As a result, the general impression has been that long-term IOP control in separate procedures is better than in combined procedures, although to date, no prospective randomized study has been performed to confirm this.

In conclusion, the key to success in the management of patients with both cataract and glaucoma is good preoperative planning. The surgeon must consider what both he and the patient have in reserve. For the patient this is the number of remaining optic nerve neurons (i.e., the degree of optic nerve damage) and the level of preoperative IOP control. For the surgeon the critical issue is what additional medication or other therapy is at this disposal, should an IOP spike occur. This might be limited by the patient's general health, previous drug intolerances, glaucoma etiology, and by the pseudophakic status postoperatively. If in doubt it is usually better to err on the side of performing a glaucoma procedure, particularly if the patient has advanced glaucoma and is thus more sensitive to poor pressure control. In all cases close postoperative monitoring is essential. Provision should be made in the initial planning for the possibility that further glaucoma surgery might be required and a virgin area of conjunctiva maintained, if feasible, for future procedures.

References

1. Savage JA, Thomas JV, Belcher CD, et al. Extracapsular cataract extraction and posterior chamber intraocular lens implantation in glaucomatous eyes. Ophthalmol 92:1506-1516, 1985.
2. Kolker AE. Visual prognosis in advanced glaucoma: a comparison of medical and surgical therapy for retention of vision in 101 eyes with advanced glaucoma. Trans Am Ophthalmol Soc 75:539-555, 1977.
3. Heuer DK, Gressel MG, Parrish RK, et al. Trabeculectomy in aphakic eyes. Ophthalmol 91:1045-1051, 1984.

4. Bellows AR, Johnstone MA. Surgical management of chronic glaucoma in aphakia. Ophthalmol 90:807-813, 1983.
5. Shields MB. Combined cataract extraction and guarded sclerectomy. Reevaluation in the extracapsular era. Ophthalmol 93:366-370, 1986.
6. Shields MB. Combined cataract extraction and glaucoma surgery. Ophthalmol 89:231-237, 1982.
7. Antonios SR, Traverso CE, Tomey KF. Extracapsular cataract extraction using a temporal limbal approach after filtering operations. Arch Ophthalmol 106:608-610, 1988.
8. Sugar HS. Postoperative cataract in successfully filtering glaucomatous eyes. Am J Ophthalmol 69:740-746, 1970.
9. Brown SVL, Thomas JV, Budenz DL, et al. Effect of cataract surgery on intraocular pressure reduction obtained with laser trabeculoplasty. Am J Ophthalmol 100:373-376, 1985.
10. Galin MA, Obstbaum SA, Asano Y, et al. Trabeculectomy, cataract extraction and intraocular lens implantation. Trans Ophthalmol Soc UK 104:570-573, 1985.
11. Oyakawa RT, Maumenee AE. Clear-cornea cataract extraction in eyes with functioning filtering blebs. Am J Ophthalmol 93:294-298, 1982.
12. McGuigan LJB, Gottsch J, Stark WJ, et al. Extracapsular cataract extraction and posterior chamber lens implantation in eyes with preexisting glaucoma. Arch Ophthalmol 104:1301-1308, 1986.
13. Simmons ST, Litoff D, Nichols DA, et al. Extracapsular cataract extraction and posterior chamber intraocular lens implantation combined with trabeculectomy in glaucoma patients. Am J Ophthalmol 104:465-470, 1987.
14. Svedburgh B, Sherwood MB. Argon laser trabeculoplasty in exfoliation glaucoma. A retrospective analysis. Dev Ophthalmol 11:116-123, 1985.
15. Schwartz AL, Kopelman J. Four-year experience with argon laser trabecular surgery in uncontrolled open-angle glaucoma. Ophthalmol 90:771-780, 1983.
16. Campbell DG, Grant WM. Trabecular deformation and reduction of outflow facility due to cataract and penetrating keratoplasty sutures. Invest Ophthalmol Vis Sci 16 (suppl):126, 1977.
17. Galin MA, Hung PT, Obstbaum SA. Cataract extraction in glaucoma. Am J Ophthalmol 87:124-129, 1979.
18. Shields MB, Simmons RJ. Combined cyclodialysis and cataract extraction. Ophthalmic Surg 7:62-73, 1976.
19. Spaeth GL, Sivalingam E. The partial-punch: a new combined cataract-glaucoma operation. Ophthalmic Surg 7:53-57, 1976.
20. Ohanesian RV, Kim EW. A prospective study of combined extracapsular cataract extraction, posterior chamber lens implantation, and trabeculectomy. Am Intraocular Implant Soc J 11:142-145, 1985.
21. Handa J, Henry JC, Krupin T, et al. Extracapsular cataract extraction and posterior chamber lens implantation in glaucoma patients. Invest Arch Ophthalmol 105:765-769, 1987.

22. Percival SPB. Glaucoma triple procedure of extracapsular cataract extraction, posterior chamber lens implantation, and trabeculectomy. Br J Ophthalmol 69:99-102, 1985.
23. Skuta GL, Parrish RK, Hodapp E, et al. Zonular dialysis during extracapsular cataract extraction in patients with pseudoexfoliation syndrome. Arch Ophthalmol 105:632-634, 1987.

Index